The Uncomplicated Guide
to
DIABETES
COMPLICATIONS
3rd Edition

EDITED BY MARVIN E. LEVIN, MD
AND MICHAEL A. PFEIFER, MD

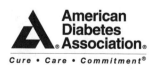

American
Diabetes
Association
Cure • Care • Commitment®

Director, Book Publishing, Robert Anthony; *Managing Editor, Book Publishing,* Abe Ogden; *Production Manager,* Melissa Sprott; *Composition,* ADA; *Cover Design,* pixiedesign, llc.; *Printer,* Victor Graphics

Printed in the United States of America
1 3 5 7 9 10 8 6 4 2

The suggestions and information contained in this publication are generally consistent with the *Clinical Practice Recommendations* and other policies of the American Diabetes Association, but they do not represent the policy or position of the Association or any of its boards or committees. Reasonable steps have been taken to ensure the accuracy of the information presented. However, the American Diabetes Association cannot ensure the safety or efficacy of any product or service described in this publication. Individuals are advised to consult a physician or other appropriate health care professional before undertaking any diet or exercise program or taking any medication referred to in this publication. Professionals must use and apply their own professional judgment, experience, and training and should not rely solely on the information contained in this publication before prescribing any diet, exercise, or medication. The American Diabetes Association—its officers, directors, employees, volunteers, and members—assumes no responsibility or liability for personal or other injury, loss, or damage that may result from the suggestions or information in this publication.

⊗ The paper in this publication meets the requirements of the ANSI Standard Z39.48-1992 (permanence of paper).

ADA titles may be purchased for business or promotional use or for special sales. To purchase more than 50 copies of this book at a discount, or for custom editions of this book with your logo, contact the American Diabetes Association at the address below, at book-sales@diabetes.org, or by calling 703-299-2046.

American Diabetes Association
1701 North Beauregard Street
Alexandria, Virginia 22311

Library of Congress Cataloging-in-Publication Data

Uncomplicated guide to diabetes complications / edited by Marvin E. Levin and Michael A. Pfeifer. -- 3rd ed.
  p. cm.
Includes index.
ISBN 978-1-58040-290-3 (alk. paper)
1. Diabetes--Complications--Popular works. I. Levin, Marvin E., 1924- II. Pfeifer, Michael A.

RC660.4.U53 2008
616.4'62--dc22
            2008024321

Contents

Introduction

Much has happened in the field of diabetes since the second edition of this book was published in 2002. The number of people with diabetes in the United States in 2008 was approximately 24 million, or 8% of the population. As this number grows, so does the number of people suffering from complications of diabetes. Today it is rare for an individual with diabetes to die of diabetic coma; most deaths associated with diabetes are actually due to complications of the disease. These complications are more likely to occur in those who have had diabetes for many years, particularly if their blood glucose levels have been poorly controlled. Fortunately, there is some preliminary data that suggests that glucose control is improving and the rate of some of the complications (kidney and eye) of diabetes may be stabilizing or (we hope) decreasing. Nevertheless, many people still suffer from the complications of diabetes. And if you're one of the individuals with a complication, it doesn't matter that the overall rate may be declining.

This third edition of *The Uncomplicated Guide to Diabetes Complications* is devoted to educating the person with diabetes about the disease and its complications, and to making that person a team member in helping to prevent these complications. Many advances have been made in the treatment of diabetes complications. Additionally, new complications related to diabetes have been recognized since the second edition was published. Therefore, thirteen new chapters and an appendix have been added. Many of the complications discussed in these new chapters have not been recognized as being associated, or related to, diabetes until recently.

Some of the most important new complications associated with diabetes are discussed in this new edition. For example, some cancers have been found to be more common in people with diabetes. These cancers are not necessarily caused by diabetes, but do have a strong association with diabetes. In fact, it has been reported that approximately 8–18% of those diagnosed with cancer also have diabetes.

Alzheimer's disease is another complication not normally linked to diabetes. But due to the aging population, Alzheimer's disease and dementia have been on the increase in the United States, and an association of Alzheimer's disease with diabetes has been documented. A chapter on this important topic has been included.

A new chapter has also been included on polycystic ovary syndrome (PCOS), a relatively common problem that is associated with irregular or absent menstruation and difficulty in achieving pregnancy. This complication is related to insulin resistance and is associated with increase in blood sugar.

Other highlights in this new edition include a new chapter on sleep disturbance, a new section on osteoporosis, and a new chapter discussing anemia.

Finally, a new appendix listing a variety of medications, both prescription and over the counter, has been included. Many people with diabetes take a multitude of pills. Some of these medications, taken in combination with your diabetes medication, can raise or lower your blood glucose. Therefore, this appendix is extremely important in helping you avoid high and low blood glucose levels that may be due to medications.

As you read this edition of *The Uncomplicated Guide of Diabetes Complications,* it will become apparent that the single most important approach to preventing diabetes complications is controlling your blood glucose. You should strive for an A1C value of less than

7%. AlC is a test that measures your average blood glucose over a period of 2–3 months. Unfortunately, only 42% of the people in the United States with type 2 diabetes have an A1C of less than 7%. It has been documented that a single percentage point drop in AlC, for example, from 8% to 7%, can reduce the likelihood of diabetes complications by approximately 40%.

To help you achieve improved blood glucose levels and prevent complications, it is important to realize that this is a team effort among you and your physician, nutritionist, diabetes educator, and all other specialists involved in your care. With that in mind, the goal of the third edition of *The Uncomplicated Guide to Diabetes Complications* is to make you and your family aware of the diabetic complications that can occur and to educate you so that you can recognize the complications and discuss their prevention and/or treatment, should they occur, with your physician and his or her team.

Because physicians like to talk in medical terminology, patients frequently have difficulty understanding them. The authors of the chapters in this edition, many of whom are experts in their specialty of diabetes, are well aware of this and have made sure the information provided is easily understood. That is why this book is called *The Uncomplicated Guide to Diabetes Complications*.

Marvin E. Levin, MD
Michael A. Pfeifer, MD

General Overview

1

Diabetes: The Facts and Figures

In a general sense, diabetes is simply abnormally high blood glucose levels, or hyperglycemia. Over time, diabetes may cause complications involving the eyes (retinopathy; chapter 12), kidneys (nephropathy; chapter 17), and nerves (neuropathy; chapters 14–16). Diabetes is also associated with an increased risk of cardiovascular disease, usually appearing in the form of stroke, heart attack (chapters 6, 7, and 11), or peripheral arterial disease (chapter 10).

Diabetes is a common, serious, and expensive condition. In 2008, approximately 24 million people—8% of the population of the United States—had diabetes. Of this population, 17.9 million were diagnosed and 5.7 million were undiagnosed. In the United States, diabetes is the leading cause of blindness (up to 24,000 cases per year), kidney failure (over 46,000 cases per year), and amputations of the feet and legs (over 71,000 non-traumatic amputations per year) in working-age adults. Diabetes is also a major cause of stroke and heart attack (the risk is two to four times higher in those with diabetes), disability (about half of all persons with diabetes reporting being limited in activity), and death (diabetes is the sixth leading cause of death in the United States). The costs attributable to diabetes in the United States alone are over $174 billion per year.

How Is Diabetes Diagnosed?

Common symptoms of diabetes include increased thirst and urination and unexplained weight loss. However, especially in cases of type 2 diabetes, symptoms are so mild they often go unnoticed for years. For many, the first sign of diabetes comes when complications of high blood glucose begin to appear, such as damage to the eyes, kidneys, and nerves, or damage to the heart and blood vessels. During this "asymptomatic" period, a fasting blood glucose level check or an oral glucose tolerance check administered by a health care provider may be the only ways to catch the condition.

According to the American Diabetes Association (ADA), there are three ways to diagnose diabetes (Table 1-1) in adults who are not pregnant, and all require that blood glucose be measured. If an initial glucose tolerance check reveals high glucose levels but there are no other symptoms, another check is recommended at a later date.

Table 1-1. ADA Criteria for Diagnosing Diabetes

1. Symptoms of diabetes plus a blood glucose level $\geq$ 200 mg/dL at any time.

2. Fasting blood glucose level $\geq$ 126 mg/dL. Fasting is defined as no food or drink (other than beverages with no calories) for at least 8 hours.

3. A blood glucose level $\geq$ 200 mg/dL 2 hours after an oral glucose tolerance check. The test should be performed using 75 grams of glucose dissolved in water.

What Are the Different Forms of Diabetes?

Before 1997, diabetes was based on a person's age at diagnosis as either juvenile-onset diabetes mellitus (JODM) or adult-onset diabetes mellitus (AODM), and clarified by type of treatment as either insulin-dependent diabetes mellitus (IDDM) or non-insulin–dependent diabetes. Unfortunately, the different forms of diabetes are very different physiologically and are not always age-specific (the type of diabetes that normally affects the young can also appear in older adults and vice versa). So, in 1997, the current classification system was introduced to recognize two major forms of diabetes: type 1 diabetes and type 2 diabetes. There a several other forms of diabetes, most significantly gestational diabetes, which affects pregnant women. However, the vast majority of diabetes cases fall under type 1 and type 2 diabetes.

In both forms of diabetes, the hormone insulin plays a large role. Insulin is produced in your pancreas and released into your bloodstream when your body senses a rise in blood glucose (usually after eating, but also in response to stress and other situations). Insulin works by moving glucose from the bloodstream into the cells of your body, which use the glucose for energy. In the case of diabetes, insulin production either stops, or it stops working as well as it once did. This breakdown in insulin is what leads to high blood glucose levels. How this breakdown happens is, in large part, what differentiates the types of diabetes.

Type 1 diabetes

Type 1 diabetes is the result of an autoimmune response that causes the body to destroy its own beta cells in the pancreas. No one is exactly sure what causes this response. The beta cells are responsible for the production of insulin, and once they are destroyed, natural insulin production stops, and blood glucose levels rise rapidly. Currently, taking external insulin, either via multiple daily injections or through an insulin pump, is the only treatment for this form of diabetes.

Type 1 diabetes accounts for around 5% of diabetes cases in the United States. Type 1 diabetes commonly occurs in childhood and adolescence, but can occur at any age. Most people with type 1 diabetes have no family history of diabetes, and obesity does not appear to play a part.

Type 2 diabetes

As opposed to the sudden and severe development of type 1 diabetes, type 2 diabetes develops at a much more gradual pace. Though not always, type 2 often begins with a condition called insulin resistance, where the body stops using insulin as efficiently as it once did. To counteract this, the pancreas produces more and more insulin to cover rising blood glucose levels. Eventually, the pancreas can't keep up with the increased demand and it begins to produce less insulin, which leads to even higher blood glucose levels. Why this process happens is still not understood, though we do know that age and/or lifestyle factors—obesity, lack of physical activity, family history, race—play large roles.

Type 2 diabetes accounts for around 95% of all diagnosed diabetes in the United States and the vast majority of the cases of undiagnosed diabetes. Type 2 diabetes occurs more frequently in women with prior gestational diabetes, which develops during pregnancy, and in individuals with high blood pressure and high cholesterol and triglycerides. Most people with type 2 have a family history of diabetes, and the condition is more common in African Americans, Hispanic Americans, Arab Americans, and Native Americans. More than 70% of those with type 2 diabetes are obese.

How Do You Treat Diabetes?

The goal of diabetes treatment is to keep blood glucose levels as close to normal as possible, while minimizing the risk of low blood glucose. According to the ADA, normal blood glucose levels are 70–90 mg/dL fasting and 120–140 mg/dL 1–2 hours after a meal. Numerous studies have demonstrated that normal or near-normal glucose control can delay or prevent the development and progression of complications affecting the eyes, kidneys, and nerves in all forms of diabetes. More recent studies have suggested that near-normal blood glucose control may delay or prevent cardiovascular disease.

Because it can be difficult to determine average glucose levels with self-monitored blood glucose checks alone, the ADA recommends regular A1C checks. A1C is a measure of the average blood glucose level over the previous 3–4 months. In those without diabetes, A1C is generally less than 6.1%. The ADA recommends that those with diabetes strive for an A1C of 7% or less, though certain risk factors may require a slightly higher goal.

The treatment for diabetes depends on the type of diabetes and the individual. Those with type 1 diabetes need insulin either in the form of multiple daily injections or through an insulin pump; there is currently no other approved treatment. The options for type 2 diabetes are a little more varied, and can include lifestyle changes, oral medications, insulin, or a combination of all three.

How Common Is Diabetes?

The number of people developing diabetes and the number of people with diabetes are increasing worldwide. By the year 2025, it is estimated that nearly 300 million persons, or 5.4% of the world's population 20 years of age and older, will have diabetes. The major part of this increase will occur in developing countries where populations are aging and becoming increasingly urbanized (which leads to increased body weight and decreased physical activity).

In 2005, 1.5 million new cases of diabetes were diagnosed in Americans aged 20 years and older. Diabetes disproportionately affected the elderly and minority populations. The incidence of diagnosed diabetes was 7.2 cases per 1,000 population in 2004.

In 2008, about 17.9 million people in the United States reported that they had diabetes. The prevalence of diagnosed diabetes increased with age.

Diabetes was the sixth leading cause of death in the United States in 2004. Overall, the risk of death among people with diabetes is about twice that of people without diabetes of similar age. Unfortunately, most death certificates don't list diabetes as a cause of death, making the actual mortality rates difficult to discern. Only about 10% of people with diabetes who die have diabetes listed as the underlying cause of death on their death certificates, and only about 40% have it listed anywhere on their death certificates. Diabetes was the underlying cause of death for approximately 73,200 Americans in 2004, and diabetes was recorded on the death certificates of approximately 224,100 Americans. In 2003, African American women had the highest death rates due to diabetes, followed by black men and white women. In 2002, heart disease and stroke accounted for about 65% of deaths in people with diabetes.

What Is the Cost of Diabetes?

In the United States in 2007, the direct cost of non-diabetes-related and diabetes-related medical care was estimated to be $116 billion.

In 1992, health care expenditures for people with diabetes averaged $13,243 compared to $2,560 for people without diabetes. In other words, health care costs for people with diabetes were nearly $10,700 higher, or more than five times larger, than for people without diabetes. Part of this difference may be because people with diabetes are older than the general population and health care costs increase with age. Still, when adjusted for age, per capita health care expenditures for people with diabetes were approximately $3,082 higher, or more than twice as high, for people with diabetes than for people without diabetes ($5,642 per person per year versus $2,560 per person per year).

This chapter was written by Kingsley Onyemere, MD, MPH, and William H. Herman, MD, MPH.

2

Pre-Diabetes

Case Study

RS is a 46-year-old African American woman with a strong family history of type 2 diabetes on both sides of her family. She has been healthy all of her life, but a routine examination found an elevated fasting blood glucose level of 115 mg/dL, indicating impaired fasting glucose (IFG). She is 5 feet tall and weighs 143 pounds, which gives her a body mass index (BMI; see chapter 33) of nearly 28, indicating that she is overweight. Her A1C (a measurement of glucose levels over a 2–3 month period) is 6.4%, and her total cholesterol is high at 278 mg/dL. Her doctor performs a glucose tolerance test to see if she has diabetes. Her 2-hour response to the oral glucose is also high at 153 mg/dL, which indicates impaired glucose tolerance (IGT). With these results, she is told she has pre-diabetes.

Would You Like to Know More?

Are you concerned that you or a loved one could have pre-diabetes? Visit *www.diabetes.org* for more information. Once there, you can learn more about prevention and treatment, check your BMI, and find answers to commonly asked questions.

What Is Pre-Diabetes?

To understand pre-diabetes, it helps to understand how one is diagnosed with full-blown diabetes. Clinically, diabetes is defined by the American Diabetes Association as a fasting blood glucose level (meaning you haven't eaten when your level is checked) of 126 mg/dL or higher or a level higher than or equal to 200 mg/dL 2 hours after ingesting a 75-gram glucose load (see Table 2-1). If your levels are higher than this, you are diagnosed with diabetes. Normal levels are less than 100 mg/dL fasting and less than 140 mg/dL 2 hours after a 75-gram glucose load. In the case of type 2 diabetes, blood glucose levels rarely progress from normal to abnormal right away (the case is different in type 1 diabetes, where an autoimmune response destroys the insulin-producing cells in the pancreas, causing blood glucose levels to often rise very quickly and dramatically). Plus, as you can see, there is a large gap between normal glucose levels and levels consistent with diabetes. This "no-man's land" in between normal and diabetes has come to be called pre-diabetes. We now know that individuals with pre-diabetes are very likely to develop diabetes over time and may be at increased risk of both microvascular complications (eye, kidney, and nerve disease) and macrovascular complications (heart disease, stroke) even before the official diagnosis of "diabetes."

Table 2-1. The Range of Glucose Levels: ADA Definitions for Normal, Pre-Diabetes, and Diabetes

	Normal Glucose Range	Pre-Diabetes	Diabetes*
Fasting Blood Glucose	< 100 mg/dL	100–125 mg/dL	≥ 126 mg/dL
2-Hour Blood Glucose following an Oral Glucose Tolerance Test	< 140 mg/dL	140–199 mg/dL	≥ 200 mg/dL

*To make a diagnosis of diabetes, a repeat test (either fasting blood glucose or oral glucose tolerance test) should be performed in most cases.

What Causes Pre-Diabetes?

We know that certain ethnic groups are more prone to develop diabetes than others, especially African Americans, Latinos, Asian Americans, American Indians, and Pacific Islanders. Genetics clearly play a role, but environment is a culprit as well. In addition, individuals with a history of polycystic ovary syndrome, gestational diabetes, and/or stress-related high blood glucose are at greater risk. A sedentary lifestyle and being overweight or obese are usually the factors that help a genetic predisposition transform into diabetes. Being overweight or obese usually results in a condition called "insulin resistance." Insulin resistance means that your cells have impaired action to insulin. Thus, more insulin is needed to get the same cellular effect as a person who is not insulin resistant. At first, your pancreas pumps more and more insulin into the bloodstream to keep glucose levels normal. Eventually, your pancreas cannot keep up with this increased demand, and blood glucose levels will begin to rise. After awhile, your pancreas becomes impaired as well and will produce less and less insulin, making the situation even worse. Blood glucose levels will continue to rise above normal into the pre-diabetes stage and, if left untreated, into the diabetes range.

What Happens if Pre-Diabetes Is Left Untreated?

The progression from pre-diabetes to diabetes occurs over many years, with a higher risk for those with both IFG and IGT compared to either alone. IFG is a fasting glucose between 100–125 mg/dL. IGT is a 2 hour glucose level of 140–199 after the 75-gram glucose test. IFG, IGT, or both are all considered part of pre-diabetes. If you have normal blood glucose, your chance of developing diabetes is less than 1% a year. In contrast, if you have either IFG or IGT, your risk is 5–10% a year. If you have both, it's even higher. Over a lifetime, approximately 80% of those with pre-diabetes will develop diabetes if left untreated. Identifying pre-diabetes gives you and your health care provider the opportunity to examine risk factors, check for complications, and implement a plan for both prevention and treatment. Coronary heart disease (see chapter 6), for example, appears to be far more common in pre-diabetes than in those with normal glucose levels, and the diagnosis of pre-diabetes may lead you and your health care provider to be more proactive with prevention strategies.

Are There Effective Treatments for Pre-Diabetes?

Over the last 10 years, multiple clinical trials from around the world demonstrated the ability to identify people with pre-diabetes, intervene with a variety of different treatments, and slow or prevent the progression to diabetes. Here we highlight the evidence surrounding some of the treatments of pre-diabetes.

Lifestyle modifications

Five separate studies—in China, Finland, India, Japan, and the United States—show the significant benefits of moderate lifestyle changes. These studies all used slightly different methods, but all focused on four things:

1. Increasing physical activity
2. Modestly lowering calorie intake
3. Lowering fat intake
4. Increasing fiber intake.

These four factors generally led to weight loss, which had the biggest effect on delaying diabetes. The methods used were not extreme, and massive weight loss was not required to gain a benefit. Participants were encouraged to lose 7% of their body weight, but by the end of the studies, most usually achieved only around 4%. Despite modest changes, these lifestyle interventions reduced the risk of diabetes by 29–67%. Although the studies were generally carried out for 3–5 years, most participants maintained weight loss after the studies were completed and diabetes rates remained drastically reduced. This represents true prevention of diabetes.

Drug therapy for pre-diabetes

Lifestyle change is an excellent therapy, but it can be difficult for some people, and drug treatment would be a useful alternative. Some studies have shown promising results, but more research is needed before we can confidently suggest medication for pre-diabetes.

The United States Diabetes Prevention Program (DPP) compared the diabetes medication metformin to lifestyle changes. Metformin is an inexpensive, well established, and well tolerated treatment for diabetes, and moderate doses of 850 mg twice daily were recommended. Around 20% of those in the program could not tolerate the drug or had contraindications, but overall, it decreased the development of diabetes by 31%. Younger individuals and those with a BMI greater than or equal to 35 appear to have the best response to metformin. Two weeks after the medication was discontinued, 25% continued to be diabetes-free, suggesting that metformin was doing more than simply treating early diabetes. The combination of metformin and lifestyle was used in the Indian DPP, but did not show any added benefit to either alone. (Metformin alone reduces risk by 26% and metformin plus lifestyle reduces by 28%.)

Other classes of drugs have also been studied in pre-diabetes. In the Study to Prevent Non-Insulin-Dependent Diabetes Mellitus (STOP-NIDDM), acarbose appeared to decrease the development of diabetes by 25%, but this protection completely disappeared after the medication was discontinued. This suggests acarbose was really just treating diabetes early rather than preventing it.

One class of diabetes medications, thiazolidinediones (TZDs), has been controversial in diabetes treatment and continues to be even more controversial in pre-diabetes. Despite causing weight gain, three representatives of this class—troglitazone, rosiglitazone, and pioglitazone—decrease the development of diabetes by well over 50%. Unfortunately, fatal liver disease prompted the removal of troglitazone from the marketplace, and rosiglitazone is under scrutiny for potential cardiovascular side effects. Neverthless, rosiglitazone decreased the risk of diabetes by 60% (while still on the drug) and 40% after the drug was stopped and washed out. Pioglitazone reduced the development of diabetes by 81% over 2.6 years of study, despite an 8-pound weight gain. It appears from preliminary data that it also improves insulin resistance and islet function in the pancreas (the area responsible for producing insulin), which could provide true protection from diabetes, but further studies are currently underway to see if this benefit persists. When considering the use of TZDs to treat pre-diabetes, you and your health care provider must balance the apparent significant reduction in diabetes with the higher cost, weight gain, increase in fluid retention and heart failure, and other possible side effects.

Weight-loss drugs have also shown a decrease in the progression of pre-diabetes to diabetes in two studies, but the side effects of the medications make it difficult to suggest their use in a prevention strategy. Nevertheless, one study used orlistat and it showed a risk reduction of 37%.

In addition, a study in Sweden showed that bariatric surgery can prevent diabetes, but it is generally considered prudent to reserve bariatric surgery for morbidly obese individuals or obese individuals with other complications (see chapter 33).

Should Pre-Diabetes Be Treated?

The evidence is indisputable that you can delay or prevent diabetes by either changing your lifestyle or following drug treatments. The risks of treatment, particularly with lifestyle change, are low, and the benefits extend beyond the prevention of diabetes to improvements in blood pressure and lipids. In addition, lifestyle change is inexpensive.

The ADA recommends lifestyle change with the goal of losing 5–10% of your body weight and engaging in 30 minutes of moderate daily physical activity. If you run an especially high risk for developing diabetes (for instance, you have IFG and IGT combined with other risk factors), metformin therapy may work well, keeping in mind that metformin therapy has been shown to work best if you are younger (less than 60 years of age) or more obese (have a BMI equal to or greater than 35). The ADA does not recommend acarbose, weight loss drugs, or TZDs for treating pre-diabetes at this time.

Back to the Case Study

RS participated in the DPP and was assigned to the lifestyle-modification group of the study. Her caregivers encouraged her to follow a healthy, low-calorie, low-fat diet and to increase her physical activity by walking 150 minutes a week. Her goal was to lose 7% of her body weight (10 pounds). Over the next few years, she complied with the lifestyle recommendations, losing 13 pounds (9% of her body weight). Her fasting glucose remained in the 95–108 mg/dL range, her A1C stayed 6.1–6.3%, and she was able to reduce her total cholesterol to 175 mg/dL.

After 8 years, however, her lifestyle changes have waned, and she has gained weight beyond her baseline to 150 pounds. Her total cholesterol has risen to 286 mg/dL. Her A1C has increased to 6.9% and her glucose tolerance test reveals a 2-hour glucose of 252 mg/dL—well within the range of diabetes. This is confirmed with a second glucose tolerance test, which reveals a fasting glucose of 148 mg/dL and an elevated 2-hour glucose.

To keep her blood glucose under control and minimize long-term complications, she has started medication therapy with 850 mg of metformin twice daily. In addition, she has started taking a statin to reduce her cholesterol levels, and an aspirin. She is encouraged to restart her lifestyle changes and to aim for her previous weight loss.

Even though she eventually developed diabetes, RS successfully delayed its onset and was diagnosed and treated early in the course of her diabetes. Early, aggressive, and appropriate management is her best opportunity to avoid the complications of diabetes.

* * * *

If you have pre-diabetes, estimates suggest that by just making modest lifestyle changes, you can delay the onset of diabetes by more than 11 years. Metformin can delay the onset of diabetes by 3.4 years. Furthermore, both can reduce your risk of diabetes-related complications such as blindness, kidney disease, amputation, stroke, and heart disease.

This chapter was written by Robert E. Ratner, MD, and Vanita R. Aroda, MD.

3

Diabetes Standards of Care

Over the last decade, the management of diabetes has undergone revo-lutionary change. High-quality diabetes care is much more widely avail-able, and many new treatments have been developed. Unfortunately, many patients and some doctors have gotten stuck in the old ways of doing things. The purpose of this chapter is to make sure that you know what you and your health care team should focus on to ensure a long and healthy life with diabetes. In the 21st century, it is reasonable for you to expect a long life without diabetes-specific complications.

The Diabetes Team

You didn't know that you were part of a diabetes team? Well, guess what? You are. Not only that, you are the captain and most valuable player. You are responsible for almost all the good plays as well as the bad ones in your personal diabetes care. You decide what you are going to eat, when and how long you'll go for a walk, whether you'll take your medicines on time, how often you'll monitor your blood sugars, and whether you'll go for your check-ups. But this is no game, it's your life. And you're participating 24 hours a day, 7 days a week, most likely for the rest of your life.

Just like any other most valuable player and captain, how well you perform in some ways is not entirely under your control. It will be determined partially by your teammates. Your teammates in this struggle of diabetes are friends, family, co-workers, your community, and very importantly, your insurance company. As captain of this team, with your coaches, you need to make sure everyone is helping you move forward and not holding you back.

Coaches

No matter how good your team, to get the most out of your efforts you need some good coaches. Everyone with diabetes should probably have at least two coaches:

1. A primary care doctor
2. A diabetes educator

You will likely need other coaches from time to time. These include:

- Pharmacist
- Nutritional counselor (registered dietitian)
- Behavior therapist (psychiatrist, psychologist, medical social worker)
- Eye care professional (ophthalmologist or optometrist)
- Foot care specialist (podiatrist)
- Shoe specialist (pedorthist)
- Diabetes specialist (endocrinologist)
- A host of others trained professionals with special expertise that can be helpful to some patients with diabetes

Remember, none of your coaches can or will take care of your diabetes. They are on the sidelines, making suggestions, teaching, helping you see where you are going wrong and what you are doing right. Just like the most valuable player and captain on any team, you need to communicate well with your coaches. Be sure they know what you feel prepared to do now and what you are willing to work on. When a team has trouble achieving goals, it's generally because the coaches and the key players are not aligned. Coaches and star athletes often butt heads. But successful teams always work out their disagreements before game time. In your diabetes care, make sure you don't leave a session with your coaches without a well-defined plan that everyone agrees is appropriate, doable, and measurable.

Measurements

Athletes and coaches measure all kinds of statistics beyond just the final score of a game. Why? To see patterns that help determine what works and what does not. Being the star of your diabetes team, you need to be aware of all the important measurements, how you personally perform, and what the expectations are to remain well. There are fourteen areas on which your team should focus in diabetes. This may sound like a lot but, fortunately, these areas are pretty simple and easy to track. Table 3-1 lists the key measurements for your diabetes care and when they should be taken. Make sure that you take the measurements and that you both know and understand the results. When you are underperforming, make sure to develop a plan to get back on track. This is the responsibility of the whole team—you, your teammates, and the coaches.

Most of the measurements are discussed in more detail elsewhere in this book. But remember—each is critically important. You could literally be dead wrong if you think that glucose or blood sugar is the only thing that is important in diabetes care.

Table 3-1. Fourteen Areas of Focus in Diabetes Measurements

Focus	Measurement	Goal	Frequency
Glucose	A1C	Less than 7.0%	Every 3 to 6 months
	Before meal, bedtime, and mid-sleep finger-prick glucose	70–130 mg/dL	As needed to ensure control and to avoid hypoglycemia
	1–2 hours after meal finger-prick glucose	Less than 180 mg/dL	As needed to ensure control
Blood Pressure	Systolic/diastolic blood pressure	Less than 130/80 mmHg	Every doctor's visit

Focus	Measurement	Goal	Frequency
Cholesterol	LDL (bad) cholesterol (fasting)	Less than 100 mg/dL for most (less than 70 mg/dL with vascular disease, hypertension, smoking, or family history of early vascular disease)	Annually; more often while adjusting treatment
	Non-HDL cholesterol (does not require fasting)	Less than 130 mg/dL for most (less than 100 mg/dL with vascular disease, hypertension, smoking, or family history of early vascular disease)	
	HDL (good) cholesterol (does not require fasting)	Greater than 40 mg/dL (greater than 50 md/dL if you are a woman)	
	Apolipoprotein B (ApoB; does not require fasting)	Less than 90 mg/dL (less than 80 mg/dl with vascular disease, hypertension, smoking, or family history of early vascular disease)	
	Triglycerides (fasting)	Less than 150 mg/dL	
Aspirin	History	Appropriate therapy	81 mg daily if vascular disease is present or over age 40 with additional risk factors
Weight	BMI	Ideal: 18.5–24.9 kg/m^2	Every visit
Kidney	Estimated GFR (eGFR) derived from serum creatinine test	More than 60 ml/min/1.73m^2	Annually
	Albumin-to-creatinine ratio	Less than 30 mcg/mg	
Feet	Complete exam	Can feel 10g filament	Annually
Eye	Dilated eye exam	Normal	Annually
Arteries	History and physical	Normal exam, no symptoms; stress testing with symptoms	Every visit
Depression	Frequency of feeling sad or blue	None or infrequently	Every visit
Tobacco	Medical history	None	Every visit
Sex	History	No concerns; contraception	Every visit
Education	History	Understand all aspects of care and complications	At diagnosis; annual update
General Health	History	Vaccines, cancer screening, liver test (ALT), etc.	At least annually

Glucose Treatment Techniques

Of all the improvements associated with the treatment of diabetes, glucose-lowering techniques have advanced the most over the last decade. We now have twelve different types of glucose-lowering techniques for type 2 diabetes. They are listed in Table 3-2, in the order they were first available for use in the United States. The table also lists the relative effect in lowering A1C (an indicator of average glucose level), whether they can produce hypoglycemia (low blood sugar) as a complication, what they do to weight, how often they need to be taken, and whether there are other concerns that are particularly notable. For some people, concerns over the safety and costs of newer medication might be the most important. For others, how often a medication needs to be taken is really critical to being able to follow the treatment plan; if you just can't remember to take medication three times a day, it will not work very well if it needs to be taken three times a day. For some, particularly those who drive or do physical labor for a living, concern over hypoglycemia and the potential for injury as a consequence might be a critical safety concern. To make sure they are in agreement, people with diabetes may need to spend significant time with their coaches carefully reviewing advantages and disadvantages of treatments.

Table 3-2. Twelve Glucose Lowering Techniques

Type of treatment	Generic name	Brand names	A1C % reduction	Can it cause a low blood sugar reaction?	What does it do to weight?	How many times a day do you need to take it?	Other concerns
Lifestyle treatment	N/A	N/A	More than 1%	No	Loss	Minimum of 30 min/ 5x a week*	
Rapid acting insulin	Regular insulin	Humulin or NovolinR	More than 1%	Yes	Gain	1–4 (injected)	Must be timed to meals
	Lispro	Humalog					
	Aspart	Novolog					
	Glulisine	Apidra					
Long acting insulin	NPH insulin	Humulin or NovolinN	More than 1%	Yes	Gain	Usually 1 (injected)	
	Glargine	Lantus					
	Detemir	Levemir					

*Check with your healthcare provider regarding the best type of exercise and length of exercise before starting. If you have nerve damage to your feet, some types of exercise may not be advisable; your HCP may suggest a heart stress test before beginning an exercise program.

Type of treatment	Generic name	Brand names	A1C % reduction	Can it cause a low blood sugar reaction?	What does it do to weight?	How many times a day do you need to take it?	Other concerns
Sulfonylurea	Glipizide ER	Generic available	More than 1%	Yes	Gain	1	May fail over time
	Glyburide	Generic available				1–2	
	Glimepiride	Generic available				1	
Biguanide	Metformin	Generic available	More than 1%	No	Neutral	Usually 2	Nausea, diarrhea
Alpha-glucosidase inhibitors	Acarbose	Generic available	Less than 1%	No	Neutral	Usually 3	Gas; must be timed to meals.
	Miglitol	Glyset					
Glitazone	Rosiglitazone	Avandia	About 1%	No	Gain	1–2	Heart failure; bone fractures; swelling in lower extremities (edema); swelling in back of eye (macular edema); rosiglitazone is also associated with increased risk of ischemic heart disease
	Pioglitazone	Actos				1	
Glinide	Repaglinide	Prandin	More than 1%	Yes	Gain	Usually 3	Must be timed to meals
	Nateglinide	Starlix	Less than 1%	Rare	Gain	Usually 3	
Amylin-mimetic	Pramlintide	Symlin	Less than 1%	No	Loss	2–3 (injected)	Nausea; may limit your ability to recover from a low blood glucose caused by another agent
Incretin agonist	Exenatide	Byetta	About 1%	No	Loss	2 (injected)	Nausea, vomiting
DPP-IV inhibitor	Sitagliptin	Januvia	Less than 1%	No	Neutral	1	
Bile resin	Colesevelam	WelChol	Less than 1%	No	Neutral	6 tablets a day; also approved for lowering cholesterol	

Lifestyle therapy

When it comes to treatment options, one thing is for certain—few diabetes teams or coaches spend enough time and effort on lifestyle therapy. Whereas drugs generally lower glucose, or cholesterol, or blood pressure, or improve heart health, or reduce depression, or whatever, physical activity and good nutrition have extremely broad benefits. There are very well-done studies that demonstrate that a serious effort on the part of motivated patients working regularly with lifestyle coaches, usually dietitians but in some cases also trainers and behavioral therapists, can lead to weight loss and improve essentially all the areas that we focus on in diabetes care.

Not every lifestyle program works, however. Those that do generally include a cluster of similar attributes:

- Frequent meetings with lifestyle coaches—every week for the first month, every month for the first three months, and every three months for life
- A structured program
- Moderately vigorous exercise such as brisk walking for 30 or more minutes at least five days a week, with strength training to provide additional benefit if needed
- Low-calorie balanced nutrition with a focus on increased consumption of vegetables, fruits, whole grains, and low-fat sources of protein (such as beans, low-fat dairy products, fish, skinless poultry, and low-fat meats) and decreased consumption of refined carbohydrates (such as white bread, high-fructose corn syrup) and alcohol

Putting It All Together—"Good CENSE"

Diabetes is a serious health condition. Most people are scared when they are first told that they have diabetes. That is natural, but, in fact, absolutely the wrong way to approach the problem. In many, many ways, the diagnosis of diabetes is an opportunity to take better care of yourself than you would have been inclined to do anyway—you will certainly be healthier knowing that you have diabetes than if you did not. You should expect to live a long and healthy life with the disease. You just have to use good CENSE.

C—Control

Diabetes is a controllable disease. But you have to control all the individual parts. Check your blood sugar at home often enough to be sure that it stays controlled between visits with your team. Routinely get A1C tests, blood pressure measurements, cholesterol tests, and have your weight monitored regularly. Achieve and maintain control of all of these components. Doing so is the most significant way to avoid complications of diabetes.

E—Evaluate

Once you have your measurements, work with your team to evaluate the numbers. These will tell you what is good and what could use work. If your numbers indicate that you have complications, it is not the end of the world. Early treatment can almost always prevent serious problems or disability. Technically, almost no one with diabetes should go blind, have an amputation, or need dialysis. Unfortunately, one overlooked complication of diabetes is depression, a complication that makes it more difficult to get your diabetes under control. Get check-ups for your kidneys, feet, eyes, arteries, and heart and for depression. Discuss whether you should have a stress test with your doctor. Take aspirin unless you can't; there are alternatives that you can discuss with your team. Bring attention to problems that you notice, particularly chest discomfort or shortness of breath that seems out of the ordinary. But even if you feel great, make sure to get your exams and tests, as early complications rarely, if ever, produce symptoms until things have gotten pretty bad.

N—No smoking

Tobacco and diabetes make a nasty combination that drastically increases your risk for heart attack, stroke, and poor circulation to the legs. It is a poor choice to smoke whether you have diabetes or not. Smoking with diabetes is like throwing gasoline on a fire. If you smoke, make a huge effort to stop. If you don't smoke, don't start.

S—Sex

Women with diabetes should not get pregnant unless they prepare and plan beforehand with their team. Good control (the "C" in CENSE) and caution with regard to the medications that you take are essential for a healthy baby. With the proper planning, women with diabetes should be able to have perfectly normal healthy babies. Without planning, tragedies can happen. If you have problems with sex, whether you are a man or a woman, recognize that sexual dysfunction is common in diabetes and can almost always be solved. Feel free to raise concerns with your team; it's guaranteed that they have heard them before.

E—Education

You are the captain and most valuable player on the team, which means much of the legwork is your responsibility. It is essential that you understand diabetes, its treatments, its complications, and how to care for yourself. Make sure not to shirk your responsibility to be the best that you can be. You've made a great first step in getting this book and reading it. You should see a Certified Diabetes Educator (CDE) regularly. Most insurance covers comprehensive initial diabetes education plus three hours with a dietitian. In subsequent years, coverage generally includes another two hours of education as well as two hours with a dietitian.

One More Thing

Because you have diabetes, your family and friends are likely to be at risk. Your family is at risk because they are related to you, and diabetes is in part a genetically determined problem. Your friends are at risk because they probably share lifestyle similarities with you that are linked to diabetes. What should you encourage all of them to do?

If your friends and family are overweight, they should be checked for diabetes with a fasting glucose test at least every three years, starting at puberty. If they are not overweight, they should be checked at least every three years, starting at age 45. A normal result is 99 mg/dL or less. If the result is 100 mg/dL or more, they should have it checked again. If both tests are 126 mg/dL or higher, they will be diagnosed with diabetes. If they have a result between 100 and 125 mg/dL, they may want to have a glucose tolerance test to further define their risk (see chapter 2). In any case, they should follow two lifestyle treatments (activity and nutrition) often prescribed to those with diabetes:

1. Moderate-intensity aerobic exercise such as brisk walking for at least 30 minutes at least five days a week
2. Reduced calorie intake designed to drop 1/2 to 1 pound per week, with a goal of losing at least 5% of body weight (for example, 10 pounds if they weigh 200 pounds)

Those two simple things will reduce their risk of developing diabetes by about 60%. And you can do them together and help each other be the best that each of you can be.

This chapter was written by John B. Buse, MD, PhD.

Acute Complications

4

DKA, HHS, and Lactic Acidosis

Case Study

MJ is 47 years old and has had type 1 diabetes for 20 years. She is suffering from an intestinal flu with vomiting and hasn't eaten in 24 hours. Because she hasn't eaten, she has mistakenly decided not to take any insulin. Now she feels really awful, dizzy, and short of breath. The vomiting continues. She calls her health care provider, who suspects diabetic ketoacidosis (DKA) and tells her to go to the emergency room immediately.

Case Study

LP is 72 years old, lives alone, and was just diagnosed with type 2 diabetes last week. He has been taking prednisone, a steroid, for 4 weeks for another serious condition. Now he is extremely thirsty and urinating often. He feels exhausted. Sensing that something is wrong, he goes to see his physician, who finds that his blood pressure is low and his blood glucose level is 925 mg/dL. By now he is sleepy and lethargic. He is experiencing a hyperosmolar hyperglycemic state (HHS).

What Is DKA?

DKA occurs when blood glucose levels rise too high, and the body becomes very dehydrated and begins to burn excessive amounts of fat for energy. This causes the body to produce ketones, acid products of burning fat. The large excess of ketones and acids give this condition the name ketoacidosis. When severe, this can be life-threatening.

What Causes DKA?

When you don't have enough insulin or it's not working right, glucose cannot get from your bloodstream into the cells. The cells send out a distress signal. Replacement glucose is made in the liver and flows into the blood. In DKA, both factors—slower exit of glucose from the blood and faster entrance of glucose from the liver—raise glucose levels in the blood. Exactly how high they can go depends on still another organ, the kidney.

The role of the kidney is complicated to explain (Figure 4-1). The kidney saves glucose, because the glucose molecule is essential to so many body functions. Normally, glucose is filtered out of the blood in one part of the kidney and returned to the blood in another part. However, when blood glucose (BG) levels rise above 180 mg/dL, the kidney cannot reclaim it all and lets the excess glucose go in the urine. This is how the kidney helps keep BG from going even higher than it already has.

The glucose must be dissolved in water to be excreted. So, your body needs more water. The glucose excreted in urine takes with it huge amounts of water and sodium chloride (salt). Sodium chloride keeps enough water in the bloodstream so that the blood pumped by the heart can carry sufficient oxygen and nutrients to every cell in the body. As more and more water and sodium chloride are lost in the urine, you become dried out (dehydrated), limiting further what the kidney can do. Thus, two of the symptoms of uncontrolled diabetes are extreme thirst and excessive urination. Finally, in DKA, the kidney excretes more fluid than you drink, and your body becomes severely dehydrated. The kidney cannot filter enough glucose out of the blood. Your BG can rise to levels of 400–1,000 mg/dL (and, although rarely, sometimes higher).

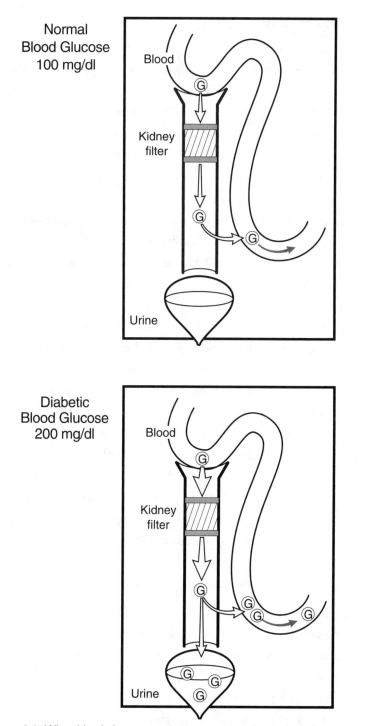

Figure 4-1. When blood glucose goes above a certain level, the kidney releases glucose in the urine.

What Does Ketoacidosis Mean?

Ordinarily, the body burns fat and carbohydrates and produces carbon dioxide and water. To keep this process going efficiently, some glucose must be added to the fuel mix; this requires insulin. When insulin either is unavailable or doesn't work properly, two things happen. First, more fat is released from storage cells and broken down for use as an energy source, but there's too much fat, and the liver can't burn it completely. The process stops at a chemical halfway point—becoming ketoacids—before carbon dioxide and water are formed (Figure 4-2). The ketoacids are made in huge quantities, and they pile up in the blood after they are released from the liver. The ketoacids are the keto in ketoacidosis. They also are excreted in your urine and can be detected by a urine ketone test, as well as by a fingerstick blood test.

Now, what about acidosis? The two ketoacids are relatively strong acids. Think of them like acetic acid in vinegar. The body cannot tolerate ketoacids for long. They must be neutralized, and the body converts them to carbon dioxide, which is exhaled by the lungs. People with DKA must breathe more rapidly and deeply to get rid of the extra carbon dioxide. Ketoacids are also changed into acetone, which is exhaled. This causes the breath to have a fruity odor. If the lungs did not get rid of the extra carbon dioxide, the high acid level of the blood would poison all the body cells, and life would cease. That's why insulin was truly a magical, life-saving drug in the first few years of its use—and it still is.

What Puts You at Risk for Developing DKA?

Not having enough insulin puts you at risk for DKA. Most cases occur in people with type 1 diabetes. In some instances, the individuals did not even know they had diabetes—for example, school-age children sent off to camp, where neither they nor their counselors recognized that frequent urination or bed-wetting could be signs of diabetes. Most people with undiagnosed diabetes have suffered

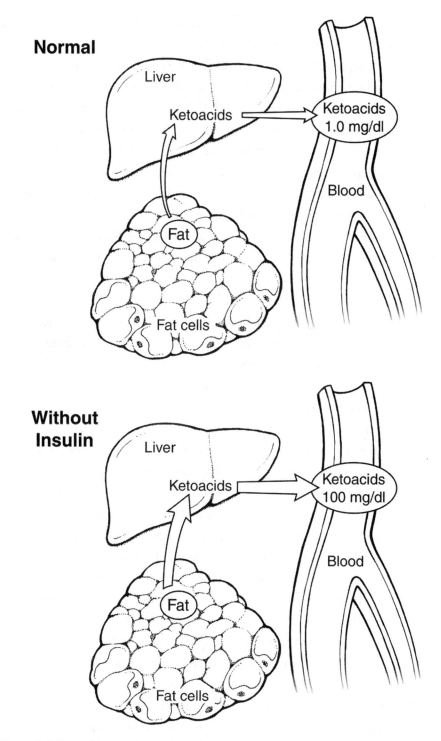

Figure 4-2. Ketoacids are a by-product of the incomplete breakdown of fat in the liver.

from frequent urination, thirst, loss of weight, and blurred vision for 4–8 weeks before they see a doctor.

People with type 1 diabetes who have an interruption in their insulin treatment get DKA. The time between stopping insulin and going into DKA varies a great deal. The quickest example occurs in those who use an insulin pump. If the catheter gets blocked or the pump stops delivering insulin for any reason, DKA can occur within 6–12 hours, because the insulin used in the pump is rapid-acting insulin, which disappears quickly from the body. (Note: This is not a reason to avoid the insulin pump, just be aware.) In contrast, DKA may take several days to develop after stopping NPH, lente insulin, ultralente insulin, insulin glargine, or insulin detemir because they hang around longer in the skin. The more years a person has had type 1 diabetes, the more quickly DKA is likely to develop when treatment is interrupted, because there are no beta cells left to provide even the small amount of insulin it takes to prevent ketoacidosis.

Even if you take all prescribed insulin doses, DKA can still happen. This is usually brought about by an illness—such as strep throat or intestinal flu. Flu is especially bad because it causes vomiting and/or diarrhea, both of which decrease body fluids and make dehydration worse. The stress of an illness or surgery causes your body to release stress hormones, including cortisone, glucagon, epinephrine, and growth hormone. Each of these opposes insulin action. Together, they raise BG and ketoacid levels. In people with type 1 who have little or no insulin reserve, DKA can develop quickly unless extra insulin is given. Those with type 2 diabetes can develop DKA even though their bodies make insulin. They have insulin resistance; their bodies are resistant to the action of insulin, and they need additional insulin to correct the elevated BG and DKA.

As in the first case study, people cause DKA by not taking insulin when they are vomiting or have diarrhea. They make the mistake of thinking that because they are not eating, their blood glucose will be low. If you don't inject insulin, your BG will rise even if you haven't eaten, because your liver will continue to make glucose.

On rare occasions, no illness can be found, but DKA still occurs. The stress causing DKA may be emotional, such as a distressing school, work, or family situation. Emotional upsets can cause repeated episodes of DKA weeks or months apart, and your physician or family may need to help you unveil the problem to yourself. You may need professional help.

DKA is more likely to occur in adolescents, who are trying to deal with the physical, psychological, and social changes of puberty in addition to diabetes. The problem is especially dangerous when it leads teenagers to stop taking insulin as a means of testing themselves, their diabetes, and their family's love and attention. Teenage girls will sometimes allow themselves to have higher-than-normal glucose levels, so they can eat whatever they want and not gain weight. The problem is that it takes very little to send them into ketoacidosis. They are seen multiple times a year in the emergency room in DKA. If the parents or doctor recognize what is happening, they can help the young person balance their responsibilities better.

Can People with Type 2 Diabetes Develop DKA?

Yes, DKA can occur in older people with type 2 diabetes. It is usually brought on by major medical illness such as a heart attack, trauma such as a hip fracture, or an emergency surgery such as appendicitis. When there is no obvious cause of DKA, your physician must look for unusual infections that may be masked by the DKA itself. These include meningitis, serious external ear infections, fungal infections in the nose, dental infections, and even rectal abscesses. Finally, adrenal or pituitary glands may secrete excess amounts of the stress hormones mentioned above. In rare cases, this may present as DKA. You might say that while DKA itself is easy to recognize, identifying its cause may take detective work by you and your diabetes care team.

What Are the Symptoms of DKA?

With few exceptions, you feel awful. Rising BG levels cause frequent urination and extreme thirst. Dehydration causes a parched tongue, weakness, and dizziness on standing. The high blood-acid level causes nausea, vomiting, and, rarely, abdominal pain so severe that it mimics diseases such as appendicitis. Diarrhea is not a symptom of DKA, and its presence may point to gastroenteritis as the illness causing DKA. You hyperventilate to "blow off" the carbon dioxide being formed from neutralizing the acid in the blood. This often gives you the sensation of being short of breath. After many hours of high BG, the brain cells also become dehydrated and function abnormally. Lethargy, sleepiness, and confusion result and can end up as coma. Someone must get you to a hospital immediately.

How Is DKA Treated?

The most pressing need is for intravenous water and salt. These are given rapidly in the first 1–2 hours of treatment to restore circulation to all body tissues. This improves blood flow to the kidneys so they can remove glucose from the blood more efficiently (Figure 4-1). More intravenous fluid is given slowly over 8–24 hours until all the body water losses have been made up. This may require as much as 5–10 quarts of fluid.

Next, you need regular or rapid-acting insulin. This is also given intravenously whenever possible to guarantee a quick and reliable effect. However, rapid-acting insulin such as lispro (Humalog) or aspart (Novolog) given hourly or every two hours by subcutaneous injection is also effective. Besides bringing BG down to a reasonable range (150–250 mg/dL), the insulin stops the release and the burning of so much fat. In turn, this stops production of ketoacids and gradually corrects the acidosis. It is important to get potassium, too. Otherwise, potassium levels may fall to dangerously low levels in the blood because the cells soak it up so quickly. A very low blood potassium level can interfere with the action of the heart. Occasionally, phosphate is given. The rarest are circumstances where magnesium falls to critically low levels in the blood and causes heart irregularities that require emergency treatment with intravenous magnesium.

The acidosis is gradually corrected by insulin treatment. Occasionally, however, the level of acid is so high that it endangers you. A sterile liquid form of baking soda may be given intravenously to neutralize the excess of acid and allow time for insulin to work. This is usually not recommended for young children, however.

Your pulse, blood pressure, and mental status are checked hourly. Blood samples to check glucose, acid levels, potassium, and phosphate are taken regularly. To prevent vomiting, no fluids are allowed by mouth. All intravenous fluids given and all urine passed must be measured and charted to be sure that you are regaining body fluids. Electrocardiograms (ECGs) are performed. It is small wonder that most people get very little rest and are often very tired and somewhat cranky the next day.

How Can You Prevent DKA?

Learn when to be concerned about DKA and how to check for it. Ask your physician to help you make a sick-day plan. Any illness, even the common cold, should trigger your and your family's early warning system. Fever, nausea, and vomiting even one time are danger flags. If you have any of these symptoms, check BG and urine ketones immediately. If BG level is less than 250 mg/dL and urine ketones are negative, take your usual insulin doses and continue to monitor BG and urine ketones every 4 hours until the illness has passed. Drink fluids of all kinds, in generous amounts. If you vomit a second time, your BG increases to more than 250 mg/dL, or the urine test for ketones becomes positive, call your health care provider immediately for advice.

You must pay attention to vomiting, because it increases your risk of dehydration. Diarrhea may add to the loss of fluids and salts. Infants and young children are particularly vulnerable to DKA because they normally begin with less fluid in their bodies. Elderly people have less kidney function to start with. You can replace lost water and salt with bouillon (one cube in 8 oz water). Gatorade or similar products or a solution of glucose, salt, baking soda, and potassium, recommended by the World Health Organization, usually works well. Small amounts of fluid taken frequently, for example, 3 ounces every 20–30 minutes for an adult, are better for you than large amounts drunk rapidly. If BG is below normal, drink high-carbohydrate fluids, such as fruit juices, regular sodas, or tea with sugar, alternating with fluids that contain salt, such as bouillon.

Some physicians provide you with prescriptions in advance for medications for nausea and vomiting, such as rectal suppositories and instructions on how to use them. Stopping the vomiting helps prevent DKA because it reduces the risk of dehydration.

The other rule is: Never stop your insulin injections because of loss of appetite, nausea, vomiting, or fear of hypoglycemia. You may need to change your insulin dose. That is why you need to check your BG and urine ketones often to navigate through this dangerous period, especially if you have signs of DKA. You may need to check every 2 hours, even in the middle of the night, and call in the results to your health care team. They should give you instructions about doses of insulin to take and instructions for future doses, depending on later BG and urine ketone test results.

When you call the doctor, have up-to-the-minute BG and urine ketone results and an estimate of how much and what kind of fluids you have drunk. If you all work together as a true team, the risk of DKA can be minimized or eliminated. If the infection is bacterial (for example, strep throat), antibiotics may speed your recovery, so get prescriptions filled immediately. Once your BG has been in a safe range (100–200 mg/dL) for a few hours and no ketones are in your urine, the danger of DKA is generally over.

What Are the Signs that DKA Is Getting Worse?

Continued vomiting, complaints of shortness of breath, and excessive sleepiness. Your doctor may note breathlessness and a dulling of mental processes by listening to you on the telephone. That's why he should talk with you and not a family member. If these symptoms appear, you need to go to the emergency room for help.

What Is Hyperosmolar Hyperglycemic State (HHS)?

Many of the things already said about DKA apply to HHS. The first H stands for hyperosmolar and is a technical way of saying that all of the chemicals contained in blood are now dissolved in much less water. Because of this, water is drawn into the blood from the body cells, and the person becomes dehydrated. The blood may become so thick that it clots easily, which can cause strokes and heart attacks.

Hyperglycemic (the second H) means that BG levels are too high. HHS has a higher average blood glucose (900 mg/dL or higher) than DKA. BG can go higher for several reasons. HHS develops more slowly and gradually. The thirsty individual seems to prefer sweet liquids with higher carbohydrate content. The function of the kidneys is more greatly reduced because the person becomes more dehydrated. And the individual or caregivers ignore or mistake the symptoms for something else and wait too long to see the health care team. By the time they do, the loss of salt and, especially, plain water from the body can be enormous.

Ketoacids are not produced in HHS and do not build up in the blood. The reason may be that these people have type 2 diabetes. They still make a small amount of insulin. The lack of high acid levels in the blood is a reason for the long delay in getting care: They are not alerted by nausea and vomiting that something is very wrong. HHS more often leads to coma (a state of unconsciousness) than does DKA. It is more life-threatening and harder to reverse.

Who Is at Risk of Developing HHS?

The typical person at risk of HHS is elderly and is often living alone or in a nursing home and may be unaware that she even has type 2 diabetes. A heart attack or an infection that has spread into the bloodstream from a site such as the urinary tract or a foot ulcer may start the process. Certain drugs can contribute to a steep rise in BG, too. Examples are prednisone or other steroids, diuretics such as hydrochlorothiazide, and anticonvulsant medication such as dilantin.

What Are the Symptoms of HHS?

You are usually more dehydrated—literally dried out—with prune-like, wrinkled skin. You are more likely to be in shock, that is, to have very low blood pressure with poor blood flow to many organs. Coma is much more frequent. The brain may be so affected by the dehydration that seizures, paralysis, and other neurological problems can occur. Many people seem to have had a stroke; yet, with complete treatment, the abnormal neurological signs can disappear completely. It may take several days. HHS is a more serious acute complication of diabetes than is DKA, and the chances of recovering from it are not as good, even with correct treatment.

What Is the Treatment for HHS?

Usually, only small amounts of insulin are required. Those with HHS need emergency fluid flowing to their tissues to get them out of shock and to restore normal blood flow to the heart, brain, kidneys, liver, and limbs. Because elderly people with type 2 diabetes usually have atherosclerosis, improving blood flow and oxygen delivery quickly is vital to prevent complete blockage of one of these narrowed major arteries. A blockage can cause a heart attack, stroke, or kidney failure.

How Can You Prevent HHS?

You, your family, nursing home personnel, and health care professionals all need to be educated about this condition. Elderly people should be tested for diabetes periodically. Paying close attention to the welfare of elderly relatives who have diabetes can prevent many cases. Aides and nurses in facilities that care for the aged must be alert to frequent urination or the abrupt appearance of incontinence. Elderly people do not experience thirst as well as younger people do, when the body needs water. They and their caregivers need to note how much fluid they drink. Don't write off a decline in mental status as "senile dementia" without checking for high BG. Likewise, don't dismiss a complaint of dizziness, especially on standing, which could signal a low volume of blood. We need to be as concerned that a person is having a "glucose attack" as we are for heart attacks and the recently coined term brain attacks. Nothing is easier or more certain to help a person with HHS than to bring down a dangerously high blood glucose level—provided treatment is started in time.

What Is Lactic Acidosis (LA)?

Lactic acidosis is a condition like DKA. Lactic acid is normally present in blood and muscle tissue as a by-product of the metabolism of glucose. When some event such as a heart attack limits oxygen to the blood and tissues, lactic acid levels can build up. LA occurring with diabetes is rare. The symptoms can be like those of DKA. The high blood acid level causes nausea and vomiting, and the person has to breathe hard to get rid of the carbon dioxide being released.

Who Is at Risk for Developing LA?

Rarely, LA will appear in people with type 2 diabetes who take metformin, a diabetes pill. Metformin (Glucophage) is an effective and safe medication for people with type 2 diabetes. If the kidneys are not functioning, however, problems can arise. For example, JD is taking metformin for his type 2 diabetes. He also has vascular disease and had dye-contrast X-rays taken yesterday. Today, the dye is causing kidney problems. Because he was not told to stop the metformin before the test, he develops LA.

Although LA is a very uncommon complication of taking metformin, it does happen. You should not be taking metformin if you have kidney disease, liver disease, alcoholism, cardiovascular disease, or if you are pregnant.

What Are the Symptoms of LA?

The symptoms of LA are nausea, vomiting, abdominal pain, shortness of breath, and lethargy. The signs are shock, severe anemia, low blood pressure, and hyperventilation. LA can have serious effects on the heart and blood circulation, affecting heart rhythm, heart rate, and blood pressure.

What Is the Treatment for LA?

As with DKA, it is important to restore fluid for circulation to provide oxygen and nutrients to all body tissues. Salt and water may be given intravenously along with a sterile form of baking soda to neutralize the acid. Using a dialysis machine to cleanse the blood of metformin and lactic acid is sometimes an effective treatment.

This chapter was written by Saul M. Genuth, MD.

5

Low Blood Glucose

How Does Your Body Naturally Avoid Low Blood Glucose?

When you eat, the rise in glucose tells your pancreas to release insulin (a hormone) into the blood. Insulin, natural or injected, opens the door to the cells and lowers the amount of glucose in the blood. There are several other hormones—glucagon, epinephrine, cortisol, and growth hormone—that work to raise blood glucose levels (Table 5-1). These hormones are released into the blood when blood glucose gets too low. They are called counterregulatory or stress hormones.

Table 5-1. Hormones Controlling Glucose Levels

Lowers Blood Glucose	Raises Blood Glucose
Insulin	Glucagon
	Epinephrine (adrenaline)
	Cortisol
	Growth hormone

Glucagon is made in the pancreas, as is insulin, but in a different type of cell. It raises glucose levels within a few minutes by causing the liver to release glucose into the blood. Epinephrine, also known as adrenaline, is made by the adrenal glands. Epinephrine works within minutes. It stops insulin release, causes cells not to respond to insulin, and also causes the liver to release glucose. When it is released in response to hypoglycemia, it causes rapid heartbeat, sweating, and a feeling of anxiety. Cortisol is released by another part of the adrenal glands and acts more slowly to raise blood glucose. Growth hormone is released by the pituitary gland. It also acts more slowly to raise blood glucose levels.

What Are the Symptoms of Hypoglycemia?

Symptoms of hypoglycemia are usually divided into those that affect the body and those that affect the brain (Table 5-2). Among the bodily symptoms, rapid and forceful heartbeat, hunger, sweating, and nausea are the most common. Most of these symptoms are related to the release of epinephrine.

Table 5-2. Symptoms of Hypoglycemia

Bodily Symptoms	Central Nervous System Symptoms
Rapid heartbeat	Light-headedness
Sweating	Confusion
Tremors	Headache
Nausea	Anxiety
Hunger	Slurred speech
	Delayed reflexes
	Seizures
	Loss of consciousness (coma)

When the brain is affected, symptoms may range from lightheadedness and anxiety to confusion, loss of consciousness, and even seizures. These symptoms occur when the brain doesn't get enough glucose. The bodily symptoms depend on how low the glucose levels go and how rapidly they are falling.

What Is Hypoglycemia Unawareness?

People who have hypoglycemia frequently may lose most bodily symptoms. This is called hypoglycemia unawareness, and it can be dangerous.

Frequent hypoglycemic episodes cause your body to gradually adapt to hypoglycemia, requiring lower and lower blood glucose levels to cause a release of epinephrine and the accompanying warning symptoms. However, your brain does not adapt to hypoglycemia, and your first symptom of hypoglycemia will often be confusion, making it more difficult for you to treat yourself, judge situations appropriately, or operate a car or machinery. For example, your blood glucose level drops and you "know" that you are low. But because your judgment is impaired, you leave your house and drive to a restaurant to get some food instead of treating yourself at home with food that is there.

Hypoglycemia unawareness can also be the result of other complications. If you have nerve damage (autonomic neuropathy), epinephrine may not be released on time, and there may be no warning symptoms. Often glucagon is also not released, so hypoglycemia may last longer (see chapter 16).

If you have hypoglycemia unawareness, check your blood glucose frequently and wear diabetes identification. You should *always* carry a source of readily absorbed glucose with you (see below). Always check your blood glucose before you drive and every 1–2 hours on long trips. You need to protect yourself and others.

Even when hypoglycemia unawareness is not present, many people find that the symptoms they develop will gradually change over the years, and generally such symptoms become much more subtle.

Do People Without Diabetes Develop Hypoglycemia?

Even if someone without diabetes fasts for 3 days, blood glucose levels won't fall to hypoglycemic levels. With prolonged starvation, levels may dip below 50 mg/dL, but this rarely happens outside of countries plagued by malnutrition.

In some people, glucose may be absorbed too rapidly from the intestine, triggering a sharp rise in insulin. The large amount of insulin rapidly sends glucose into the cells, but no more glucose comes in from the intestine, and there is an imbalance. Low blood glucose occurs. This low usually lasts a few minutes up to an hour or two and stops because counter-regulatory hormones stimulate the liver to release more glucose into the blood. Additionally, the low glucose level shuts off further insulin release. If you have this type of hypoglycemia, avoid eating a lot of carbohydrate at one meal so you don't have a sharp rise in blood glucose. Eating high-fiber foods and small snacks between meals may help.

Do Diabetes Pills Cause Hypoglycemia?

Sulfonylureas and meglitinides can cause low blood sugar.

Sulfonylureas

Sulfonylureas stimulate the pancreas to release insulin (Table 5-3), and they can cause hypoglycemia. This may occur 2–3 hours after a meal if the sulfonylurea causes the pancreas to release too much insulin. Don't skip a meal or take too much medication. This hypo-

Table 5-3. Medications Used to Treat Diabetes

Stimulates More Insulin	Insulin Sensitizers	Slows Glucose Absorption
Sulfonylureas	Biguanides	alpha-Glucosidase inhibitors
Tolbutamide (Orinase)	Metformin (Glucophage)	Acarbose (Precose)
Chlorpropamide (Diabinase)	Thiazolidinediones	Miglitol (Glycet)
Tolazamide (Tolinase)	Rosiglitazone (Avandia)	
Glyburide (generic)	Pioglitazone (Actos)	
Glipizide (generic)		
Glipizide-GITS (Glucotrol XL)		
Glimepiride (Amaryl)		
Meglitinides		
Repaglinide (Prandin)		
Nateglinide (Starlix)		
Exenatide (Byetta), injectable		
DPP IV inhibitors		
Sitagliptin (Januvia)		

glycemia is usually mild and is detected by symptoms or checking blood glucose. Treat by eating a rapidly absorbed carbohydrate source (see below). Prevent this from happening again by reducing the dose of medication or eating a snack between meals.

People taking the longer-acting medications chlorpropamide and glyburide can have prolonged hypoglycemia. Prolonged hypoglycemia occurs in older people who may skip meals, and it may last for many hours, or more than a day. Treatment is to eat carbohydrate immediately, but hospitalization may be necessary. Those with kidney failure or impairment taking the other sulfonylureas may also develop hypoglycemia.

Meglitinides

Two drugs that act like sulfonylureas and can cause hypoglycemia are repaglinide (Prandin) and nateglinide (Starlix). They act rapidly, so they must be taken with a meal. However, nateglinide does not cause hypoglycemia if no food is eaten.

Two new drugs can potentially cause hypoglycemia also. Exenatide (Byetta) is taken by injection twice daily and works by increasing insulin secretion, as well as by decreasing glucagon secretion and delaying intestinal absorption of glucose. Sitagliptin (Januvia) is taken orally and has similar effects. In early studies, neither has been reported to cause hypoglycemia, but because of how they work, they have the potential to do so. At this point, these two new drugs are generally given along with other diabetes medications and rarely alone.

Other oral agents—metformin, acarbose, miglitol, thiazolidinediones

People who take metformin (Glucophage), acarbose (Precose), rosiglitazone (Avandia), or pioglitazone (Actos) should not experience hypoglycemia. However, if you take one of these pills with a sulfonylurea or with insulin, you can develop hypoglycemia.

Anyone taking acarbose or miglitol must treat hypoglycemia with pure glucose tablets and not juice, candy, or table sugar. These medications will not allow your body to properly metabolize sugar into glucose.

Also keep in mind that combination pills can contain one of the medications mentioned above. If your combination pill contains a sulfonylurea or meglitinide, it may cause hypoglycemia.

What Causes Hypoglycemia in People Taking Insulin?

For those taking insulin, hypoglycemia can be caused by either taking too much insulin, eating too little food, skipping a meal, or exercising more than planned.

Although the usual times of insulin action are listed in Table 5-4, these times vary from one person to another, making lows quite possible. You may find there is a variation, depending on where you inject insulin—absorption is fastest from the abdomen and slowest from the buttocks—and whether there is any scar tissue at the site of injection. If you exercise within 30–60 minutes of the injection, blood flow to the legs and arms is increased; if you inject in your legs, the insulin may be more rapidly absorbed than you expect, causing low blood glucose. Exercise will also make your body use more glucose while the muscles are working harder and making your body more sensitive to insulin.

Table 2-4. Types of Insulin

Type	Onset (h)	Peak (h)	Duration (h)
Rapid-acting			
lispro	5–30 min	1/2–1	1–3
aspart	5–30 min	1/2–1	1–3
glulisine	5–30 min	1/2– 1	1-3
Regular	1/2–1	2–3	3–6
NPH	2–4	4–10	10–16
Detemir	2–4	10–16	14–24
Glargine	2–4	Peakless	24

Finally, people sometimes mistakenly inject insulin into muscle instead of fat, especially if they inject in areas where there is little fat, such as the arms. This causes a more rapid absorption of insulin with peaks that do not match the later food intake, thereby resulting in hypoglycemia.

How Do You Adjust Insulin and Food for Exercise?

You'll need to keep records of blood glucose levels and exercise so you and your doctor can see your patterns. Here's an example of what to do. A 16-year-old patient takes 12 units of NPH in the morning before breakfast and 8 units of NPH before supper. When he knows he has basketball practice after school, he lowers his morning dose of NPH by 4 units and his evening dose of NPH by 2 units. He also decreases his lunch rapid-acting insulin by 2 units and his supper rapid-acting insulin by 1 unit. He has learned that this helps prevent hypoglycemia during practice and later that evening. Exercise can lower glucose levels for up to 24 hours. He knows that, so he'll eat a bigger bedtime snack than usual. He also carries glucose tablets with him in case his game is more vigorous or longer than expected.

How Do You Treat Hypoglycemia?

When you have symptoms or get a low blood glucose reading, eat 15–20 grams of carbohydrate right away. Wait for 15–20 minutes and then check your blood glucose level to be sure it has risen enough. If it hasn't, eat another 15–20 grams of carbohydrate.

Can You Prevent Going Too Low When Driving?

Check your blood glucose before driving and every 2 hours on long trips. Always have something to eat where you can reach it in the car. By the time you feel low, your nervous system reaction times are decreased, and your ability to respond quickly is not good.

Pull off the road. Get in the passenger seat, eat, check your blood glucose, and wait at least 20–30 minutes until your blood glucose has risen to over 80 and you are feeling normal before driving again. The last thing to do when you feel low is to decide that you are almost home (or to the restaurant or store) and drive the rest of the way. That is a sure way to have an accident.

What Can Others Do to Help with Hypoglycemia?

The rule for helpers: Never force juice or food into the mouth of an unconscious person. If you are unconscious or unable to eat, you need an injection of glucagon. Ask your doctor to prescribe it, and teach friends or family members how to give it. If you do not respond, they should call 911.

What Can You Do About Nighttime Hypoglycemia?

The only sign that you have this problem may be elevated glucose levels in the morning or waking up drenched in sweat. You may also remember vivid dreams or nightmares and wake up with a headache in the morning. Checking your blood glucose at 3:00 A.M. can detect middle-of-the-night lows. These may be eliminated by reducing your evening dose of NPH or by changing the time you take it. Another approach would be to switch to glargine, which tends to cause less nighttime hypoglycemia than NPH. If you take rapid-acting insulin at bedtime, reduce the dose. A snack at bedtime may help. Try one of the cornstarch-based bars made for this situation.

This chapter was written by Mark E. Molitch, MD.

Chronic Complications

6

Heart Disease

Introduction

There is an important association between diabetes and heart disease. Just as diabetes can affect organs such as the kidneys, nerves, blood vessels, and eyes, it can also affect the heart. Adults with diabetes are three times more likely to die of heart disease than patients without diabetes, and 65% of all deaths in patients with diabetes are due to heart disease. Many studies have shown that keeping blood glucose in good range reduces your chance of developing heart (cardiac) complications.

What Is Heart Disease?

The heart is a muscle that pumps blood to the lungs and to the body. It requires oxygen and electrical stimulation to work properly. The heart moves blood from the veins in the body through valves in the right side of the heart and up to the lungs, where the blood gets loaded with oxygen. Once filled with oxygen, the blood then moves into the left side of the heart, through valves, and out to the organs in the body. The pumping of the heart is stimulated by electrical impulses in the heart itself (the natural "pacemaker" that everyone is born with).

Good heart pumping function requires valves that do not leak, correctly timed electrical impulses, heart muscle strength, and a continuous supply of oxygen from blood. The heart muscle itself gets oxygen through blood flow from the coronary, or heart, arteries. These arteries lie on the outside of the heart and bring blood to the heart muscle itself. The term "heart disease" can refer to diseases of the heart muscle itself, the coronary arteries that feed oxygen to the heart, the valves, or the electrical system.

More about Coronary Artery Disease

Coronary artery disease (CAD) refers to the reduction or stoppage of blood flow to the heart muscle because of blockages inside the arteries that supply the heart. These blockages reduce the supply of oxygen and nutrients to the actual heart muscle, and this can cause either a heart attack or damage to the muscle, which reduces the strength of the heart muscle pump.

The most common cause of artery blockage is called atherosclerosis, or hardening of the arteries. Cholesterol and fatty deposits can build up inside the artery over many years, resulting in a blockage. In addition to long-term damage to the lining of the artery, deposits can also cause blood clots to form inside the artery that can cause further acute blockage and accelerate the onset of a myocardial infarction (heart attack).

What Are the Risk Factors for Developing CAD?

Risk factors for developing CAD are outlined in detail in chapter 7. In general, they are divided into three categories:

- **Nonmodifiable**—These are things you can't change, such as age, gender, and family history.
- **Modifiable**—These are things you can control, such as cholesterol, blood pressure, blood glucose, and smoking.
- **Partially modifiable**—Diabetes falls under this category, because it is a risk factor that you can't eliminate, but controlling diabetes makes a big difference in reducing complications.

People with pre-diabetes (impaired glucose tolerance or mildly elevated blood glucose levels) are also at risk for developing heart disease, so early recognition and treatment of diabetes helps reduce the risk of long-term complications. The risk of developing CAD increases with the length of time you have had diabetes. After 20 years of diabetes, you are ten times more likely to develop heart disease. Also, people with diabetes are more likely to have other cardiac risk factors such as hypertension (high blood pressure), obesity, and an unfavorable cholesterol profile that includes high triglycerides (fats) and low HDL (good cholesterol).

Risk Factors for Heart Disease (CAD)

Nonmodifiable
  Age
  Gender
  Family history
Modifiable
  High cholesterol
  High blood pressure
  Smoking
Partially modifiable
  Diabetes

Secondary (but still important!) risk factors
  Obesity
  Lack of exercise
  Hostile personality

How Do I Know if I Have CAD?

Blockages in the arteries that are severe enough to limit the blood flow to the heart muscle (usually 70% blockage or greater) can cause symptoms called angina. Typical angina is described as a "pressure-like" feeling in the chest, with radiation down the left arm or up to the neck, jaw, or shoulder. Other symptoms that can accompany the chest pressure include a sweaty or clammy feeling, shortness of breath, or nausea. In some patients, the angina is not typical pain, but can be felt as indigestion or upper abdominal pain, back pain, or right arm pain. The symptoms usually come on with exercise and go away with rest, but occasionally can occur during sleep or in times of emotional upset.

People with diabetes may have a difficult time determining symptoms of CAD. Because many may have a "faulty warning system" (little or no symptoms at all) from nerve damage, diabetes may affect the perception of pain. In some cases, the only warning sign of heart disease may be shortness of breath.

Symptoms that only occur with exercise and go away with rest, and last less than 10 minutes are called stable angina. If these symptoms begin to occur more frequently, last longer, or occur at rest, they may be warning signs for an impending heart attack, also called acute coronary syndrome.

Symptoms of Coronary Artery Disease

Chest pressure
Under breastbone
Radiation to shoulder, arm, or jaw
"Tightness" or "pressure"
Worse with exercise
Better with rest
Can come on with emotional stress
Shortness of breath
Nausea
Can occur along with indigestion
Syncope (fainting)
Can be caused by an irregular heart rhythm

How Can My Doctor Tell if I Have CAD?

Making a diagnosis of CAD can include a review of your symptoms, a physical exam, and testing. Patients who have "classic" symptoms (pressure below the breastbone that travels to the arm or jaw, comes on with exercise and goes away with rest, and is associated with nausea, sweating, and shortness of breath), are more likely to have coronary artery disease than those with less typical symptoms. But even having typical symptoms does not mean that the patient has true CAD.

Unfortunately, a physical exam can offer few clues about the presence of CAD. Fluid on the lung or in the legs may point to heart failure, but in general, the physical exam in a patient with CAD may be completely normal.

However, the doctor may do some further testing to determine whether you have CAD. The following tests may produce more conclusive results:

- Electrocardiogram (ECG)—This is a 5-minute test that involves putting electrical leads on your chest and generating an electrical picture of the heart. This can provide valuable clues about the heart. Approximately 35% of heart attacks cause no symptoms (they are "silent"), but may show up on an ECG. Coronary blockages that have not yet caused any damage do not usually show up on an ECG alone.

- Stress testing—Your doctor may want to do a stress test that requires your heart muscle to obtain more oxygen in order to look for CAD. Stress testing involves 1) stressing the heart either with exercise or chemicals, and 2) measuring either the heart function (with an ultrasound or echocardiogram) or the blood flow (with thallium, an imaging agent). The stress test provides valuable information to your doctor. By looking at the result of the stress test, including how long you exercise, how high your heart rate and blood pressure get, what symptoms you are having, what your ECG looks like, and the results of the thallium scan or echocardiogram, the doctor can determine whether you have coronary heart disease or not. Although the test is not 100% accurate, it can give your doctor valuable information concerning whether you have artery blockages or not.

Chemical Stress Test

Chemical or pharmacologic stress tests (mentioned earlier in this chapter) are useful in patients who cannot exercise due to orthopedic problems (such as arthritis), vascular problems (blockages in the leg arteries), lung problems (such as asthma or emphysema), or a heart electrical problem (left bundle branch block, or LBBB). A chemical stress test can be done with

● adenosine or dipyridamole as the chemical "stressing" agent, followed by thallium as the imaging agent to look at the blood flow to the heart, or
● dobutamine as the chemical "stressing" agent, followed by echocardiography to look at the pumping function of the heart.

What happens if the stress test results are not positive?

In most cases, your doctor will start medication to control symptoms and reduce your risk factors. Your doctor may also recommend a test called a cardiac catheterization, sometimes called a coronary angiogram. This procedure involves inserting a tiny catheter (a small, hollow plastic tube) into a blood vessel in the groin, or occasionally in the arm artery and threading it up into the heart. Dye is then injected into the catheter, and X-ray pictures are taken to outline the pumping function of your heart and the arteries to see whether there is blockage.

Depending on the result, your doctor may decide to treat you with medication, open up the artery blockages using a balloon or stent, or possibly recommend open-heart bypass surgery.

What Are the Medications Used to Treat CAD?

Treatment for Coronary Artery Disease

Medications
    Aspirin
    Nitrates (nitroglycerin)
    Beta-blockers
    ACE or ARB
Catheter-based therapy
    Balloon angioplasty
    Stenting
Surgery
    Coronary Artery Bypass Graft Surgery

Aspirin

Aspirin is an essential medication for people with CAD. It works by altering the "stickiness" of *platelets*, which are small elements that cause blood clots. Aspirin is very useful if you have CAD, are having a heart attack, or need to undergo balloon angioplasty or stenting (see below).

Nitroglycerin

Nitroglycerin is a medicine that helps dilate the heart arteries to get more blood to the heart muscle and is often used to reduce the symptoms of angina. You can take nitroglycerin under the tongue to dissolve quickly, as a long-acting daily pill, or in skin patch or paste form. Side effects of nitroglycerin include headaches or, occasionally, lightheadedness.

Beta-blockers

Beta-blockers (β-blockers) reduce the symptoms of angina by lowering the heart rate (pulse) and blood pressure, and thus the workload, of the heart. Commonly used β-blockers include propranolol (Inderal), metoprolol (Lopressor or Toprol), atenolol (Tenormin), or carvedilol (Coreg). β-blockers are also very useful in controlling rhythm problems. Many studies have shown that giving β-blockers to people who have had heart attacks or congestive heart failure improves survival rates.

Although β-blockers are very useful drugs, they can have significant side effects, such as dizziness from the slowed the heart rate or lowered blood pressure. Importantly for people with type 1 diabetes, β-blockers can sometimes mask the symptoms of low blood glucose, so you need to asses the risk/benefit ratio with your health care team.

Angiotensin-converting-enzyme inhibitors and angiotensin-receptor-blockers

Angiotensin-converting-enzyme (ACE) inhibitors or angiotensin-receptor-blockers (ARB) are very useful in the treatment of people with heart disease, especially if they have had a heart attack or congestive heart failure. There is also evidence that they may reduce kidney complications caused by diabetes. ACE inhibitors and ARB reduce the workload of the heart, improve pumping function, and lower blood pressure. For people with depressed heart function, these medications clearly prolong survival.

If you have had kidney failure, or have a narrowing in the kidney artery (renal artery stenosis) or high potassium levels, you should avoid ACE inhibitors and ARB. A common side effect of ACE is dry cough, but this is less of a problem with ARB. Commonly used ACE inhibitors include lisinopril (Zestril, Prinivil), quinapril (Accupril), captopril (Capoten), enalapril (Vasotec), and ramipril (Altace). Common ARB include valsartan (Diovan), losartan (Cozaar), candesartan (Atacand), or irbesartan (Avapro).

What if Medication Alone Is Not Enough?

If your coronary angiogram reveals blockages, your doctor may recommend opening up the blockages with balloon angioplasty or stenting or may recommend open heart surgery.

Angioplasty is a procedure done in a cardiac catheterization laboratory, much like an angiogram. Instead of just taking a picture of the artery, however, the cardiologist will insert a thin wire through the catheter, and then a deflated balloon is advanced over the wire down the artery across the blockage. The balloon is inflated and this widens the passageway for the blood to flow. In many cases, the doctor will then place a small metal tube called a stent across the blockage and expand the stent against the artery wall to hold it open. Stents are placed inside the artery permanently. If only a balloon is used, it is removed at the end of the procedure.

There are two types of stents: non-drug-eluting (bare metal) and drug-eluting. The drug-coated stents are embedded with a drug designed to prevent the formation of scar tissue, which could clog up the stent and create a blockage. Drug-coated stents require a year of treatment with an antiplatelet drug (a type of blood thinner), but bare metal stents only require 2–4 weeks of the drug. Common antiplatelet agents are clopridogel (Plavix) and ticlodipine (Ticlid). If you develop an allergy to these drugs, a drug called cilostazol (Pletal) could be used.

What if I Have Too Many Blockages for Stents?

If you have extensive blockages, open-heart bypass surgery, called Coronary Artery Bypass Graft (CABG) surgery, will probably be the best option. Studies have shown that if you have diabetes and extensive blockage, you'll fare better with open-heart bypass surgery than with angioplasty. During this operation, the breastbone is cut open, and the heart is exposed. The surgeon bypasses blockages in coronary arteries by sewing veins taken from the leg or arteries from inside the chest wall to the heart above and below the coronary artery blockages. In this fashion, blood is able to flow into the heart muscle, "bypassing" the blockages. This operation takes several hours and requires nearly a week's stay in the hospital, as well as a recovery period of 1–2 months, to allow healing. Risks of CABG include bleeding and infection, and diabetics sometimes heal more slowly than non-diabetics. The overall complication rate is relatively low even in diabetics (5–8%), unless other problems are present.

What Is a Heart Attack?

Most people are familiar with the term "heart attack," but the actual mechanisms at work may be a mystery. The term heart attack, or myocardial infarction, refers to death of heart muscle tissue from a sudden loss of blood flow, which restricts blood, oxygen, and nutrients from reaching the heart muscle. This usually occurs when there is a preexisting cholesterol buildup in the coronary artery. During a heart attack, the cholesterol buildup suddenly cracks open, resulting in bleeding or hemorrhage and the formation of a blood clot. Once the blood clot closes off the artery, death of heart muscle begins to occur.

How will I know if I'm having a heart attack?

Typical signs of a heart attack include a severe and crushing pressure-like pain under the breastbone that spreads to the left arm, shoulder, or jaw, accompanied by profuse sweating and shortness of breath. Occasionally, the pain can seem like a bad case of indigestion accompanied by nausea (these symptoms are more prevalent with women).

If you are having a heart attack, it is critical to seek medical attention immediately! Half of the people who die fom a heart attack do so within the first hour. If you feel you're having a heart attack, take aspirin (one 325 mg adult aspirin, or four baby 81 mg aspirin) and immediately call 911.

Symptoms of a Heart Attack

Crushing chest pain
> Below the breastbone
> Spreads to the neck, jaw or arm
> "Pressure" or "tightness"
> Doesn't go away

Profuse sweating
Nausea/vomiting
Shortness of breath
Palpitations
Fainting or near fainting
Severe case of indigestion

People with diabetes may have different symptoms during a heart attack or, because diabetes affects the sensory nerves of the heart, no symptoms at all. Occasionally, the only sign of a heart attack will be shortness of breath. One potential sign of a heart attack in a diabetic may be a sudden difficult-to-control blood glucose level. Because you are more likely to be at risk of a heart attack, your doctor may want to do prospective testing to help predict whether you are at risk for a heart attack before it happens.

What will they do when I get to the hospital?

A heart attack is an important priority to hospital staff. You will immediately be placed on a monitor, have an intravenous line (IV) placed in the vein in your arm, and receive oxygen. An ECG will be done. Medications will be given, including aspirin, nitroglycerin, and beta-blockers. In some cases, if the ECG shows a heart attack, you will be given an intravenous medication called a "clot-buster" drug (such as tissue-plasminogen-activator, or TPA) to dissolve the blood clot causing the heart attack. In many cases, you will be taken urgently to the cardiac catheterization laboratory for a coronary angiogram and possible balloon angioplasty to open up the blockage.

If it is not clear whether or not there is a heart attack on the ECG, blood will be drawn every 6–8 hours to measure cardiac enzymes. These are substances released into the bloodstream after a heart attack occurs. It takes 4–6 hours after a heart attack starts for these enzymes to appear in the bloodstream. The results of these blood tests will help your doctor determine whether heart damage has occurred, even if it doesn't show up on the ECG.

What Is Congestive Heart Failure?

Congestive heart failure (CHF) is a condition in which a weakened heart muscle cannot pump enough blood to meet the needs of the body's organs. Symptoms include fatigue, difficulty exercising, shortness of breath, leg swelling, and especially fluid retention.

CHF can be the result of a lack of blood to the heart muscle because of blockage, damage to the heart muscle from heart attacks, problems with the heart valves being too leaky or too narrow, or problems with the heart muscle itself (due to a variety of things, such as alcoholism, obesity, or viral infection). Successful treatment involves finding and treating the underlying cause, and the use of medications.

Symptoms of Congestive Heart Failure

Shortness of breath
- When exercising
- When reclining
- Awakening because of breathing difficulty

Inability to exercise

Swelling or weight gain
- Feet/ankles
- Abdomen

Palpitations

People are sometimes said to have CHF if they have a stiff, vigorous heart. This condition is called "diastolic dysfunction" (as opposed to "systolic dysfunction" from a weakened heart muscle). A stiff heart cannot relax, and this leads to a buildup of pressure and fluid, causing shortness of breath. This form of CHF is a bit of a misnomer because, although we call it "congestive heart failure," the heart is not failing at all.

What is the connection between diabetes and CHF?

People with diabetes have an increased chance of developing CHF because other cardiac problems associated with diabetes (high blood pressure, CAD, etc.) can also cause heart failure. Studies have shown that the risk of developing CHF is four to five times higher in people with diabetes, even if all of the other risk factors are taken into account.

How will my doctor diagnose CHF?

By analyzing your reported symptoms. People with heart failure will report generalized fatigue or tiredness, and inability to exercise. There might be shortness of breath, especially if exercising or lying down. Fluid retention can cause your feet, ankles, and occasionally abdomen to swell.

If symptoms point to CHF, a physical exam is useful. The doctor may detect fluid in the lungs with a stethoscope, or find swelling in the feet or ankles due to fluid accumulation. A heart noise called a "third heart sound" might be heard. Occasionally, a murmur or irregular heart rhythm may be detected.

Other useful aids in the diagnosis of CHF include an ECG and a chest X-ray. Your doctor will usually also perform an echocardiogram, which is an ultrasound picture of the heart. This test reveals information about the size, shape, and pumping function of the heart, the valve function, and the presence of a pericardial effusion (fluid around the heart).

How will my CHF be treated?

If CHF is due to a stiff heart muscle (diastolic dysfunction), medications to relax the heart and slow down the heart rate will be used. If CHF is due to a weakened heart muscle (systolic dysfunction), medications include the following:

- Digitalis (Digoxin)—improves the force of contraction of the heart
- Diuretics (water pills)—help to get rid of excess fluid buildup
- ACE or ARB—help the heart pump by blocking hormones released by the kidney that cause constriction of the arteries and retention of salt and water
- Beta-blockers—help to reduce the workload of the heart by reducing blood pressure and heart rate, and help reduce the tendency for rhythm problems
- Nitroglycerin—useful for dilating coronary arteries

Both ACE/ARB and beta-blockers have been shown to improve the survival of people with CHF. Although digoxin and diuretics have not shown this, they do help improve the symptoms of CHF.

Are Diabetic Medications Bad for My Heart?

In general, diabetic medications are safe for your heart. However, a couple of oral medications in the class of drugs known as the thiazolidinediones do warrant consideration.

- Pioglitazone (Actos) may contribute to the development of congestive heart failure in susceptible people by causing fluid retention.
- Rosiglitazone (Avandia), in a study published by the *New England Journal of Medicine,* has been associated with a significant increase in the risk of heart attacks. Because of this, the Food and Drug Administration (FDA) ruled that the medication must carry a "black box" warning

cautioning that the drug may cause or worsen heart failure. However, they felt that the drug was safe enough to remain on the market, pending further research.

What Other Things Can I Do to Improve My Heart Health?

There are three hallmarks of good heart health—diet, exercise, and control of risk factors. People with diabetes should follow the American Diabetes Association guidelines for healthy eating, similar to those proposed by the American Heart Association: limit fat to 30% of caloric intake (preferably 10–20%), reduce saturated fat, and focus on healthy carbohydrates, such as vegetables and whole grains. Keep your body weight at recommended guidelines. Regular exercise (minimum of 30 minutes of aerobic exercise at lease three times a week and preferably every day) will help control blood glucose, blood pressure, cholesterol, and weight.

Ways to Stay Healthy

- Control risk factors
- Maintain good blood glucose levels
- Maintain blood pressure in the recommended range
- Keep cholesterol profile within guidelines
- Exercise daily
- Keep weight within the recommended guidelines
- Stop smoking
- Take all prescribed medications faithfully
- Eat a nutritious diet
- Keep a positive outlook
- Get regular physical exams and report symptoms to your health professional

Regular visits to your doctor are essential to making sure you receive the most up-to-date information and treatment, improving both your long-term outcomes and continued heart health.

Careful attention to the control of other risk factors can also help improve your heart health. Your blood pressure goal should be 120/70 mmHg, and you should pay attention to cholesterol guidelines, which have become more stringent. Finally, stop smoking. Quitting now is critical: the combination of smoking and diabetes is a serious obstacle to good heart health.

What's in Store for the Future?

The field of medicine changes rapidly, almost on a daily basis. There are constantly new drugs being developed for diabetes, coronary heart disease, and congestive heart failure. New devices and techniques are being developed for the treatment of coronary artery blockages. Surgical improvements are reducing the complications of CABG surgery. New guidelines are being developed to reduce the impact of cardiac risk factors on the development of heart disease.

Every day, the treatment of heart disease expands and improves. Coupled with the expanded knowledge and preventative care of people like you, the future looks optimistic.

This chapter was written by Patricia L. Cole, MD, FACC.

7

Risk Factors for Heart Disease

Introduction

As medical advances allow people to live longer and more fulfilling lives, the rate of heart and cardiovascular problems rises as well. *Atherosclerosis*, the build-up of cholesterol-containing plaques in the walls of blood vessels, is the hallmark of cardiovascular disease. It causes narrowing of blood vessels, impairs their ability to dilate, and raises the risk of blood clotting. With time, this buildup can result in heart attacks, strokes, blindness, kidney failure, and amputation.

While the risk of these illnesses is present in nearly everyone, people with diabetes have a risk of cardiovascular problems that is more than double that of the general population. In fact, studies have shown that if you have diabetes, your chance of having a first heart attack is the same as that of someone who has already had a heart attack. Cardiovascular disease is the leading cause of death in people with diabetes.

While diabetes itself is a risk factor for the formation of atherosclerosis, you also have a greater incidence of the many other conditions that increase the risk of cardiovascular disease. These include high blood pressure and high cholesterol. To make matters worse, these conditions increase your risk exponentially and not simply additionally. These can be frightening concepts, but they are not foregone conclusions. It should be the goal of every person with diabetes, partnered with their health care team, to control the factors that pose these risks.

High Blood Pressure

Hypertension, or high blood pressure, causes an undue strain to be placed on the heart and also contributes to the formation of atherosclerotic plaques. (See chapter 9.) As such, hypertension is a risk factor for cardiovascular disease in everyone, with or without diabetes. Due to the already high risk of complications in those with diabetes, however, the goals for blood pressure control are even more aggressive for you than for people with high blood pressure alone. Lowering your blood pressure directly lowers your risk for heart disease, and current recommendations are to keep your blood pressure lower than 130/80 mmHg. There's also evidence that lowering your blood pressure even further may reduce your risk even more.

If you have mildly high blood pressure (systolic 130–139 mmHg, diastolic 80–89 mmHg), making lifestyle changes such as losing weight, exercising, eating a low-sodium diet, and drinking less alcohol may be all you need to get your blood pressure under control. If lifestyle changes don't work, or your blood pressure is higher than 140/90 mmHg at the time of diagnosis, you'll need to take medication. Medication therapy will probably include an angiotensin-converting enzyme (ACE) inhibitor or an angiotensin-receptor blocker (ARB), with additional medications as needed to get your blood pressure under control. Talk to your dietitian about the amount of salt you should have in your diet.

It should be noted that ACE inhibitors and ARB may be helpful for people with diabetes even if you have normal blood pressure. (See chapter 17.) Discuss the specific risks and benefits of each medication with your health care team to determine which medications are most appropriate for you.

Blood Glucose

High blood glucose levels, or hyperglycemia, can damage your blood vessels. Even in people who don't have diabetes but have higher than normal glucose levels (e.g., pre-diabetes), these increased glucose levels are associated with higher rates of cardiovascular disease. While the mechanism behind this has not been clearly defined, hypergly-cemia may increase the risk of vascular complications by causing an increased build-up of cholesterol plaques in blood vessels. This dam-age can affect small arteries, such as those in the eye, as well as larger arteries, such as those in the heart.

Controlling your blood glucose is therefore essential to lower-ing your risk of heart disease. As a result, it's recommended that you keep your fasting blood glucose between 80 and 120 mg/dL (though ideally less than 100 mg/dL), and your A1C less than 7%. You can do this through a combination of diet, exercise, and medi-cations. Modifying your lifestyle also improves many of the other risk factors for cardiovascular disease.

Blood glucose medications can come in the form of oral pills, insulin, or other injectable medications. You may need to take more than one type of medication to control your blood glucose, which often becomes harder as you grow older. If you start with oral medications, you may eventually need insulin injections. This isn't a failure of therapy; it's simply the nature of diabetes. Discuss your treatment options with your health care team to develop an effective strategy for lowering your risk for hyperglycemia.

Cholesterol

With diabetes, you are at risk for many types of cholesterol abnor-malities—higher low density lipoprotein (LDL, the "bad cho-lesterol," greater than 70 mg/dL), lower high density lipoprotein (HDL, the "good cholesterol," less than 40 mg/dL in men or 50 mg/dL in women), and high triglycerides (higher than 150 mg/dL). (See chapter 8.) Even if you have normal LDL cholesterol lev-els, you may be at a greater risk because, more than likely, you have a small, dense form of LDL cholesterol that has a higher tendency to cause atherosclerosis.

Achieving healthy cholesterol goals can significantly decrease your risk of cardiovascular complications. Studies have shown that you run a much higher risk of death and nonfatal complications of cardiovascular disease if you have poorly managed lipids. While it's recommended that you maintain an LDL level of less than 100 mg/dL, recent studies have suggested that even lower cholesterol levels may provide a greater benefit. If you have diabetes and heart disease, it's recommended you achieve an LDL of less than 70 mg/dL. Secondary goals are to maintain an HDL level of greater than 40 mg/dL in men and 50 mg/dL in women, and a triglyceride level of less than 150 mg/dL.

The best way to control your cholesterol is through diet, exercise, and medications. All of these steps are part of the optimal treatment plan. A diet low in cholesterol and saturated fats is a must. Alcohol (in moderation, not in excess) and exercise may mildly increase your HDL cholesterol. Medications for cholesterol include statins, fibrates, and niacin. Each of these may be prescribed for a specific reason, and the benefits and side effects of each should be discussed with your health care team. Interestingly, it has been shown that statins provide benefits to people with diabetes even when they have "optimal" cholesterol levels, so it may be beneficial to consider statins even if your levels are normal. Ongoing studies are evaluating whether achieving even lower levels of LDL cholesterol with medications may yield further benefit. Similarly, current clinical trials are examining whether raising the level of HDL cholesterol after achieving very low levels of LDL cholesterol may help even more.

Smoking

Smoking is the number-one preventable cause of death in the United States. About one-fourth of American men and women are smokers, with the ratio about the same for people with diabetes. Just like other risk factors for cardiovascular disease, if you smoke and you have diabetes, you run a higher risk of cardiovascular problems compared to smokers who do not have diabetes. This is true not only for death due to heart attacks, but also for the nonfatal cardiovascular complications of diabetes.

There are a number of ways nicotine has been linked with cardiovascular problems and diabetes. It has been suggested that it impairs insulin activity, resulting in poor blood glucose control. Smoking is also associated with higher blood pressure, higher LDL cholesterol levels, lower HDL cholesterol levels, and increased blood clotting, all of which increase your risk for atherosclerosis and heart attacks.

Unfortunately, it's difficult to quit smoking, and helping people quit remains one of the most challenging areas in medicine. While there are many possible approaches, the key to a successful outcome begins with your desire to quit. Once this goal is established, the options for treatment include counseling, nicotine replacement via patches, gum, or spray, and medications such as bupropion (Wellbutrin). A new medication, varenicline (Chantix), may also help. If you smoke, talk to your health care team about your smoking habits. Being open and honest can help establish a team approach to quitting, which drastically improves your chances of quitting. Generally speaking, using multiple methods at the same time often leads to the best results.

In addition to active smoking, secondhand smoke can also be harmful. In some studies, passive tobacco exposure has been found to carry even more risk, since you can't control how much smoke you inhale. Several communities throughout the United States, and throughout the world, are attempting to ban smoking in public places. If you have diabetes or other risk factors for heart disease, it is important that no one in your household smokes.

Obesity

Obesity not only increases your risk for developing diabetes, but also increases your risk for cardiovascular disease. Unfortunately, it is also one of the greatest concerns in public health. In the United States, it is estimated that 65% of the population is overweight (body mass index [BMI] of 25–29) or obese (BMI higher than 29). (See chapter 33 for more information on BMI.) Weight gain can exacerbate hypertension, has negative effects on cholesterol levels, and causes insulin resistance, all of which promotes atherosclerosis.

Losing weight and treating obesity require a multifaceted approach. Talk with a nutrition expert to determine your dietary goals. As a general rule, seek out foods that are low in cholesterol and saturated fats. Exercise programs are also essential to a weight-loss program, but need to be discussed with your heath care team to determine any safety issues. If you're cleared for exercise, shoot for 30 minutes of sustained vigorous exercise (jogging, biking, or anything that breaks a light sweat) daily. Keep in mind that lifestyle changes that help you lose weight also improve other cardiovascular risk factors.

If lifestyle factors alone aren't successful, there are medications being developed to treat obesity. Each has its own list of benefits and risks (see chapter 33).

For extreme degrees of obesity (BMI greater than 40), sometimes referred to as morbid obesity, or for obesity with diabetes and a BMI of 35 or greater, bariatric surgery is a potential option. There are two major operations that can be performed:

- A gastric band, in which the initial part of the stomach is made smaller, causing a sense of fullness after only small portions of food are consumed, or
- A bypass procedure, in which a portion of the stomach and intestines is bypassed in order to minimize the amount of food that is absorbed.

Surgery for obesity is certainly a serious decision and must be made by you and your health care team only after other weight-loss methods have proven to be ineffective.

Genetics

Genetics determine not only your gender and appearance, but also the factors that contribute to cardiovascular disease. It seems that our genetic information can contribute to the development of hypertension, cholesterol abnormalities, obesity, diabetes, and cardiovascular disease.

Researchers have found specific genes that are linked to conditons such as hypertension or that cause cholesterol abnomalities. Similarly, obesity and diabetes may run in families, and researchers have identified genes that may predispose you to conditions like diabetes and heart disease. Unfortunately, you can't change your genes. Fortunately, you can do things about other risk factors that contribute to a genetic predisposition. A family history can be a strong motivational tool for more aggressive risk factor modification and treatment. In years to come, as we learn more about the way genes affect heart disease and diabetes, we will be able to develop specific testing and improved therapies.

What Other Therapies Can Control Risk Factors?

Aspirin

Aspirin has long been recommended for those with heart disease or for people who have suffered a heart attack or stroke. Study after study has demonstrated the benefit of a daily aspirin (81–162 mg) to fight cardiovascular disease. Since people with diabetes and no history of a cardiovascular event are at the same increased risk of a cardiovascular event (heart attack, stroke) as peple without diabetes who have had a cardiovascular event, most people with diabetes should be taking a daily aspirin with their doctor's approval.

Omega-3s

Taking omega-3 fatty acid supplements to reduce cardiovascular risk remains controversial. A large study led by Oxford University is underway to determine the affect of omega-3 fatty acids in people with diabetes. This study is also examining how much benefit daily aspirin may provide to people with diabetes with respect to cardiovascular risk. The American Heart Association recommends that people with cardiovascular disease take at least 1 gram of omega-3 fatty acids supplements each day. This is probably a reasonable recommendation for people with diabetes, as well.

Reducing stress

The role of mental stress, anxiety, and depression in cardiovascular disease is controversial, but it has been suggested that factors such as hypertension are adversely affected by mental health. Furthermore, intensely stressful situations, such as natural (or unnatural) disasters, have been associated with an increased risk of heart attack. Ultimately, improving your mental health, with or without the aide of a professional, is probably good advice.

Reducing environmental factors

No one knows how environmental pollution can affect your heart health, though this is an emerging topic of study. While it has not been definitively proven, there is evidence that greater exposure to pollutants and chemicals can increase cardiovascular events. The reasons for this are far from clear, and research is ongoing in this new field.

Conclusion

More than ever before, people with diabetes have many options for treating of high blood glucose. It is important, however, to keep in mind that high blood glucose is not the only factor affecting your heart health. Many of these other factors can be addressed by changing your lifestyle, taking medications, or both, allowing you to lower your risk of cardiovascular events. By decreasing these risks, you have the opportunity to live your life free of the number-one cause of death and discomfort in both people with diabetes and those without. If you already have complications of diabetes, modifying your risk factors still decreases the chance of further problems down the road.

This chapter was written by Amar Krishnaswamy, MD, and Deepak L. Bhatt, MD, FACC, FSCAI, FESC, FACP.

8

Cholesterol and Other Blood Fats

What Is Cholesterol?

Cholesterol and other blood fats are molecules called lipids. Blood fats include triglycerides, and they actually form the fatty tissue in the human body. Fats do not mix well with water, and they have to be packaged with water-soluble proteins to form lipoproteins, so they can be transported in the blood. Cholesterol and fats have several important functions:

- To form insulation around nerves
- To make bile, which is necessary for absorbing fat and fat-soluble vitamins
- To serve as an important source of energy

The cholesterol that the body needs is made mostly in the liver. The rest comes from what you eat.

What Are Saturated Fats?

These are fats that are hard at room temperature and are found in animal products such as beef, veal, lamb, pork, butter, cream, and whole milk. They are also found in shortening, coconut oil, and palm oil. If you eat too much of these substances, they are stored as fat and also increase the production of cholesterol in your body.

What Are Polyunsaturated and Monounsaturated Fats?

These are oils that are liquid at room temperature. The oils that contain polyunsaturated fats include sunflower, soybean, and corn. Monounsaturated fats are in canola and olive oils, nuts, and seeds, and they actually lower cholesterol. However, even these so-called good oils cause weight gain when you eat too much of them.

What Are the Different Types of Cholesterol?

Cholesterol is packaged into a substance called lipoproteins to be transported in the blood. Based on the way the cholesterol and protein are packed together and the amount of cholesterol that the lipoproteins contain, they can be classified into different kinds—high-density lipoprotein (HDL), low-density lipoprotein (LDL), and triglycerides.

What are high-density lipoproteins, or HDL?

These fats are made in the liver and intestine and contain very little cholesterol. They collect excess cholesterol from the blood and blood vessels and transport it back to the liver, where it is broken down. HDL is sometimes called the "good" cholesterol. The higher your HDL level, the better. The American Diabetes Association (ADA) recommends that you aim for an HDL level greater than 40 mg/dL for men and 50 mg/dL for women.

What are low-density lipoproteins, or LDL?

These lipoproteins contain a very high concentration of cholesterol and carry it from the liver throughout the body. This form of cholesterol is also the culprit responsible for the buildup in the walls of the arteries that leads to atherosclerosis (hardening of the arteries). Some people call it the "bad" cholesterol. The higher the concentration of this form of cholesterol in the blood, the greater the chance of developing coronary heart disease (CHD). A desirable level of LDL depends on whether you already have CHD and whether you have other risk factors that would predispose you to developing

CHD. In individuals with diabetes or heart disease, it is recommended that LDL levels be below 100 mg/dL. In some high-risk individuals, an LDL level below 70 mg/dL may be recommended.

What are triglycerides?

These are a form of fat that is carried in the blood but is mostly stored in fat tissue. The ADA's goal is a level less than 150 mg/dL. Some people think that high triglycerides are an important risk factor for CHD in women. Very high levels (greater than 1,000 mg/dL) are dangerous and can cause pancreatitis (inflammation of the pancreas). They can also manifest as a skin rash that may look like small pimples on the palms or buttocks. This is condition is usually called eruptive xanthoma (see chapter 22).

How Can I Tell Whether I Have High Cholesterol?

Unfortunately, in the early stages, it is a silent disease, much like high blood pressure. You often find out about high cholesterol when you start having chest pain or, worse still, after a heart attack. Rarely, with some hereditary forms of high cholesterol, people develop "bumps" on the skin and tendons at the elbow and ankle, and a physician might notice these during a physical exam. It is therefore important to have your blood tested at regular intervals to measure your cholesterol.

When Should I Be Tested for High Cholesterol?

Cholesterol testing is recommended for all individuals over the age of 20. It should be tested every 2 years if you have desirable cholesterol levels and more frequently if your levels are abnormal or you have other risk factors. The test is called a lipoprotein profile and requires you to fast beforehand. Fasting means you may not have anything to eat or drink except for water, black coffee, or tea without milk, cream, or sugar for 9–12 hours before the test, which should be done first thing in the morning.

What Makes Cholesterol High or Low?

The factors that can affect your cholesterol levels are heredity, age, gender, diet, weight, exercise level, alcohol intake, cigarette smoking, hypertension, and diabetes.

Heredity

Your genes can influence your cholesterol levels. If your parents have high cholesterol levels, you probably will, too.

Age and gender

Cholesterol levels increase with age. Women are protected by estrogen until menopause, but women with diabetes don't have this protection. Men older than 45, women older than 55, or postmenopausal women at any age should consider themselves at higher risk for heart disease, especially if they have diabetes.

Diet

Foods high in cholesterol and saturated fat raise your LDL levels. In fact, it is believed that eating high-fat foods is the reason for the high incidence of heart disease in the U.S.

Weight and exercise

Excess weight, which is usually in the form of fat, increases LDL levels. Losing weight not only decreases your LDL and triglyceride levels, it increases your HDL levels. You can get the same benefits from regular physical activity.

Alcohol

Small quantities of alcohol can raise your HDL, the good cholesterol. One serving (5 ounces of wine, 12 ounces of beer, or 1 1/2 ounces of spirits) per day may give you beneficial effects on this good cholesterol. Red wine may have the added benefit of having antioxidants also. However, drinking too much alcohol can increase your triglyceride levels and cause liver damage. Alcohol should not be your main defense against heart disease.

Other factors

In addition, the following are risk factors for heart disease on their own:

- Cigarette smoking
- High blood pressure
- Diabetes

What Are the Benefits of Lowering Cholesterol?

Several research studies have been conducted to see whether lowering your cholesterol leads to a reduction in the number of heart attacks. In patients who already have CHD, lowering cholesterol clearly prevents second heart attacks and lowers the risk of dying from one. In these studies, for patients with diabetes, the benefits of lowering cholesterol are even more dramatic. The same holds true even for people without previous CHD. One major study followed 4,000 patients for 5 years. It found that by lowering LDL cholesterol with a group of drugs called "statins," there was a 42% reduction in the number of deaths from heart attacks and a 37% reduction in the chance of having a heart attack.

What Does Your Cholesterol Mean to You?

Since diabetes puts you at greater risk for CHD, you want your cholesterol levels to be as close to normal as possible. Your total cholesterol level should be less than 200 mg/dL. Your HDL should be 40 mg/dL or more, and the higher the better on this one (see Table 8-1). If you have diabetes, your LDL should be less than 100 mg/dL or less than 70 mg/dL, depending on what your health care team recommends. Triglycerides should be less than 150. The best ways to achieve desirable blood fat levels are with a balanced meal plan and daily exercise. If nutrition therapy and exercise do not lower LDL enough, you'll probably need drug therapy as well.

What Changes Can You Make in Your Diet?

Changes in diet help reduce cholesterol and are one of the most effective means of reducing your weight. The best—and perhaps only—way to get a meal plan that fits you and your lifestyle is to see a registered dietitian (RD) or nutritionist and work together.

More than likely, you need to reduce the amounts of saturated fat and cholesterol in your diet—and perhaps eat more monounsaturated fat.

How Do Weight Control and Exercise Affect Your Cholesterol Level?

Physical activity helps reduce weight, increase the good HDL levels, and improve blood glucose and blood pressure levels. Weight loss may lower your total cholesterol level.

When Will Your Physician Begin Drug Treatment?

If your LDL level remains above your goal after 6 months of your best efforts at meal planning and exercise, then drug treatment will be considered. You must continue with a good diet and exercise program even when you begin drug therapy. These drugs can have side effects, and you should be closely followed by your physician. The drug classes that are commonly used are statins, ezetimibe, bile acid resins, nicotinic acid, fibric acid derivatives, and hormones.

Table 8-1. Desirable Cholesterol Levels

Type	Cholesterol Level (mg/dL)
Total cholesterol	<200
LDL cholesterol	<100

Statins

These drugs inhibit the enzyme that controls the rate at which cholesterol is produced by the liver. They also improve the ability of the liver to remove LDL cholesterol from the blood. They apparently stabilize the plaque that lines the arteries, helping to prevent ruptures that lead to clots and heart attacks.

Currently, there are six statin drugs in the U.S. market designed to lower both total cholesterol and LDL cholesterol: lovastatin (Mevacor), pravastatin (Pravachol), simvastatin (Zocor), fluvastatin (Lescol), atorvastatin (Lipitor), and resuvostatin (Crestor). All are equally effective in bringing LDL levels down by about 20–60%. These drugs are given as a single dose at bedtime. Effects are seen in about 4–6 weeks, which is why your blood test should be repeated at about this time. Serious side effects are rare. Mild gastrointestinal symptoms, including abdominal cramps, gas, and constipation, usually go away after the first few weeks. Periodic lab tests are done to watch for changes in liver function. Rarely, some people may develop soreness and weakness of muscles. If this develops, you must stop your medication immediately and see your doctor.

Zetia

A relatively new medication that works differently from statins is ezetimibe (Zetia). It works by reducing the amount of cholesterol absorbed by the body. It is used by individuals who cannot take a statin medication or when a statin alone is unable to reach target cholesterol levels. A combination of simvastatin and ezetimibe is available as Vytorin.

Bile acid resins

These agents bind cholesterol in the intestines, and this combination is then eliminated in the stool. The bile acid resins lower LDL cholesterol by about 10–20%. Cholestyramine and colestipol are the two main drugs available in this class. They can be combined with statins for an additive effect on cholesterol reduction. Their greatest advantage is their safety profile, because they are not absorbed into your system. Bothersome side effects include constipation, bloating, and gas. These side effects can be avoided by taking the drug with meals and with large quantities of water. They can also cause your triglyceride levels to increase, so this will need to be watched. In addition to binding to cholesterol, bile acid resins interfere with the absorption of other medications taken at the same time. The other medications should be taken at least 1 hour before or 4–6 hours after the resin.

Nicotinic acid

Nicotinic acid is often avoided because it increases blood glucose levels. It is a B vitamin and has several beneficial effects, such as causing a 10–20% reduction in LDL cholesterol and a 20–50% reduction in triglyceride levels. It also raises HDL levels by about 15–30%. This drug is inexpensive and available without prescription. Because of potential side effects, don't use it without a doctor's supervision. The immediate-release form is preferred. Start the dose low and raise it slowly. A common side effect is flushing, which can be reduced by taking aspirin first. Discuss this with your doctor.

Fibric acid derivatives

Gemfibrozil (Lopid) is the fibric acid derivative available in the U.S. and is mainly effective in lowering triglyceride levels by about 20–50%. Another medication in this class is fenofibrate (Tricor).

This chapter was written by Aruna Venkatesh, MD, and Laurinda Poirier, RN, MPH, CDE.

9

High Blood Pressure

High blood pressure is often called hypertension. Unfortunately, if you have hypertension and diabetes your risks for kidney, heart, and cardiovascular disease are higher.

Case Study

Mr. ST is a 55-year-old Caucasian male who is a successful salesperson and was diagnosed with diabetes 5 years ago. Additionally, during the last couple of visits to his doctor, his blood pressure had been elevated, and a urine analysis showed his kidneys were spilling proteins. No pharmacological treatment has been started yet (besides his diabetes medications). During his college years, he was relatively active and was a member of the football team, but later in his life, as his workload increased, his physical activity progressively declined. Mr. ST's day typically starts around 7 A.M. with a breakfast consisting of orange juice, toast, eggs, sausage, and coffee with cream. He has a doughnut or pretzel for a snack around midmorning, eats a sandwich for lunch, and has dinner while watching TV in the evening.

His family history is concerning. His father has type 2 diabetes, his mother has hypertension, and an older brother had a heart attack at age 42. Mr. ST has never been admitted to the hospital. He is 5 feet 7 inches tall and weighs 200 pounds.

Dr. JR: Mr. ST, your blood pressure today is 150/90 mmHg. You told me that this is not the first time someone recorded an elevated blood pressure reading.

Mr. ST: For the last couple of months, I have had high readings at my doctor's office. At first, I was not too concerned because the readings were close to what I considered normal. However, later, I learned that healthy blood pressure in not the same for every person. Is this correct?

Dr. JR: Well, for someone with diabetes, blood pressure at or above 130/80 is considered high blood pressure, or hypertension. Have you been following your blood pressure readings at home?

Mr. ST: Yes, I recently got an ambulatory monitor, and I brought the results with me today. I started checking at home because it seems like I only have high blood pressure when I visit the doctor's office.

Dr. JR: Well, what you suggest is something called "white coat hypertension," a term used when someone has high blood pressure readings in the clinic but normal blood pressure at home. In your case, based on the readings you brought today, your problem is truly hypertension, since it seems your readings are high at home as well.

Mr. ST: Is high blood pressure common?

Dr. JR: It is a very common problem. One in three American adults (over 65 million people) has high blood pressure. Diabetes is also common, affecting almost 24 million people in the United States. Among those, about 73% also have high blood pressure.

Mr. ST: Is there any specific cause for high blood pressure?

Dr. JR: Usually, we talk about primary and secondary hypertension. Primary, sometimes called essential hypertension, does not have a clear cause, but it often accompanies diabetes. Secondary hypertension means that there is a clearly identifiable cause behind the high blood pressure. For example, it is being caused by a tumor in the adrenal glands or a narrowing of the kidney arteries, just to name a couple.

Mr. ST: What is the next step?

Dr. JR: First, I am going to ask you some questions:

1. Are you taking any medication, prescribed or over the counter? This is important to know, as some medications may either raise blood pressure or interfere with blood pressure medications. For example, over-the-counter cold medicines and appetite suppressants may raise your blood pressure. Commonly used painkillers (such as ibuprofen and naproxen) affect your kidneys and can cause interactions with blood pressure medications. Certain medications for depression may also affect your blood pressure.

2. Have you been told that you have high cholesterol? Do you have any recent lab results?

3. Do you smoke? Smoking cigarettes is bad enough, but if you have diabetes, it can be even worse.

4. Do you have heart disease, kidney disease, or eye disease? Have you ever had a heart attack? Have you ever had a cardiac stress test, and if so, do you have the results?

5. Do you get leg pain or cramps when you walk short distances? This may be a sign of narrowing of the arteries in your legs, called peripheral arterial disease (PAD).

6. Can you describe your dietary habits? Do you add salt to your foods? Do you eat a lot of canned foods and processed meats (which usually have a lot of salt)?

7. Do you exercise? What type of physical activity do you do?

8. Have you gained or lost weight recently? If so, why?

9. Have you felt any numbness or tingling in your hands or feet?

10. Do you have impotence problems?

11. Have you had problems with you urine?

12. Do you ever feel dizzy when you stand up?

13. Do you snore? This may be a sign of something called obstructive sleep apnea, a condition in which overweight or obese people may have periods during the night when they stop breathing. This can affect blood pressure, so detecting this sleep apnea is very important.

14. Have you noted problems with your eyes?

(*Note to reader:* You may wish to bring answers to these questions with you if and when you talk about your blood pressure with your doctor.)

Questions Dr. JR Asks Established Patients

Mr. ST was a new patient to Dr. JR, so there some were questions that were better suited for a later time. With an established patient, Dr. JR would also ask:

1. What treatments have you received in the past? Have you followed these treatments? Do you know how well you control your high blood pressure and diabetes?

2. Have you had any adverse effects from medications? If so, what were they?

3. Have you had an exam that checks for protein in the urine?

Dr. JR: Now that we've gone over some of your medical history, it's time for a physical exam.

Mr. ST: What are you looking for in the physical examination?

Dr. JR: There are a number of things:

- I will take your height and weight.
- I will take your blood pressure readings in different positions (standing, sitting, and lying flat). Getting readings while you're in different positions is important because medications and diabetes may cause abrupt changes in blood pressure when a person goes from lying flat to the standing position. This is called orthostatic hypotension and it is important to recognize, as it can cause you to get dizzy and even fall down.
- I will check your retinas (the back part of your eyes) with the opthalmoscope, looking for damage to blood vessels from diabetes and high blood pressure.
- I will look and listen to your neck. Distended veins in your neck might mean heart failure. I will listen for bruits, a sound that might be produced when the arteries that carry blood to your brain are narrowed by artery disease.
- I will examine your heart, looking for signs of enlargement and failure. The heart undergoes hypertrophy (thickening of its wall) as a response to high blood pressure. This can help the heart cope with high blood pressure in the beginning, but in the long run, heart hypertrophy is harmful and can lead to heart failure.
- I will also listen to your lungs to check for congestion that usually accompanies heart failure.
- In the abdomen, I will check again for bruits (like I did in the neck), because this may represent narrowing of the renal arteries that may, by itself, cause elevated blood pressure. After listening to your abdomen, I will try to feel any masses or enlargement of your kidneys. In the lower part of your abdomen, I will examine your bladder. Long-standing diabetes may damage the nerves in your bladder, making it difficult to fully empty your bladder.

- In your legs and feet I will check for diminished pulses, which can reflect narrowing of the arteries. I will also check your feet for ulcers or calluses and test your sensation. This foot exam needs to happen at every visit—many complications can be prevented by a simple foot exam.

* * * *

The physical exam does not reveal any abnormalities that suggest Mr. ST has had high blood pressure for a long time.

* * * *

Dr. JR: The normal physical examination is a good sign. But before beginning a treatment, I will request a series of blood tests, including:

- Serum creatinine (a marker of kidney function)
- TSH (a thyroid test)
- Electrolyte levels that may point to hypertension caused by excess or reduced production of certain hormones
- CBC (complete blood count) to check for anemia
- A1C to measure your blood glucose levels over the past 2–3 months
- Fasting blood lipids profile to detect abnormalities in your cholesterol levels (cholesterol, HDL, LDL, and triglycerides)
- Randomly collected spot urine sample to detect leaking of proteins in the urine (*albuminuria*), which can reflect not only damage to the kidney but also damage to the blood vessels

We will repeat some of these tests 6–12 weeks after treatment begins to see the effects of medication, especially on your blood lipids. These are tests that you should repeat yearly, but the type of tests and how often you have them should be based on the damage to your organs and how you respond to the treatment. You may need other specialized tests or consultations.

Mr. ST: Will I need to see any specialists?

Dr. JR: More than likely. Fortunately, the physical exam did not find any evidence of organ damage, so that's not an issue at this point. I will refer you to an ophthalmologist (eye doctor) for now. A yearly eye exam is recommended for adults with diabetes.

It would also be a good idea to see a registered dietitian (RD). An RD can help design a meal plan that not only meets your nutrition requirements, but will also allow you to lose weight and control you high blood pressure and lipids.

Additionally, a registered nurse clinician specially educated and certified in diabetes education (CDE) will teach you how to check your blood glucose and blood pressure at home and help you deal with specific situations.

Mr. ST: Why didn't I feel any symptoms of high blood pressure?

Dr. JR: Most people don't have symptoms. When symptoms do appear, they are usually a sign of organ damage. This is why it is important that your doctor screen for hypertension periodically, whether during annual physical exams, employment physicals, or ordinary visits to your doctor for some other cause. Certainly, if you have a family history of heart disease, kidney disease, diabetes, or hypertension, you need routine screening.

Mr. ST: What treatment do I need now?

Dr. JR: There are a few approaches I'll recommend. The first, and most important, is lifestyle modifications.

Mr. ST: What do you mean by lifestyle modifications?

Dr. JR: I mean what and how much you eat, as well as how much you exercise. Just losing a few pounds can have significant health benefits. While eating healthy meals is essential, exercise is as important as food. The American Diabetes Association recommends at least 150 minutes a week of moderate-intensity aerobic exercise and/or at least 90 minutes a week of vigorous aerobic exercise (keeping in mind that you don't rest for more than two consecutive days). Additionally, you should do some resistance exercise at least twice a week.

What you do isn't necessarily as important as how much you do it. Aerobic exercises include walking, bicycling, jogging, swimming, water aerobics, and many sports. Resistance exercises include weight lifting and exercises using weight machines.

However, before you start any exercise program, *get medical advice!* I would like you to see a cardiologist who may decide if you need a stress test done to check your heart before you start exercising. If you have any damage to the nerves in your feet, some types of exercise may need to be avoided.

Remember, you should start slowly, progress gradually, and immediately report any symptoms, such as chest pain or shortness of breath, and check your feet carefully after you exercise each time.

Mr. ST: I'm not too eager to take medications, and my brother told me about "non-pharmacological treatments." What exactly are these?

Dr. JR: "Non-pharmacological" treatment refers to interventions aimed at treating a medical condition without using drugs. In the case of high blood pressure and diabetes, they include healthy eating habits ("dieting"), regular physical activity, and smoking cessation—many of the lifestyle modifications we were just discussing.

Mr. ST: Then can I just do non-pharmacological treatments and avoid medication?

Dr. JR: Usually, a person who has diabetes with a blood pressure value higher than 130/80 but less than 140/90 can try just lifestyle modifications for up to 3 months. But if your blood pressure isn't at goal (less than 130/80) within this period, it's best to start treatment with medications.

Because, Mr. ST, your current blood pressure is higher than 140/90, you'll need both lifestyle modifications and medications. Keep in mind that the medications don't make the lifestyle changes any less important. If you have a healthy diet combined with regular physical activity, it is easier to control your blood pressure, which means the numbers of medications and the dose sizes you need would be smaller.

Mr. ST: Well, since it sounds like I'm going to need medication, I'm curious about how you choose the right drug combination. Are specific drugs suited for people like me?

Dr. JR: The combination of diabetes and hypertension, which you have, creates a special situation. This combo puts you at a greater risk of organ damage than does either condition alone. This leads to some extra considerations when choosing medications for people like you. There are several available medications for blood pressure control, but we need to focus on medications that specifically lower your risk of death from cardiovascular disease.

First, let's discuss some medications proven to clearly benefit people with diabetes—angiotensin-converting enzymes (ACE) inhibitors and the angiotensin-receptor blockers (ARB). These medications block what is known as the renin angiotensin–aldosterone system (RAAS) and blocking this system lowers blood pressure. These medications can slow the progression of diabetic kidney disease and control protein spillage in the urine (albuminuria). They also lower your risk of cardiovascular events, such as heart attacks. ARB and ACE inhibitors do not negatively affect blood glucose control and do not raise blood lipids, but these drugs do have side effects. There is some evidence that they may specifically help protect your eyes and nerves as well. In rare instances, they can worsen kidney function in people with narrowing of both renal arteries. Therefore, we would need to monitor your serum creatinine and potassium levels. Cough is also a common side effect of ACE inhibitors, though not of ARB.

The second medication class to consider is diuretics, though the only medications in this class that would be worth exploring for high blood pressure are thiazides. Thiazide diuretics in low doses (25 mg per day or less) have few side effects and generally work well for people with diabetes. Because diuretics can cause potassium loss, you would need frequent blood potassium tests, and you may need potassium supplementation.

We could also consider beta-blockers. Usually these are used under special circumstances, for instance, when a person with diabetes has coronary artery disease (heart attacks or myocardial infarctions) and heart failure.

Calcium channel blockers (CCB) are another option for blood pressure control, and, like thiazides, they have also been shown to decrease the rate of "bad" cardiovascular events in people with diabetes. CCB would not affect your blood glucose levels or your lipid levels either.

Considering all of these options, I should mention that people with diabetes usually need several blood pressure medications to control hypertension. Current recommendations are that one of those medications should be an ACE inhibitor or an ARB. If another medication should be added to your regimen, and beta-blockers aren't necessary, a thiazide is usually a good option.

There is another option as well. The Food and Drug Administration recently approved a new class of blood pressure medication called aliskiren (Tekturna). This medication inhibits a substance called renin and consequently lowers blood pressure. At high doses, diarrhea can be a side effect. Studies are still ongoing concerning any cardiovascular benefits in patients with diabetes

Mr. ST: All this talk about drugs makes me wonder how much lifestyle changes can really lower blood pressure.

Dr. JR: Clinical studies using a low-sodium meal plan called the DASH diet (rich in fruits, vegetables, and low-fat dairy products and with reduced saturated and total fat) have shown to lower systolic blood pressure by 11.4 mmHg and diastolic blood pressure by 5.5 mmHg when followed by people with high blood pressure.

Another study called TOMHS (Trial of Mild Hypertension Study) showed that lifestyle changes alone reduced average blood pressure from 141/91 to 130/83 mmHg for 234 participants after a year of intervention.

Mr. ST: Is it useful for healthy normal people to follow lifestyle changes?

Dr. JR: Of course it is. It would make everyone healthier and happier. The DPP (Diabetes Prevention Program) study demonstrated that dietary changes and exercise prevented the development of diabetes in a group of 3,234 people at risk for diabetes.

Mr. ST: Can you explain to me why the combination of diabetes and hypertension is so dangerous for me?

Dr. JR: I'm glad you asked. I mentioned before that this combo can damage your organs such as your heart, blood vessels, brain, retinas, nerves, and kidneys.

Let's talk about cardiovascular disease. The risk to your heart and blood vessels is doubled when you have diabetes and hypertension. This includes coronary heart disease (which produces heart attacks), heart failure, and peripheral vascular disease, causing poor circulation in your arms and legs that can end in amputation, especially if you have nerve damage in your feet. The risk of stroke is increased two- to fourfold in people with diabetes, but hypertension increases the risk by six times. Thus, the risk of stroke is substantial when you have both diseases.

Eyes are another target of both diabetes and high blood pressure. Patients with both diseases are definitely at higher risk for optic nerve damage and glaucoma. Retinopathy is twice as likely to occur when the average systolic blood pressure is 145 rather than 125 mmHg. Good control of hypertension can go a long way toward preserving your eyesight.

Remember that kidneys can be damaged by diabetes, too. This is called diabetic nephropathy and is currently the main cause leading to dialysis in America. Hypertension speeds up the progression of this complication. Controlling your hypertension and getting your blood glucose under control can prevent the progression of nephropathy.

So, as you can see, controlling hypertension is a key factor in preventing some of the most dreadful complications of diabetes.

Mr. ST: I have read on the Internet and heard from some friends that blood pressure medication can affect my sex life. Is that true?

Dr. JR: Well, I should first mention that diabetes and hypertension can cause erectile dysfunction (ED) all on their own. Diabetes and hypertension can damage blood vessels and nerves, including those in the penis. This damage can cause ED. Similarly, diabetes and hypertension can result in decreased vaginal lubrication, decreased libido, and difficulty in achieving an orgasm. Controlling blood pressure and diabetes can help prevent these complications in both men and women.

With that said, your concern about the medications is valid, but it should not stop you from taking them at this time—their benefit is too great. Additionally, not everyone experiences these side effects, and not all the medications affect sexual life in the same way. If you note a problem in the future, we can adjust your medication to minimize the problem.

Mr. ST: That's reassuring. Now that I am ready to start treatment, what can I do to ensure my treatment is successful?

Dr. JR: Maintaining a long-term effective treatment regimen is not possible without continued commitment from you, your family, and your primary care doctor. Aside from your primary physician, other health care practitioners such as nurses, pharmacists, podiatrists, dietitians, and ophthalmologists, can play vital roles in education and support of you and your family.

I would encourage you to master the skills you need for self-care and to follow the treatment plan we are going to develop together. I'll try to make the instructions simple and clear. I'll also write them down so that you can refer to them later.

Mr. ST: Why do so many treatment programs fail?

Dr. JR: Simply put, most fail because people don't make lifestyle changes or take their medications. Sometimes this is because drugs are too expensive, instructions are not clear, instructions are not written down, people aren't educated well enough, or physicians won't work as a team with their patients.

One helpful strategy is to write a personal "treatment contract" with realistic short-term goals. The doctor and patient can review these goals periodically, taking care not to be judgmental if the program isn't working. Patience and perseverance are the rules for success.

By the same token, a successful patient-education program should be tailored to the individual and be culturally sensitive. The diabetes educator must pay attention to the ethnic, religious, and regional issues of the patient. Adults need hands-on, active learning. Further, the family should be involved at every stage of the management. They can help record the results of blood glucose and blood pressure monitoring in a simple-to-use log book. A log book should be kept and reviewed periodically with the provider to make treatment decisions. Providers should also keep patients aware of available community resources and programs at workplaces and health care institutions.

Mr. ST: I've already bought a blood pressure instrument for home, but how do I know I have the right instrument? And how do I interpret the numbers?

Dr. JR: Well, Mr. ST, the "gold standard" for blood pressure measurement devices is the mercury sphygmomanometer, but this device is not easy to use and is usually only available at your doctor's office.

Currently, there are several electronic models that you can use at home. The ideal monitor is one that is consistent, accurate, easy to use, and affordable. Your current machine should be checked against the one that we used in my office periodically to make sure yours is accurate. Whatever instrument you use, make sure you choose an appropriate cuff size, place the arm at the level of the heart, and rest well before taking measurements. Blood pressure readings vary at different times of the day. In addition, physical activity, stress, caffeine, tobacco, and alcohol can influence readings. It is better to stay away from electronic finger models because there are more factors that can interfere and give false readings.

Regarding the numbers, as I told you before, your blood pressure readings should be below 130/80.

Mr. ST: We've covered what we plan to do for me. Are there special considerations for people in other demographics? Like my parents or wife, for example?

Dr. JR: Children and pregnant women are usually treated by specialists. The elderly also need extra consideration, but don't often require specialists. Just like middle-age people with diabetes and high blood pressure, elderly patients, even over 85 years old, benefit from control of their hypertension and diabetes.

However, certain considerations are in place when treating elderly patients. They can metabolize drugs differently, causing more prolonged effects. They may also have trouble taking medication regularly because of memory loss or existing medication regimens that require a lot of drugs.

Additionally, many elderly people have orthostatic hypotension (extreme changes in blood pressure caused by standing up), which means medication dosages may need to be decreased. Wearing elastic stockings may help in this situation.

Mr. ST: I've heard that some people just have high systolic blood pressure. Do you recommend treating them?

Dr. JR: Yes, even though for many years doctors were hesitant to treat elevated systolic pressure (the higher number of a blood pressure reading) alone. Clinical data now show that systolic hypertension on its own can affect cardiovascular health, especially in people with diabetes. The medications available are the same ones that we have already discussed. The treatment can be started with small doses of a thiazide diuretic. If a second drug is needed, I would recommend an ACE inhibitor.

Mr. ST: What promise does the future hold for a patient with hypertension and diabetes?

Dr. JR: Every day we learn more about what causes diabetes and hypertension and how these conditions affect our bodies. Nowadays, we have treatments for blood pressure that also affect the development of diabetes, such as the ACE inhibitors and ARBs, and we have new treatments available for controlling blood pressure, such as Aliskiren. We also have sophisticated new medications that improve blood glucose using hormones produced in the gut, such as exenatide (Byetta) and sitagliptin (Januvia). With the ongoing intensive worldwide research focused on diabetes and hypertension, the future appears promising.

The chapter was written by Camila Manrique, MD, Guido Lastra, MD, and James R. Sowers, MD.

10

Peripheral Arterial Disease

Case Study

TL is a 65-year-old male who has had type 1 diabetes for 25 years, a prior heart bypass, and a long history of foot problems due to nerve-related disease (neuropathy) in his feet. His podiatrist has previously treated his foot ulcers but now notices that for 6 weeks the right foot ulcer has not been healing. TL was referred to a vascular surgeon for examination and recommendations. Examination shows that the ulcer under the ball of his foot behind his big toe goes down to the bone. TL does not have any pulses in that foot. He was sent for a blood pressure cuff exam of his legs and feet to assess the lack of blood flow in the foot and to see where the blockage(s) might be. The blood supply was 1/3 normal to that foot. TL has some kidney disease, and to limit the risks of giving dye that can damage the kidney function, a Magnetic Resonance Imaging Arteriogram (MRA) was performed to give further detail about blockages and whether there were options for a procedure to increase the blood supply. This scan showed widespread disease in the arteries in the calf with a good artery down in the foot. Two options were proposed to the patient. The first is an arterial bypass from his knee to his foot using a vein. Because of his age, this may prove to be a more durable choice. However, some of his vein was used for the prior heart bypass, so a less invasive option can also be considered. This would involve opening up one or more of the diseased arteries in his calf through a groin puncture using balloons, stents, or a device to scrape out the plaque attached to a catheter. Although this is better tolerated by patients with multiple medical problems, success is not always possible and the result does not last as long as a bypass.

What Puts You at Risk for Developing Peripheral Arterial Disease?

Peripheral arterial disease (PAD) is a condition that involves plaque buildup in the arteries of the body. It commonly occurs in the legs and can remain unnoticed until a part of the blood vessel becomes so narrowed that blood supply to the foot gets very low. The case study above is a good example of PAD in a person with diabetes. PAD is twenty times more common in people with diabetes. Other behaviors that increase your risk include:

- Smoking
- Lack of exercise
- Obesity
- High blood pressure
- Increased lipid levels (including cholesterol)

Women and men are equally at risk. How long you have had diabetes and your family history can affect your risk. This is not just a disease of the elderly. Recognizing the disease and its symptoms is important and must be treated.

How Is PAD Different for People with Diabetes?

PAD in people with diabetes can affect several areas in the leg but it more commonly occurs in the calf arteries between the knee and foot. Checking for pulses in the leg and foot may not be enough to rule out the presence of PAD (Figure 10-1). This is because diabetes can make the arteries rigid and hard from heavy calcium in the walls (called Mönckeberg's sclerosis). The blood pressure in the leg can be falsely elevated because the arteries are not compress-

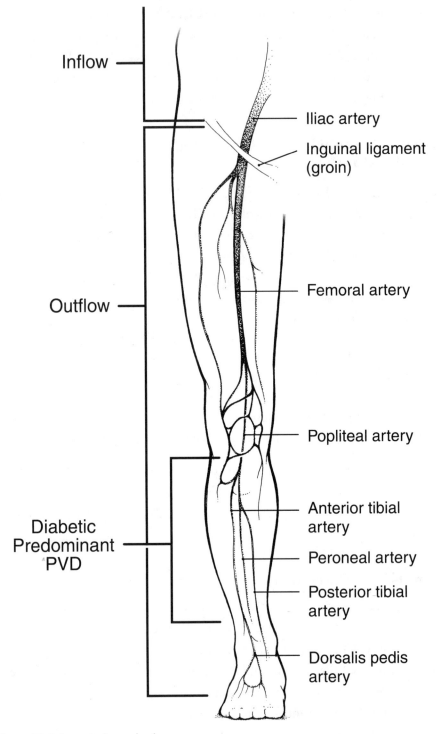

Inflow

Outflow

Diabetic
Predominant
PVD

Iliac artery

Inguinal ligament
(groin)

Femoral artery

Popliteal artery

Anterior tibial
artery

Peroneal artery

Posterior tibial
artery

Dorsalis pedis
artery

Figure 10-1. Leg arteries and veins.

ible due to the calcium. Nerve damage (neuropathy) contributes to this, making it difficult at times to feel the pulse even though there is circulation there. A better tool to assess the flow of blood to the foot is a toe pressure test, because the toe arteries aren't as affected by these conditions. Measuring oxygen in the skin of your feet is another option.

Approximately 40–60% of all amputations in the United States are performed on people with diabetes. An ulceration of some form precedes more than 85% of these amputations. However, PAD is not the only factor leading to ulcers. Other factors include:

- Injury or cracks in the skin
- Repeated trauma from lack of sensation (due to neuropathy)
- Tissue swelling (edema)
- Medical problems such as congestive heart failure
- Uncontrolled infection

What Are the Symptoms of PAD?

The symptoms of PAD are different from person to person, but can include:

- Coolness of the foot
- Loss of hair on the leg and foot
- Skin color change on your foot or calf to white or red
- Calf or thigh pain when walking or climbing stairs
- Pain in the foot that develops after going to bed at night
- Ulcers or wounds that heal very slowly or not at all
- Black areas on the foot (gangrene)

Leg pain from PAD, sometimes referred to as claudication, generally occurs gradually over a period of time, and you may notice that you get cramping in your calf, buttock, or thigh when walking. For some people with diabetes, impaired-circulation pain to the lower legs can feel like an aching in the foot that feels better when the area is supported. This discomfort is from decreased blood supply to the muscles of the leg or foot. Walking faster or up an incline may intensify this pain.

It should be noted that leg pain can have many causes, not just PAD. Other causes of leg pain include:

- Nerve irritation
- Arthritis
- Herniated disk
- Tarsal tunnel syndrome
- Neuropathy

Sometimes more than one of these problems can exist at the same time.

Fortunately, claudication and leg pain do not automatically lead to amputation. In fact, only 10–15% of people reach the point where amputation is necessary. Prevention and treatment are the keys to avoiding limb loss. If cramping while you walk occurs within 1/2 to 1 city block or interferes with your lifestyle or work, you should schedule a vascular consultation. Feeling pain while you are resting and/or experiencing any tissue loss are especially serious situations and need immediate attention.

How Is PAD Diagnosed?

Careful physical examination by a trained specialist must be performed to assess impaired circulation to the legs and feet. Your doctor will inspect your skin for loss of hair growth, any changes in skin and nail texture, the pallor of your foot when elevated or redness when it hangs down, and temperature changes compared to your other foot. Feeling for pulses in your leg or listening via a Doppler ultrasound can give valuable information as well.

If pulses in your leg are low or even absent, your doctor will probably perform a Doppler arterial test to measure pressures in your legs from your thigh to your foot. Your doctor will then compare these pressures to those in your arms and the opposite leg. Additional testing includes ankle-arm blood pressure ratios, toe pressures, waveform analyses, pulse-volume recordings, laser Doppler, transcutaneous (skin) oxygen determination, and MRA (like the one done in the case study above). If results are still unclear, the more invasive contrast arteriography (CT) scan (a dye study that creates a picture of your anatomy) can be considered. Talk to your physician or vascular surgeon for more information on the procedures mentioned here.

How Does the Doctor Decide What to Do?

Once the clinical evaluation and diagnostic work up is performed, your doctor can recommend treatment. Your underlying medical problems should be taken into account when deciding which procedure to perform. The newer, less invasive procedures have become more common, especially if you are elderly or have other medical conditions to consider, and technology has advanced so the results have improved. However, they usually do not last as long as the "gold-standard"—open surgical bypasses. Further, they require the administration of dye, which can be a problem if you have kidney disease. Intravenous fluids and a medication called N-acetylcysteine can be administered before and after the procedure to minimize damage to your kidneys, but your kidney health remains a consideration.

After your assessment, you and your doctor can decide whether a minimally invasive procedure, a bypass, or an amputation is the best course of action. If an open surgical bypass is the best option, improving any other medical conditions can improve your outcomes (for instance, getting your blood glucose levels under control).

What Needs to Be Done to Prepare for a Procedure?

A team approach with close communication among all parties involved is important. All active medical issues need to be evaluated and addressed by your health care team. It's routine to assess heart health beforehand with procedures such as electrocardiogram (ECG), echocardiogram (echo), or even stress testing and nuclear imaging. Occasionally cardiac catheterization, coronary angioplasty, and even cardiac bypass are necessary in preparation for the lower extremity procedure. If there is active infection, this must be controlled before surgery. Using antibiotics and removing dead infected tissue are important.

What Techniques Are Used to Treat PAD?

The location of the blockage, its length, and degree of calcium in the arteries will play a role in what your physician suggests. It is best to have a surgeon or vascular specialist who is comfortable with various techniques. If the blockage is in your aorta or iliac arteries above your groin, a less invasive choice, such as angioplasty or stenting, may be the best option. If your blockage is at or below your groin, angioplasty, stenting, atherectomy (laser or rotational), endarterectomy, or bypass surgery are options.

Minimal or less invasive procedures

Advances in technology, plastics, and optics have permitted the development of newer techniques labeled endovascular, so called because the procedure is performed on the inside of the artery from a remote location. The oldest and most commonly used is percutaneous transluminal angioplasty (PTA). This uses a small balloon to "crack the plaque" in the interior of an artery to make more room. Sometimes, usually if the angioplasty didn't work as well as planned, your team will decide to place a stent (circular wire mesh) or stent-graft (covered mesh) in the artery to maintain blood flow. A newer therapy is atherectomy (removing the plaque) with a blade or laser.

How well these less invasive techniques hold up over the long run is still being determined, though they have shown some benefits in certain patients in the short term. Successful results depend on a lot, including:

- The amount of calcium in the artery, which makes the plaque very hard and difficult to manage
- Whether the artery is completely or only partially blocked

- The length of blockage or disease of the artery being treated
- The location of blockage

Larger arteries that are only partially blocked and those with short lesions tend to do better. For example, the iliac arteries above the groin do well with these procedures. In fact, angioplasty and stenting results in this location have been as good as surgical bypass. The same cannot be said for the smaller vessels in the calf, which are the more commonly affected arteries in people with diabetes who have PAD.

Endarterectomy

This is a more invasive surgical procedure in which an incision is made over the blocked artery and the blocked portion is "cleaned out" directly. In non-PAD situations, this procedure is often performed on the carotid artery in the neck. However, it is effective in cases of PAD where blockages are limited to a very specific location, usually in the groin where the procedure can improve blood flow to the lower body.

Open bypass surgery

As mentioned above, when open bypass surgery is the best option, the first course of action is to improve any other medical conditions you may have. How long this takes varies from person to person and the severity of the conditions. Once any other factors are under control, three important details affect the outcome of the surgery and can affect how long your bypass will be effective.

1. The inflow, or source of blood supply, has to be adequate
2. The outflow, or the "run off," of the artery to the planned target site must be determined.
3. The graft, usually a vein but occasionally a substitute for vein, has to be in good condition to act as a tube connecting the inflow and outflow.

So, if the plan is to improve blood flow to your foot, and blockages are in your calf and thigh, your surgeon will create a bypass from the groin artery (femoral) to the foot artery (dorsalis pedis) using a vein from your inner leg. After the surgery, you may be asked to take medication such as aspirin to help keep the graft open.

Bypasses for the legs and feet are complex procedures and should only be considered if your leg or foot is at risk of amputation or your ability to walk is dramatically limiting your lifestyle and ability to live independently. Nonetheless, a bypass to the foot artery may be the only hope to heal ulcers. Results with these bypasses, even 5 years after surgery, show that limbs can be saved in 87–92% of cases.

What are the drawbacks of bypass surgery?

All things considered, an aggressive approach to saving limbs is in your best interest, and bypass surgery remains the "gold-standard" in most cases. However, the recovery from bypass surgery takes longer than less invasive approaches, and for the elderly and those with advanced medical conditions other than PAD, including many with diabetes, bypass surgery can simply be too invasive to consider. Fortunately, the advancement of less invasive endovascular therapy has given hope in cases where bypass surgery is not an option.

This chapter was written by Palma Shaw, MD, and Gary W. Gibbons, MD.

11

Stroke

Case Study

A 65-year-old woman with a history of type 2 diabetes, hypertension, and high cholesterol went to her physician when earlier that day she had experienced an episode of "drooping" of the right side of her face, weakness in her right arm, and difficulty with her speech that lasted 15 minutes. She reported a blood glucose level of 180 mg/dL after the episode. Her physician told her that he was glad she had come for evaluation so quickly. He listened to the carotid arteries in her neck and to her heart and performed a neurological examination. He heard a left carotid bruit (a soft, whooshing sound) over the artery in her neck. He recommended further testing, including a carotid artery ultrasound; a complete blood evaluation that included blood glucose, cholesterol, and triglycerides; and a brain computed tomography (CT) scan. He started her on aspirin, which can prevent clotting.

Diabetes and Stroke

An ischemic stroke is caused by a lack of blood supply to an area of the brain because of blockage of a blood vessel either in or leading to the brain. Diabetes increases your risk of having an ischemic stroke by approximately two to three times, and this increased risk applies whether you have type 1 or type 2 diabetes. It is estimated that at least 25% of all ischemic strokes are related to the effects of diabetes alone or in combination with high blood pressure. Persons with diabetes may have other associated conditions that further increase the risk of ischemic stroke.

People with diabetes tend to have more severe disabilities after a stroke, a higher frequency of another stroke, and a higher risk of death after a stroke than the general population. However, your risk of a stroke can be reduced by knowing the warning signs and by identifying risk factors, other than diabetes, that you can do something about. There are medications and a surgical procedure called carotid endarterectomy (where a surgeon removes a clot in the carotid artery in the neck) that can be used to reduce the risk of stroke in appropriate situations.

What Are the Signs and Symptoms of Stroke?

Your brain requires a constant supply of blood circulated from the heart to the brain arteries. When there is an interruption in this blood supply to an area of the brain, that area stops functioning properly. There are certain warning signs and symptoms that this is happening, and these symptoms are similar for a temporary transient ischemic attack (TIA) or a permanent lack of blood supply, otherwise called a stroke.

A TIA, which is illustrated in the case study above, is a clear warning sign of a possible impending stroke. A TIA usually lasts 5–15 minutes and then resolves. It differs from a stroke in one regard—its symptoms are short and reversible. Pay attention to the signs of a TIA, because if you are treated quickly, your risk of a subsequent stroke is reduced.

There are typical warning signs of a TIA or stroke (see box). One of these signs is sudden weakness or numbness in your face, arm, or leg, usually on one side of your body. Rarely, both sides of the body may be affected at the same time. The weakness may feel like heaviness or clumsiness in your arm and/or leg. There may be weakness on one side of the face, often described as "drooping." You

Warning Signs of a Stroke

- Sudden weakness or numbness of the face, arm, or leg on one side of the body

- Sudden dimness or loss of vision, particularly in one eye

- Loss of speech or trouble talking or understanding speech

- Unexplained dizziness, unsteadiness, or sudden falls, especially with the presence of any of the above symptoms

- Sudden, severe headaches with no apparent cause

may experience sudden dimness or loss of vision, particularly in one eye. People often describe this as a "fog," "haze," or "scum" over the eye. Loss of vision may progress from the top to the bottom in one eye. You may have trouble pronouncing words clearly. Some people have trouble understanding words that are spoken, trouble expressing themselves, or difficulty in both areas. You may have trouble reading or writing. You may suddenly become dizzy (vertigo), unsteady, or rarely, suddenly fall down. Finally, a sudden, severe headache with no other apparent cause can be a warning of a stroke.

Low blood glucose (hypoglycemia) can sometimes mimic a stroke or cause a seizure with paralysis. This usually clears up quickly after the low blood glucose is treated, but in some cases the symptoms may last for several days. Extremely high blood glucose and hyperosmolar hyperglycemic state (a condition caused by extremely elevated glucose levels) can also be mistaken for a stroke if you become disoriented and confused.

What Are the Causes of Stroke in a Person with Diabetes?

Strokes can be divided into ischemic stroke and hemorrhagic stroke. An ischemic stroke is the most common type of stroke, accounting for approximately 80–85% of all strokes. This type occurs when blood flow to the brain is interrupted due to blockage of an artery or arteries (Figure 11-1A). There can be many reasons for an artery being blocked, the most common of which is atherosclerosis of large and medium-sized arteries, which occurs more commonly, advances more rapidly, and is present at a younger age in people with diabetes. Due to the systemic nature of atherosclerosis, survivors of a TIA or stroke are at increased risk of a recurrent stroke or ischemic event in other parts of the vascular system, a phenomenon termed "cross risk."

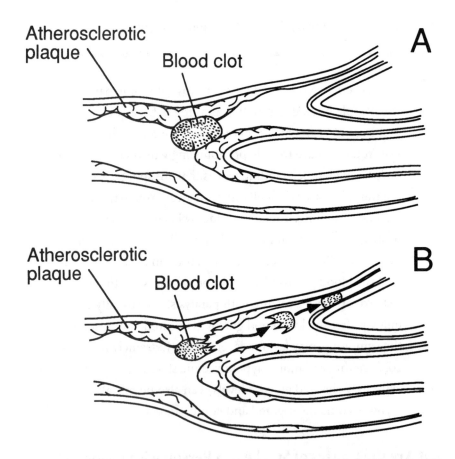

Figure 11-1. A. In an area of atheroslerotic narrowing of a blood vessel, a blood clot can form and block off the blood vessel, often leading to a stroke. **B.** A blood clot can originate in the area of an atherosclerotic plaque or it can travel from the heart to the blood vessel. A piece of the clot can break off and lodge in a smaller artery, causing a stroke.

Another cause of ischemic stroke, called cardioembolism, is often due to the development of a clot in one of the chambers of the heart that breaks loose and lodges in an artery of the brain. Other conditions that contribute to this type of stroke are

- atrial fibrillation (an irregular heart rhythm due to rapid and ineffective beating of the atria of the heart),
- a prior heart attack,
- history of rheumatic fever with heart abnormalities,
- or congestive heart failure.

If you have diabetes, a heart attack (which can go unrecognized) or a heart that is not contracting properly can lead to this type of stroke.

Ischemic strokes are also often caused by small-vessel occlusive disease, predominantly found among patients with arterial hypertension and diabetes.

Finally, an abnormality in the way the blood clots can also lead to strokes in people with diabetes. This may be due to changes in clotting factors, changes in platelet stickiness and clumping, or changes in the way red blood cells alter their shape as they travel through your blood vessels. The end result is that red blood cells can clot more easily than normal. This is especially true if you have diabetic kidney disease (chapter 17).

How Does Your Physician Diagnose Stroke and Determine the Cause?

Your doctor will more than likely initially diagnose a stroke based on a sudden onset of symptoms. Testing to detect a stroke includes a brain CT (or CAT) scan or magnetic resonance imaging (MRI) of the brain. A CT scan of the brain quickly creates several images of the brain to help your doctor determine whether the stroke is caused by bleeding (hemorrhage) or blockage (ischemia). MRI produces a three-dimensional image of the brain without the use of radiation. This test can identify small areas of stroke in places the

CT may not show, such as the brain stem, the cerebellum, and deep in the brain. Newly developed MRI techniques can detect ischemic brain tissue within minutes after the stroke begins. An MRI takes longer than a CT to perform and may not be appropriate for people with certain illnesses or those with severe claustrophobia.

A carotid artery scan is an ultrasound of the neck arteries that can determine whether there is narrowing or total blockage of the carotid arteries in the neck. A carotid ultrasound is noninvasive, fast, and inexpensive, but it requires meticulous technique and is highly dependent on the skill of the person doing the test.

Angiography (visualization of the blood vessels) may be performed with a CT scan, or it may be done by inserting a catheter into a blood vessel. Computed tomographic angiography (CTA), with its unlimited projection angles and three-dimensional display, allows superior assessment of the degree of arterial blockage and the degree of ulceration and calcification of the arterial walls. Catheter cerebral angiography, which requires a catheter to be inserted in an artery, has the highest spatial resolution of any these tests, but it is expensive and carries a very slight risk of stroke.

You may also receive cardiac testing, including an electrocardiogram (ECG), to check for an abnormal cardiac rhythm, or an echocardiogram, which is an ultrasound of the heart done to check for any clots in the chambers of the heart or other abnormalities that could be the source of a stroke.

In people with diabetes, blood tests for glucose, cholesterol, and triglycerides are particularly important. These basic tests attempt to determine a cause of the stroke, which directs your physician toward the appropriate treatment to prevent another stroke.

What Happens After You Have a Stroke?

After an acute stroke, you are admitted to the hospital, preferably to a stroke unit under the care of a neurologist. Patients who are treated within 3 hours of ischemic stroke should be considered for tissue plasminogen activator, an intravenous medication that dissolves clots. It is only for people who have suffered an ischemic stroke (not a brain hemorrhage), and there are strict guidelines for its usage.

After the initial treatment, you may need to see an endocrinologist, internal medicine physician, or family physician for diabetes or high blood pressure treatment. Depending on the type of neurological impairments present after the stroke, other health care professionals may be brought in, including a dietitian, speech pathologist, physical therapist, occupational therapist, and recreational therapist. You may need intensive rehabilitation under the care of a physician specializing in physical medicine. It is also important to be evaluated and quickly treated for any depression that may be present.

How Can You Prevent a Stroke?

There are three approaches you can take to prevent either a first stroke or recurring strokes:

- Modify your risk factors (at least those you can change)
- Try medical therapy
- Have surgery

Risk factors that you can't change

Age. Age is the greatest risk factor for stroke. Almost 75% of strokes occur after age 65. In fact, the risk more than doubles each decade after age 65.

Gender. While men are at a greater risk for stroke than women at most ages, stroke continues to be a major cause of death in women, and the risk begins to even out once someone reaches his or her eighties. Factors such as smoking, especially while using birth control pills, are contributing to higher rates of stroke in women. Also, women with diabetes are at higher risk of stroke than men with diabetes.

Race. African Americans are approximately 60% more likely than Caucasians to have a stroke. It is likely that both genetic and environmental factors play a role in this imbalance. African Americans are also more likely to have a cluster of contributing conditions (diabetes, hypertension, high blood cholesterol, obesity) than are whites. The higher rate of obesity in African Americans, Latinos, and American Indians causes their risk of developing diabetes to increase significantly, which may be one factor leading to an increased stroke risk.

Family history. Heredity can play a role in your risk of developing stroke. This is particularly true if many people in your family have high blood pressure, diabetes, or high cholesterol.

Risk factors that you can change

High blood pressure. High blood pressure is one of the single biggest risk factors for stroke. Hypertension, or blood pressure of 140/90 mmHg or higher, affects more than 50 million people in the United States. People with diabetes have a 40% higher rate of high blood pressure than those who do not have diabetes. If hypertension is combined with other risk factors, such as obesity, high blood lipids, smoking, or diabetes, the risk of stroke rises significantly. Fortunately, treating hypertension has been shown to work. In fact, successful treatment of hypertension has contributed to the overall decline in the number of strokes and deaths from strokes in recent years. If you have diabetes, your blood pressure should be at least less than 130/80 mmHg. Some experts recommend that your blood pressure should be below 120/80 mmHg.

High blood lipids. Try to get your total cholesterol and triglyceride numbers under control. High cholesterol can worsen atherosclerosis, which can lead to stroke. Lipid-lowering agents may slow and even reverse the formation of atherosclerotic plaque.

Heart disease. There are many different forms of heart diseases that can increase your risk of stroke. Some of the more common are heart attack, congestive heart failure, rheumatic heart disease, artificial heart valves, and atrial fibrillation or other heart-rhythm disturbances.

Tobacco. Cigarette smoking dramatically increases your risk of stroke. If you do smoke, you need to quit as soon as possible. Men who smoke have a 40% greater chance of having a stroke than do nonsmokers. Women who smoke have a 60% greater chance of having a stroke compared with nonsmokers. If you're a woman who smokes and uses birth control pills, your risk of stroke is 22 times higher than a woman who does neither. Smoking or exposure to secondhand tobacco smoke also increases your chances of developing atherosclerosis, which can lead to stroke.

Alcohol. Heavy or binge drinking is strongly associated with stroke. Drinking alcohol increases your blood pressure levels, which increases your risk of stroke. Elimination or reduction of alcohol consumption is recommended in heavy drinkers. You should drink fewer than one drink (12 ounces of beer, 5 ounces of wine, or 1.5 ounces of spirits) a day if you're a non-pregnant woman (and none if you're pregnant), and fewer than two drinks if you're a man.

Drugs. Drugs including cocaine, LSD, amphetamines, diet pills, and ergot derivatives can increase blood pressure and cause stroke. Substances in these drugs can also have toxic effects on your blood vessels, which can lead to stroke. Additionally, birth control pills have been shown to increase your chances of having a blood clot that could lead to a stroke.

Blood glucose control. Tight glucose control is recommended to prevent stroke. Out-of-control glucose levels can lead to complications in both small and large blood vessels, which may then increase your risk of stroke. The presence of diabetic complications such as coronary artery disease, heart disease, disease of the blood vessels in the legs (peripheral arterial disease), diabetic kidney disease (nephropathy, microalbuminuria), and disease of the blood vessels in the eyes (retinopathy) has been linked in some studies to a greater stroke risk. That's why it's so important for you to stop smoking and to control your blood pressure and your blood glucose to minimize your risk of stroke (see box).

Obesity. Obesity has been strongly linked with several major risk factors for stroke (such as high blood pressure, diabetes, and high blood lipids). It is thought that abdominal obesity, rather than general obesity, may be more related to stroke risk. If you are overweight and have had either a stroke or TIA, you should lose weight.

How to Reduce Your Risk of Stroke

- Know the warning signs of stroke and obtain emergency treatment if they occur.

- Pay attention to the modifiable risk factors, including high blood pressure, high cholesterol, and heart disease. Avoid tobacco, alcohol, and recreational drugs.

- See your physician regularly. Follow treatments for high blood pressure and heart disease and any treatment given to you by your physician for prevention of stroke.

Medical treatments for stroke

Modification of risk factors such as high blood pressure, diabetes, high cholesterol, cigarette smoking, and obesity are fundamental to stroke management. In addition, there are several other medical therapies available for the prevention of stroke or recurrent stroke and these medications generally fall into two categories: platelet antiaggregants and anticoagulants.

Platelet antiaggregants. Antiplatelet therapy is an integral component of secondary stroke prevention. It is highly effective in reducing the risk of recurrent vascular events and is recommended over oral anticoagulants (such as warfarin) for non-cardioembolic strokes.

Platelet antiaggregants work by preventing blood platelets from sticking together and forming clots. The most commonly used drugs in this category are aspirin, clopidogrel (Plavix), and sustained-release dipyridamole plus aspirin (Aggrenox). Aspirin has been used for several decades, and studies have shown that it reduces the risk of nonfatal stroke by 30%, the risk of nonfatal heart attack by 30%, and the risk of death by 15% compared with groups taking a placebo. Aspirin has the advantages of being inexpensive, generally safe, and well tolerated by most individuals. The most common side effects are gastrointestinal irritation or bleeding. In 1998, the FDA recommended a dose of 50–325 mg/day. The appropriate dose for you should be recommended by your physician, though low doses appear to be as effective as higher doses and have fewer side effects. If you are allergic to aspirin or cannot tolerate it, ask your doctor for an alternative.

Clopidogrel is modestly more effective than aspirin in reducing the combined risk of stroke, heart attacks, and heart-related death if you have atherosclerotic heart disease. Generally speaking, it is well tolerated. Recent studies show that there is no benefit to combining clopidogrel with aspirin in the general stroke population and in fact, the combination of the two medications was associated with an increased risk of bleeding complications. However, the benefits of such dual therapy (aspirin plus clopidogrel) outweigh the risks for those with a history of acute coronary syndrome and those with coronary stents.

The combination of low-dose aspirin and high-dose dipyridamole in a modified dose (Aggrenox) reduces the risk of fatal and nonfatal stroke for those who have previously had a stroke. The main side effects of this compound are headaches and upset stomach.

Anticoagulants. Anticoagulants, or blood thinners, such as warfarin (Coumadin) are another therapy to prevent stroke or recurring strokes. In general, anticoagulants are used if a stroke was caused by cardiac clots that break loose and lodge in the brain arteries.

Warfarin (Coumadin) prevents the blood from clotting by reducing the production of some of the clotting factors in the liver. It is especially useful for those with atrial fibrillation and mechanical heart valves. It may also be used after some types of heart attack to prevent stroke.

The main potential side effect of warfarin is bleeding, either into the brain or at other sites in the body. The degree of thinning of the blood needs to be carefully and frequently monitored with blood testing. Check with your physician about foods and medications that can affect your warfarin dose.

Surgical and other treatments for stroke

There are a couple of options, though the most common is carotid endarterectomy, which was mentioned earlier in the chapter. In this procedure, the carotid artery in the neck is opened and the layer of plaque (buildup) in the artery is removed. If you've had a TIA or mild-to-moderate stroke where there is 70–99% narrowing of the carotid artery on the same side as the symptoms, this surgery is highly beneficial. Certain patients with 50–69% narrowing of the carotid artery also benefit from the procedure. However, carotid endarterectomy is not helpful for those who have experienced symptoms of a stroke but have less than 50% narrowing or 100% blockage of the carotid artery.

Like most invasive procedures, carotid endarterectomy is not recommended if you have a high risk for surgical complications, such as existing poor heart or lung function.

This chapter was written by Jose Biller, MD, FACP, FAAN, FAHA, and Betsy B. Love, MD.

12

Eye Disease

Case Study

A 35-year-old man with type 1 diabetes has had blurred vision off and on in his right eye. One week ago, he noticed a floating "cobweb" that eventually went away, but now his vision seems worse. He describes difficulty with depth perception, especially when trying to add cream to his coffee.

He visits his ophthalmologist, who explains that the sudden onset of floating "specks" or "webs" may be a harmless consequence of aging of the vitreous gel, the material that normally fills the cavity of the eye. However, since he has diabetes, these symptoms may be caused by a hemorrhage in the eye. Therefore, the ophthalmologist will dilate the pupil in order to examine the vitreous gel and the retina.

Case Study

A 60-year-old woman with a 17-year history of type 2 diabetes complains of slowly worsening vision. It is beginning to affect her ability to type and read e-mail. Stronger reading glasses have not improved her sight. These symptoms may be attributable to a variety of abnormalities, including increasing cataract or retinopathy due to diabetes. While examining her eyes with a special lens, an ophthalmologist noticed a swelling in the center of the retina, the area known as the macula. He explains to her that this swelling in the retina is the cause of her worsening vision and a consequence of her diabetes.

Introduction

Diabetes can damage your eyes and affect your vision. One of the most feared complications of diabetes is vision loss. Some of the effects of diabetes are mild or short term, such as blurred vision that comes with poor blood glucose control. However, certain long-term complications can be sight threatening, even when your vision appears to be normal.

Diabetes is the leading cause of new-onset legal blindness in the United States. Eye disease can occur in patients with either type 1 or type 2 diabetes. The onset of damage and the development of symptoms may vary considerably and be quite delayed in some people. Most vision loss can be prevented or delayed by:

- Keeping your blood glucose levels as close to normal as possible
- Receiving regular eye examinations and prompt treatment by an ophthalmologist with experience in diabetic eye care

Because there is usually no pain associated with diabetic eye disease, most people do not have their eyes examined as often as they should. Regular, life-long eye care is one of the most important elements of managing your diabetes. *Visit an eye-care specialist at least once a year even if your vision hasn't changed.* When diabetic eye disease is caught in its early phases, treatment can be highly successful. Current treatments such as laser surgery can prevent more than 95% of severe vision loss from proliferative diabetic retinopathy and more than 50% of moderate vision loss from diabetic macular edema (swelling of the macula, the central portion of the retina).

It is important to have an understanding of how diabetes can affect your vision, how the ophthalmologist will evaluate your eyes to detect retinopathy, and how a treatment plan will be developed.

How Do Your Eyes See?

Your ability to see begins with your eyes and is completed in your brain. The eye (Figure 12-1) functions like a camera. Light passes through the transparent structures of the eye, such as the cornea, lens, and vitreous gel, and is focused by the cornea and lens upon the retina. The retina consists of receptors and nerve cells that line the back of the eye and functions much like film in a camera. The retinal receptors (rods and cones) convert the image carried by the rays of light into an electrical signal that is transmitted along the optic nerve to the visual center in the brain, known as the visual cortex. Here, the image is interpreted and perceived as sight. Other nerves control the movement of your eyes, adjust its focus, or alter the pupil size.

Any abnormality in this visual pathway, including changes within the eye, the optic nerve or brain, may alter the clarity of your vision. Scars on the cornea, clouding of the lens of your eye

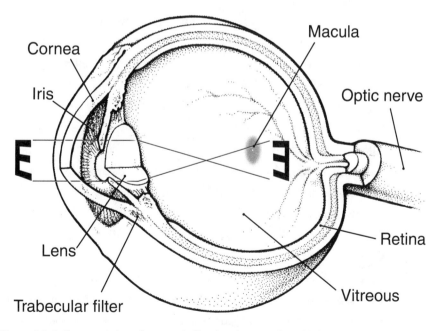

Figure 12-1. Cross-section of an eye indicating the macula, which is responsible for seeing details and color vision.

(such as cataract), or cloudiness in the vitreous gel of the eye can interfere with light reaching or being focused on the retina.

Changes to your retina can also damage vision, since it plays a critical role in vision. The retina can be divided into two zones:

- The macula, or center of the retina, is responsible for seeing fine details, such as reading, knitting, or identifying road signs, as well as recognizing colors
- The remainder of the retina, known as the periphery, is responsible for panoramic or peripheral field of vision, as well as vision in low levels of light, such as night vision

Either or both of these zones can be damaged by diabetes and obviously, any disease that affects your retina will ultimately affect your vision.

How Does Diabetes Affect the Retina?

Damage to the retina from diabetes is called diabetic retinopathy. The principal changes involve retinal blood vessels. The retina consists of many small blood vessels, and uncontrolled glucose levels over time can damage these small blood vessels.

In some eyes, blood vessels become weakened, balloon out, and become porous, allowing fluid or blood to leak into the retina which causes swelling of the retinal tissue. This is known as retinal edema. These changes in blood vessels and the swelling that results are called nonproliferative retinopathy.

In other eyes, blood vessels may become occluded so that areas of the retina receive less blood and therefore less oxygen and nutrients. This loss of nourishment is called ischemia. These affected areas of the retina stop working. The ischemic areas of the retina cause the release of growth factors that create new blood vessels. The growth of these vessels is called proliferative retinopathy. While this may seem to be nature's attempt to heal in response to a problem, it actually leads to devastating complications. The new blood vessels grow on the surface of the retina, on the optic nerve, and even on a structure in the front of the eye known as the iris, but unfortunately, do not nourish the damaged areas of the eye. In addition, the abnormal new vessels are extraordinarily fragile and tend to spontaneously bleed into the fluids of the eye. They also often carry with them scar tissue. In all of us, the vitreous gel naturally shrinks with aging, but this happens earlier in patients who have diabetes. If you have proliferative retinopathy, the shrinkage of the gel pulls on these blood vessels, causing hemorrhaging in front of the retina and into the gel itself. This blood blocks the path of light, preventing it from reaching your retina. It therefore causes a blurred image, and you may see floating material that can vary from simply a few specks to a large dark spot that blocks your central vision.

Without treatment, the proliferative retinopathy continues, resulting in the growth of more blood vessels and more scar tissue. This scar tissue is potentially very damaging to the retina. As the gel shrinks, it can pull on the scars, which then pull on the retina and cause it to rip or detach. The visual receptors, known as the rods and cones, in the retina stop working when they are detached from the cells beneath them, and the result is blank areas in your vision. Detachment of the retina results in further loss of retinal nutrition, which then leads to additional growth of new blood vessels in other locations, such as the iris. New blood vessels in this location can lead to a severe form of glaucoma known as neovascular, or new vessel, glaucoma.

What Is Macular Edema?

A common cause of vision loss in patients with diabetic retinopathy is macular edema, and it can occur both with nonproliferative and proliferative retinopathy. Blood vessels damaged by diabetes become porous and allow fluid to leak into the retina. This swelling is known as edema. The macula is the central area of the retina, and edema in this zone is called diabetic macular edema (DME). If the edema involves or threatens the very center of the macula, it is called clinically significant macular edema (CSME). Since the macula is responsible for detailed vision, people with macular edema may experience visual blur for both near and distant objects and may not be able to see colors normally. Those with uncontrolled type 2 diabetes are especially likely to develop macular edema. Because many people have type 2 diabetes, macular edema accounts for most cases of vision loss from diabetes.

What Puts You at Risk for Developing Retinopathy?

The two principal risk factors for developing retinopathy are how long you have had diabetes and your level of blood glucose control. Other medical conditions, such as high blood pressure, kidney disease, high cholesterol/abnormal levels of blood-fats, and pregnancy can add to your risk. While you cannot control how long you have had diabetes, controlling hypertension, blood lipid levels, and, most importantly, blood glucose levels is extremely important. Because eye disease can occur without causing symptoms, it is very important for you to have yearly eye examinations.

What Can You Do to Prevent or Control Retinopathy?

Control your blood glucose levels and blood pressure. People with type 1 and type 2 diabetes who control their blood glucose can significantly reduce their risk of developing retinopathy or delay its onset. This will reduce their need for treatment or surgery. You are wise to try to keep your blood glucose levels as close to the target set for you as possible.

What Are the Symptoms of Retinopathy?

All retinopathy begins as nonproliferative and causes vision loss by creating swelling of or loss of circulation to the macula. Depending on the severity of these changes, you may have no symptoms at all, or you may notice varying degrees of blurred or lost central vision. If the condition becomes proliferative retinopathy, when the fragile new blood vessels break and cause hemorrhage in front of the retina or into the vitreous gel, symptoms may include floating lines or webs. For those with large hemorrhages, vision may be reduced so that the eye can only distinguish between light and dark.

The symptoms resulting from changes in your retina vary from person to person. Some patients have no symptoms, while other patients may have blurred vision or fluctuating vision, floating webs, distortion of straight lines, or dramatic loss of vision to the level of light perception. Distortion may be a sign of macular edema, but can also be caused by scar tissue on the retina. Floating webs may be simply age-related changes involving the gel, but they can also indicate vitreous hemorrhages. Major losses of vision, like a shade in front of your eyes, can be due to vitreous hemorrhages or retinal detachment. It is important to recognize these symptoms and have your eyes examined promptly.

Keep in mind that you may have serious sight-threatening retinopathy even though you have no symptoms and your vision may still measure 20/20 (normal vision). This is why annual eye examinations are so important. An exam to determine whether you need glasses or a change in your old prescription for glasses is not enough. You need a comprehensive examination of your eye, including dilation of your pupil, in order to fully evaluate the retina. Ophthalmologists are skilled in conducting this examination, but be certain that you ask your doctor to do a dilated exam.

What Happens at Your Eye Examination?

It is very important that you see an eye care specialist who has experience with diabetic retinopathy. A complete examination should include:

- Measurement of your level of vision
- Evaluation of the movement of your eyes
- Refraction to determine your need for glasses
- Glaucoma screening

- Cataract evaluation
- Evaluation of changes in color perception or night vision
- Most importantly, dilation of your pupils to examine your retina

Examining your retina to detect retinopathy may require different techniques from those used in a routine eye exam. Dilation of the pupil allows the eye care specialist to see your entire retina, as well as the vitreous gel. A number of examination techniques may be used, including the handheld ophthalmoscope, the indirect ophthalmoscope, which is worn on the physician's head, as well as a device called a slit-lamp, which is actually a microscope.

Does an eye exam cause damage or pain?

Having your eyes examined and your pupils dilated causes no harm to retinal tissue. Right after completing the examination, you may experience a brief spell of blurred or dim vision, or may notice an alteration of colors. Following dilation, vision may seem blurry, particularly for near work, but will typically return to normal in a few hours as the effects of the drops have waned. Overall, the examination of the retina is not painful, although you will notice that the ophthalmologist's need for bright lights may cause slight discomfort at first.

Are There Other Tests for Diagnosing Retinopathy?

Other diagnostic techniques that may be useful include photography, fluorescein dye angiography, ultrasonography, and optical coherence tomography.

Fluorescein angiography

Fluorescein angiography is a technique in which photographs are taken of the retina while a fluorescent dye flows through its blood vessels. It requires dilation of the pupil, as well as an intravenous injection of the dye (typically an injection into a vein in your hand or by your elbow). A fluorescein angiogram is particularly useful in determining the extent of nonproliferative retinopathy and in particular, the location of points that are leaking. In general, this procedure is not necessary to detect proliferative retinopathy, which usually can be diagnosed by routine examination techniques. However, there are instances in which hidden zones of proliferative retinopathy can only be detected by means of angiography.

Following the test, you may notice that your vision is temporarily blurred or dimmed, or that you see peculiar colors for a few moments, but this usually passes quickly. The fluorescein dye has a brownish-yellow color, and following injection you may notice a slight yellow or tan appearance to your skin and to the whites of your eyes, lasting about 24 hours. The injected dye is cleared rapidly by way of your urinary system, resulting in a peculiar color to your urine. Fluorescein dye is nontoxic to the kidney and can be safely used, even in patients who have diabetic kidney disease, including those patients who require dialysis.

You should be aware that the injection of any medicine or dye can be associated with complications, including allergic reactions. However, these are very uncommon with fluorescein angiography. When the dye is first injected, you might feel a sensation of nausea, lasting only a few seconds. Patients who are allergic to the dye may be able to undergo future dye testing with appropriate preoperative medication and careful medical supervision.

Ultrasonography

Using reflected sound waves, ultrasound builds a picture of an area of the body that cannot be observed directly. It can be used to evaluate the back portion of the eye in people who have opacities in the eye, such as advanced cataract or hemorrhage in the vitreous gel. It may allow the physician to discover a retinal detachment or scar tissue on the surface of the retina. It does not provide a view of the retina itself. The ultrasound provides information that helps the eye care specialist understand alterations in the retinal structure and is particularly helpful in those who have chronic vitreous hemorrhage. It is used both for diagnosis, as well as to help plan vitrectomy surgery. There are no known side effects of ultrasonography.

Optical Coherence Tomography

Optical Coherence Tomography (OCT) is a non-invasive method of obtaining cross-sectional images of the retina, particularly in the macula. The high resolution of these images allows accurate measurement of retinal edema caused by leaky diabetic vessels. Your ophthalmologist can use this information to detect subtle macular edema and to precisely follow treatment to determine whether it is effective. OCT may also reveal subtle scar tissue on the retinal surface that may be responsible for swelling of the retina and it can often detect areas where your retina has detached. There are no known side effects of optical coherence tomography.

What Is the Treatment for Nonproliferative Retinopathy?

Two of the most important components of nonproliferative retinopathy treatment are controlled blood glucose levels and controlled blood pressure. If further action is needed, there are a number of nonproliferative retinopathy treatments available. Laser treatment is considered the "gold standard" for management of macular edema. The laser may be used to directly treat points of leakage or may be applied in a scattered fashion to absorb edema and to aid in the delivery of oxygen to the damaged tissue. A fluorescein angiogram is often used to map those areas that require treatment. Since over time new zones of leakage can develop, you may require a series of treatments. Other treatment options include medications that are directly injected into the vitreous gel of the eye. These medications are used in an attempt to reduce leakage from retinal vessels. In severe cases, when both laser and medical treatments have failed, some ophthalmologists may recommend a surgery called vitrectomy. During a vitrectomy, the gel of the eye is removed and replaced by a clear fluid, and any tractional membranes or scar tissue can be peeled from the surface of the retina in an effort to reduce the macular edema.

In the near future, there may be even more treatment options. A number of oral medicines are being studied that aim to reduce leakage from diabetic blood vessels. Implants of slow-release medications into the cavity of the eye are also being researched. It is hoped that these techniques will prevent or reduce macular edema from diabetes.

What Is the Treatment for Proliferative Retinopathy?

Proliferative retinopathy is treated with laser, cryotherapy (freezing), and vitrectomy (removal of the vitreous gel). The choice of method depends on multiple factors. Some patients have proliferative retinopathy only, without macular edema. Other patients have a combination of nonproliferative retinopathy causing macular edema, as well as proliferation. Some patients with proliferative disease may have associated hemorrhage, and others may have scar tissue affecting the retina. Some patients may have cataracts obscuring the view of the retina. Occasionally, patients may have new vessels growing on the iris as well, threatening to cause a severe form of glaucoma. Each of these factors must be weighed by the ophthalmologist to determine the best course of treatment.

Laser treatment

Laser treatment is currently the preferred method for managing proliferative retinopathy. The goal of the laser is to destroy the ischemic areas of the retina that promote the growth of new blood vessels. Laser can also be used to directly destroy some abnormal blood vessels, if the blood vessels are on the surface of the retina, away from the macula. This is called *focal laser treatment*. However, if the blood vessels are on the surface of the optic nerve, direct laser treatment can potentially damage this critically important nerve. When this is the case, a "scatter" treatment is used on the surrounding areas of the retina. Destroying these unhealthy zones of the retina not only inhibits the production of new blood vessels, but it may also increase the oxygenation of the remaining retina. This scatter, or panretinal, laser treatment involves the application of 1,000 to 2,000 laser spots to the peripheral retina and is typically applied over multiple sessions to reduce the chance of excessive swelling in the retina.

Laser surgery is generally performed in the ophthalmologist's office as an outpatient procedure. The eye is anesthetized with drops. A contact lens can then be comfortably placed on the eye, similar to the lens used for retinal examination. This lens holds your lids open and allows the ophthalmologist to examine the retina and to focus the laser light on the areas that require treatment. The laser applications are usually placed in rapid sequence. The ophthalmologist carefully avoids the normal large blood vessels, the optic nerve, and the macula, confining the treatment to zones of abnormal surface blood vessels, as well as to the zones of ischemia. Depending on the degree of treatment required, the number of treatment sessions may vary.

Anesthesia for Laser Surgery

Many people are worried about pain, discomfort, or not being able to comply during laser surgery, and understandably so. It is very important for you to remain still during treatment. For most, this is easily accomplished by staring at a target with the eye that is not being treated. If you cannot remain still, or if anesthetic drops in your eyes are not enough to provide you with comfort, then local anesthesia can be injected around the eye. In general, laser treatment creates very little discomfort. However, depending on the amount of treatment required, some patients may experience a localized discomfort during treatment, or a post-treatment headache.

Immediately after treatment, patients may notice blurry vision, though for most this is temporary. Some patients may notice a reduction in side or night vision, however most patients do not find this troubling.

Laser treatment may have to be modified to fit your individual case. For instance, if you have macular edema as well a proliferative retinopathy, your ophthalmologist will want to treat the edema and leakage first and the blood vessel growth later. For those who have scar tissue on the surface of the retina, your ophthalmologist may have to subdivide treatment into multiple sessions to avoid the areas of scar tissue and to minimize further damage. People with cataracts can be challenging, since the cataract may make it difficult to examine the retina and possibly block the laser light from reaching the retina. Occasionally, cataract surgery is necessary as a first measure, but it is generally best to start retinal treatment before cataract surgery and then re-evaluate the eye and complete laser treatment through the clear view afforded after the cataract has been removed.

Laser Treatment and Vitreous Hemorrhage

If you have a *vitreous hemorrhage*, or bleeding into the vitreous gel in your eye, along with proliferative retinopathy, laser treatment may be difficult. Your ophthalmologist will probably advise you to sleep with the head of your bed elevated, reduce activity, and avoid any bending that lowers your head below your heart. Taking these steps allows gravity to settle your hemorrhage in the lower portion of your eye and makes it possible to examine and treat the upper portions of the retina. As time goes on and the hemorrhage settles, larger and larger areas of your retina may become visible and therefore accessible for treatment. Something to note—since your brain flips the image it receives from the eye, you may see floaters and debris in the upper portion of your vision as your hemorrhaging settles into the lower portion of your eye.

Something to keep in mind—the photoreceptors of the retina (rods and cones) in the areas that are treated are destroyed by the treatment, and thus laser scars typically appear as blank spots in your field of vision. However, these blank spots generally don't bother you because they are quite tiny and typically located far from the central area that is responsible for our detail vision or because they involve areas that have compromised circulation (ischemia), which have already spontaneously ceased to function.

Cryotherapy

Cryotherapy uses freezing temperatures to destroy the abnormal retinal tissue and is sometimes used to manage proliferative retinopathy. It allows treatment of the far edges of the retina that may be difficult to reach with laser surgery. Cryotherapy may be used in those who have previously had complete laser treatment but have persistent new blood vessels and bleeding.

While cryotherapy was commonly used in the past, vitrectomy (see below) is often used instead. Cryotherapy, however, still has useful applications, such as in those who have hemorrhages that prevent laser treatment, yet are not candidates for vitrectomy surgery.

Vitrectomy

Vitrectomy surgery is generally reserved for people who have proliferative retinopathy that has led to hemorrhage or a detachment of the macula. These conditions don't necessarily mean a vitrectomy is necessary—many such hemorrhages will spontaneously clear and allow treatment with a laser. But if you have chronic vitreous hemorrhage that doesn't clear up on its own, or your condition has worsened to the point that you cannot carry out your normal daily functions, vitrectomy surgery may be the best option.

Vitrectomy is typically performed as an outpatient procedure in a darkened operating room. It requires either a local anesthetic or general anesthesia (you may prefer general anesthesia if it will be a long surgery, you are anxious and unable to tolerate being awake during surgery, or you're claustrophobic). Once you are anesthetized, microsurgical techniques are used to remove the central core of the vitreous gel, which may be opaque from hemorrhage or may be pulling on the underlying retina. Delicate instruments are used to cut and remove the vitreous, which is simultaneously replaced with a clear fluid similar to the natural liquids in your eye. Surgery may include removing scar tissue from the surface of your retina, clearing out any hemorrhage, coagulating new blood vessels, and/or completing laser treatment.

In general, vitrectomy surgery has long-lasting benefits for those with proliferative retinopathy. Once your retinopathy has been stabilized by vitrectomy, it typically remains stable for the remainder of your life. It would be uncommon for you to develop recurrent proliferation or bleeding later on. Following surgery, you may have a small persistent hemorrhage, or you may bleed again right after surgery, but these conditions generally clear up on their own. A small minority will experience repetitive bleeding or regrowth of scar tissue that requires a repeat vitrectomy.

Vitrectomy surgery, like any other surgical intervention, has inherent potential complications. Sight-threatening complications are relatively rare. However, it is common for cataracts to develop quickly in the eye that received the vitrectomy. Therefore, you should be aware that an additional surgical procedure, cataract extraction, may be required in an eye that has undergone successful vitrectomy.

What Do You Need to Do After Having Treatment for Retinopathy?

The most important thing you can do before and after any kind of treatment for retinopathy is to control your blood glucose and blood pressure levels. Specific postoperative instructions will vary, but the following information is generally useful.

Laser

After laser treatment, you may or may not need any eye medications. Some people will need a brief course of eye drops to reduce inflammation. Pain after the operation is typically minimal and only rarely needs to be treated with oral pain relievers. If you just receive anesthetic drops at the time of treatment, you usually will not require a patch on your eye. However, if a local anesthetic is injected, the eye may require a patch until the anesthetic wears off.

Cryotherapy

After treatment, the outer surface of the eye is often swollen and may appear red for 1–2 weeks. You may need eye drops for inflammation. Depending on the degree of treatment required, you may feel some headache after the procedure. Oral pain medications will usually treat your pain adequately. After the first day, you will probably not require any other pain medicines.

Intraocular injections

After an intraocular injection of medicine, your eye may feel irritated. You may notice that it feels dry or scratchy and tears up more than usual. This is usually caused by the cleansing solutions, rather than the injection itself. These symptoms typically clear up by the following day. Depending on the medicine injected, you may see an increase in the amount of "floaters" and debris until the injected medicine settles out of your field of vision. As a general rule, discomfort is minimal, and pain medicines are not usually necessary. Occasionally, you may see a small amount of blood on the white surface of the eye. This is harmless and typically clears up in several days. Your doctor may prescribe antibiotic drops for you to use for several days, hoping to reduce the risk of infection.

Vitrectomy

Vitrectomy is now generally done as an outpatient procedure. A variety of medications may be required after surgery, including drops to dilate the pupil, prevent infection, and reduce inflammation. Depending on the extent of surgery, you may require pain medication, given either by mouth or by injection, though oral pain medicines are usually enough.

After the operation, your lids may be somewhat swollen, and the tissues of the eye itself may appear swollen and red. This typically will go away over 3–4 weeks. While your eye is swollen, you may not be able to wear a contact lens. However, as the eye heals, you can resume wearing your lens. Depending on what was found in surgery, you may be asked to maintain a certain head position, often to help clear a small amount of hemorrhage that often is present in the eye following surgery. By sleeping with the head of your bed elevated and avoiding bending, this will typically settle by gravity to the lower portion of your eye.

If a gas bubble is used as part of the surgery, you may be asked to position yourself in such a way to allow it to rise and press against treated areas of the retina. This positioning is required until the gas is absorbed and replaced by the aqueous fluid of the eye. *Do not fly in any aircraft until the gas bubble is gone! Also, if you need another general anesthetic during the postoperative period, you must tell your physician about the presence of gas in your eye.* A general anesthesia can still be done safely, but the anesthesiologist must know in advance that a gas is in the vitreous cavity of your eye. This will allow the anesthesiologist to use anesthetic agents that will not interfere with the gas bubble. Depending on your vision in the other eye and requirements for transportation or work, you may need to remain inactive following surgery, including taking a leave of absence from work.

How Does Vision Change After Treatment for Retinopathy?

Anyone who undergoes laser treatment, cryotherapy, or vitrectomy may potentially experience changes in his or her vision. If you've been treated with a laser for macular swelling, there is a rare chance you may notice tiny blank spots in your field of vision caused by the laser. However, these are usually so small they are not troublesome. After scatter laser treatment, some may notice a decrease in night vision or peripheral vision, a temporary decrease in central vision, or, rarely, an overall slight permanent reduction in vision. Difficulty focusing on near objects is also a common occurrence after scatter treatment, but it generally goes away after several days to weeks.

It is not possible to predict how your vision will be improved after laser treatment or vitrectomy. This is because there are many causes for loss of vision, and you may have several of them. For instance, treating macular edema or abnormal blood vessels will not alter the age-related development of cataract. Removal of hemorrhage by vitrectomy will clear the path for light to reach the retina, but the health of the underlying retina cannot be determined until surgery is complete. It is the health of the underlying retina that ultimately determines the potential of the retina to see.

Some fear that laser treatment or surgery will harm their vision, and this often causes them to delay therapy. Although there are potential risks in any form of treatment, *the benefits of treating diabetic retinopathy greatly outweigh the risk of treatment.* If you do not get treatment, diabetic retinopathy is usually progressive and sight-threatening. Treatment with laser and vitrectomy has been proven to benefit vision greatly. Do not wait until you've lost your sight— detecting retinopathy just as it reaches a treatable stage is the most important factor in preventing vision loss.

Are There Causes of Vision Loss Other than Retinopathy?

There are many ways that diabetes can alter your vision. Some of these changes are temporary, while others can be progressive and permanent. While the principal damage from diabetes is due to retinopathy, not all vision loss from diabetes is due to its effect upon the retina.

Refractive changes

Uncontrolled blood glucose levels can blur your vision. Frequently, higher levels of blood glucose can cause you to be temporarily more near-sighted—your distance vision will become blurred, while your near vision actually seems somewhat clearer. Some people even find they no longer require reading glasses. However, such changes in vision are temporary and often fluctuate with the level of blood glucose. This type of visual blurring may be the first symptom that leads to the diagnosis of diabetes. Because the focus of your eye will change with the level of your blood glucose, some patients will need to have the strength of their glasses or contact lenses modified repetitively until their blood glucose levels are under control.

Corneal surface abnormalities

The cornea is the clear front part of the eye. It allows the light to penetrate into the deeper layers of the eye, but it also helps to focus the light to bring a clear image to the retina. The surface layer of the cornea, known as the epithelium, is made up of several layers of cells. This superficial layer is susceptible to being scraped or scratched in any patient, but is more easily disrupted in those with diabetes. Such abrasions of the surface layer can cause painful blurring of vision; however, they generally heal without long-term visual consequences. If you have diabetes, this healing process can take longer and even after the healing is complete, symptoms may recur. Until the healing is complete, your ophthalmologist may recommend ointments or mild antibiotic drops to lubricate the surface of your eye, prevent infection, and keep it comfortable. You may also need to wear an eye patch or, occasionally, a special contact lens known as a "bandage lens" to allow the healing to occur. Contact lens wearers who suffer such abrasions or erosions should refrain from the use of their contact lenses until their ophthalmologist confirms that the corneal surface is completely healed. As a rule of thumb, stop wearing your contact lenses any time the eye feels irritated, becomes red, or has a discharge until you are evaluated by your ophthalmologist.

What Are Cataracts?

Cataract is a term used to describe any clouding of the lens of the eye. Cataracts generally affect people 60 years of age or older, and most cataracts progress gradually. If you have diabetes, cataracts tend to develop at a younger age and progress more rapidly. It is not unusual for people with diabetes to develop cataracts in their 30s or 40s, and the progression of the cataract can be dramatically fast. Cataracts specifically related to diabetes are sometimes caused by very poorly controlled blood glucose levels.

What are the symptoms of cataracts?

Symptoms of cataracts may include:

- Dimming of vision
- Difficulty reading
- The need for brighter lights while reading
- Difficulty driving
- Occasionally, car headlights may have a star-burst or sparkler effect

What is the treatment for cataracts?

Regrettably, cataracts cannot be treated medically at this time. If cataracts prevent you from performing the necessary tasks of your daily life, the only option may be a outpatient procedure during which the affected lens is surgically removed from the eye and an artificial lens is then implanted in its place. Generally, the surgeon will leave a thin film of tissue, called the lens capsule, in place; this holds the newly implanted lens in its proper position.

It is a common misperception to think that cataract surgery can be performed with a laser. Cataract removal actually requires a surgical procedure. However, after surgery, the lens capsule that has been left in place may become cloudy much like the original cataract. This condition is known as an "aftercataract." It is routinely treated by means of a special laser that creates a permanent, clear hole in the center of the capsule. The laser used for this type of treatment is different from the laser used to treat diabetic retinopathy and is typically done by the cataract surgeon.

Following cataract surgery, you may still need glasses for reading, distance, or for both. Most artificial lenses focus the eye at only one distance, and so the addition of glasses gives you flexibility to focus at different distances. Some new artificial lenses are now being developed that may allow focusing at multiple distances.

What Is Glaucoma?

Glaucoma is a condition in which the pressure inside the eye causes damage to the optic nerve. As a person with diabetes, you are more likely to develop glaucoma than someone without diabetes. The eye constantly produces and drains a fluid known as the aqueous. This fluid is not a component of our tears and does not come to the outer surface of the eye, but instead is absorbed into the bloodstream. The balance of production and drainage determines the pressure within your eye.

If you have proliferative diabetic retinopathy, blood vessel growth and scarring can affect the tissues that regulate the drainage of this aqueous fluid. This leads to an increase in eye pressure, since the fluid continues to be produced but cannot leave. The increased pressure then compresses the delicate optic nerve fibers and can cause permanent damage to your optic nerve.

There are other forms of glaucoma that are not related to retinopathy, and these can affect anyone, whether they have diabetes or not. These types of glaucoma fall into two categories—open-angle glaucoma, which becomes common as we age, or the rarer narrow-angle glaucoma. Therefore, even if you do not suffer from retinopathy, a glaucoma test is typically performed during your routine eye examination.

What is the treatment for glaucoma?

Treatment for glaucoma depends on the type of glaucoma. For glaucoma related to proliferative retinopathy, treatment usually involves laser to eliminate the zones of vessel growth affecting aqueous drainage. If the treatment can be accomplished before permanent scarring occurs, your eye pressure may be returned to normal. However, if your filtering system is permanently obstructed by scar tissue, you may need surgery to create a new passage for fluid to drain from the eye.

Open-angle glaucoma is typically treated simply with eye drops, and if that doesn't work, laser treatment to the filtration area. For those with narrow-angle glaucoma, laser treatment can be used to create a small opening in the colored portion of the eye known as the iris, thereby allowing fluid to pass to the drainage channels. This is called a laser iridotomy,a and it usually will either prevent or cure angle closure.

Can Diabetes Affect the Optic Nerve in Other Ways?

Diabetes can damage blood vessels, sometimes even causing them to close. The optic nerve is susceptible to this effect and may be damaged when it does not receive an adequate blood supply. It may then recover, but the initial injury may result in vision loss to both the peripheral and central vision.

If the nerve pathways carrying the image from your retina to your brain don't get adequate blood, you can also suffer vision loss. This loss of circulation is typically called a stroke.

Sometimes, a clot or other particulate material may block a blood vessel briefly and then move on. This may cause a temporary loss of some or all of your vision that will then clear as the blood flow is restored. If you experience a symptom like this, you should bring this to the attention of your doctor in order to determine its cause and to hopefully prevent it from recurring.

What Causes Double Vision When You Have Diabetes?

Diabetes can sometimes cause double vision. The position of our eyes is controlled by six muscles connected to each eye. While each eye has its own muscle and nerve supply, the movements of both eyes are coordinated so that they maintain focus simultaneously on a given visual target. Diabetes can damage our blood vessels and therefore impair the flow of nutrients to these nerves. If the nerve is impaired by lack of blood supply, the muscle that it controls will not move properly, and the coordination of the two eyes will not be in sync. Under these circumstances, the two eyes will be focused on two different targets, and the brain will get two distinct images, resulting in double vision.

If you're experiencing double vision, you may be asked to wear an eye patch to eliminate one of the two images. Sometimes an optical device called a prism can be added to a spectacle lens in an attempt to align the two eyes. As a general rule, the nerve regains its function over several months, and the eyes again track together. Rarely, surgery on an affected muscle is necessary to realign the eyes so that they can maintain a single image and track together.

In some cases, double vision can be the first sign of a serious or life-threatening condition. Immediate eye examination and careful evaluation by a doctor familiar with diabetic eye disease are therefore critically important.

What Does It Mean if You Temporarily Lose Your Vision Completely?

This is often the result of a vascular occlusion—something obstructing the blood flow in the main artery feeding your retina. The main symptom is a sudden and profound loss of vision that can vary in how long it lasts. The obstruction is usually caused by debris in your bloodstream known as an embolus. This embolus travels along with the circulation until it reaches a blood vessel whose diameter is too small to allow the material to pass forward. This material then blocks the blood vessel and causes varying degrees of obstruction of blood flow beyond the point of blockage.

"Amaurosis fugax" is the term used to refer to this transient loss of vision due to the temporary blockage of circulation. People with amaurosis fugax typically lose the upper or lower half of their vision or even all vision itself. The symptoms typically are temporary, and vision will suddenly return to its prior levels. Even though these symptoms may be temporary, they are very important and should be brought to the attention of your physician.

Does Physical Activity Affect Retinopathy?

In general, physical activity and exercise do not affect those with macular edema or nonproliferative retinopathy. If you have proliferative retinopathy, particularly if you have vitreous hemorrhage, some types of physical activity may cause new blood vessels to be more likely to rupture, leading to more hemorrhaging. Those with scar tissue on the surface of their retina may be at greater risk of retinal tear or detachment should they suffer a severely jarring injury like you would find in contact sports. In the course of your comprehensive eye examination, your ophthalmologist can determine whether such risk factors are present and can recommend what levels of exercise are appropriate for you.

Does Pregnancy Affect Retinopathy?

Women who do not have diabetes beforehand will occasionally develop diabetes for the first time during pregnancy. This is known as gestational diabetes and usually does not affect eye health. However, for those who do have diabetes before pregnancy, it has been established that pregnancy can worsen retinopathy. Thus, an eye examination during the first trimester is highly recommended. The ophthalmologist can then determine the need for, and frequency of, any subsequent follow-up visits.

If mild diabetic macular edema should develop during pregnancy, it usually does not require treatment, as it usually returns to normal after delivery. However, if the edema can possibly threaten vision, laser treatment can be performed during the pregnancy.

Proliferative retinopathy should be followed very closely during pregnancy, since it may progress more rapidly. The ophthalmologist may choose to treat proliferative retinopathy with the same laser treatment recommended for a person who was not pregnant. For those who have proliferative retinopathy at the time of delivery, there is a theoretical risk of increased vitreous hemorrhage from the strain associated with labor. If this is the case, a Caesarean section rather than vaginal delivery may be the better option.

It is important to know that diabetic retinopathy on its own is no longer a reason to terminate a pregnancy. However, your obstetrician will encourage you to tightly control your blood glucose and blood pressure throughout your pregnancy in order to minimize your risks.

What Can You Do to Reduce Your Risk of Vision Loss?

You must take an active role in your own eye care. The best way to prevent severe diabetic retinopathy is to control your blood glucose and blood pressure levels. You should also undergo regular comprehensive eye examinations at a frequency recommended by your ophthalmologist. The frequency of such examinations may vary depending on the level of retinopathy and the presence of other medical conditions. It is important for you to maintain good control of other medical conditions including kidney disease, hypertension, and blood lipid levels.

In conclusion, with regular and lifelong eye examinations, with early recognition and treatment of retinopathy, severe vision loss can be prevented in more than 98% of people with diabetes.

This chapter was written by Bradley T. Smith, MD, and M. Gilbert Grand, MD.

13

The Genetics of Eye Disease

Introduction

We hear much in the news of late about "The Human Genome" and the myriad discoveries regarding its sequence, organization, and impact on health. What is the connection between these observations and your risk for disease? What about your children's risk? Are these observations relevant to whether you will develop complications to your diabetes, such as diabetic eye disease? If so, what can you do about it? You can't change genes, can you? These and many other questions are natural consequences of this explosion in genetic information. In this chapter, we discuss just what the human genome is and some of its implications for how your diabetes may progress and also what that might mean for your relatives. However, we should note that although this chapter will focus on eye disease in diabetes, the concepts detailed in this chapter are also true for the other complications of diabetes (nerve disease, kidney disease, and cardiovascular disease).

Family Members Share Genes

Among the great characteristics of humans is our natural curiosity about how things work and are organized and how we all fit together. This includes everyday observations that we all make regarding the weather, or our curiosity about how planes fly, or our wonder at the incredible diversity around us. It also includes observations about our families, where we say things such as, "She has her mother's eyes," or, "He's the spitting image of his grandfather." These latter observations reflect the fact that blood relatives will share similar genetic backgrounds. In fact, parents and offspring share one-half of all their genes identically. Similarly, individuals share an average of one-half of all their genes with each of their brothers or sisters. With our grandparents, we share one-fourth of our genes identically. Even first cousins share one-eighth of their genes. For these reasons, biological relatives will tend to resemble one another, often being similar in height or weight, or in eye, hair, or skin color, or even in certain behaviors. The more closely related we are to someone, the more likely it is that we will share such similarities.

If this sharing of genes among relatives leads to similarities in things such as our appearance, what if we share the same forms of genes that are involved in diseases? Just as with other traits, we can share similar traits like blood pressure, cholesterol, or glucose levels. For this reason, brothers, sisters, or children of someone with type 2 diabetes are approximately three times more likely to develop type 2 diabetes themselves than someone who does not have such a close relative with diabetes. This same principle can carry over to the development of the complications of diabetes, so that if your brother develops diabetic retinopathy and you also have diabetes, then your risk for diabetic retinopathy may go up. Genetic similarities may also lead to similarities in response to treatments. For example, if your sister's diabetes is well controlled with a particular glucose-lowering drug, you might respond similarly; knowing this might save some of the trial and error that might be needed to find the best treatment strategy for you.

If Your Brother or Sister Develops Diabetic Retinopathy, What Are the Implications for You?

For a long time, we have known that there seem to be some individuals who are particularly prone to the development of diabetic eye disease (retinopathy) or other diabetes complications. At the same time, there are some individuals who seem to be resistant to the development of complications. What is it that is different about these individuals? It may be that they are either genetically suscep-tible or genetically resistant. Studies of families have begun to show just how significant it is for individuals with diabetes when their brother or sister develops diabetic retinopathy.

Among the classic types of family studies are those examining twins. Identical twins share ALL of their genes in common. This is why they are so similar. One study examined 37 pairs of identical twins who all had type 2 diabetes. In 35 of these pairs, either both twins had diabetic retinopathy, or neither had it. In 31 identical twin pairs where both had type 1 diabetes, 21 pairs were classified in the same retinopa-thy category. These observations point out two things. First, twins with diabetes are similar when it comes to retinopathy. This suggests that if your brother or sister develops retinopathy, then your risk of develop-ing it also goes up. However, it also means that if your brother or sister does not develop retinopathy, then you might actually share some protective genes. Second, the fact that not all the twins are the same for retinopathy indicates that genes are not the only factor producing retinopathy. Even if there is a genetic propensity to develop diabetic retinopathy, it does not mean that developing retinopathy is inevita-ble—other factors may modify one's risk of retinopathy.

How Much Does Your Risk Go Up if a Family Member Has Severe Retinopathy?

Recent work has shown that it is not so much retinopathy itself that is similar among relatives, but rather the more severe forms of retin-opathy that are more common across relatives. This has been shown in follow-up studies of the Diabetes Control and Complications Trial (DCCT) for type 1 diabetes, and also among Mexican Americans with type 2 diabetes. The DCCT was instrumental in showing how critical good glucose control is for preventing diabetic retinopathy. There appear to be some individuals, however, who are more prone to developing severe retinopathy, and it is the severity of the disease that seems more likely to cluster in families. This was also observed among

Mexican Americans with type 2 diabetes, in whom brothers or sisters of someone with more severe retinopathy showed an increase of 75% in their risk of having more severe retinopathy, compared to brothers or sisters of someone who had either mild retinopathy or no retinopathy at all, even when analyses took the duration of diabetes and the degree of glucose control into account. This means that someone with diabetes who had a brother or sister with more severe retinopathy was almost twice as likely to develop more severe retinopathy than someone who had a brother or sister with mild retinopathy or none at all.

This evidence does not mean that the more severe forms of retinopathy cannot be prevented; what it does mean is that if you have a close blood relative who develops severe diabetic retinopathy, then you should redouble your efforts to control your own blood glucose. Even if a close relative has severe retinopathy, controlling one's own blood glucose is extremely important for reducing the risk of retinopathy and its progression.

Is Diabetic Retinopathy Different in Those with Type 1 or Type 2 Diabetes?

Family studies and other evidence indicate that the diabetic retinopathy seen in those with type 1 diabetes and those with type 2 diabetes is similar. In both cases, it is clear that prolonged exposure to higher blood glucose levels can lead to the development of diabetic retinopathy. Of those who have had diabetes for 15–20 years, nearly all of those with type 1 diabetes and as many as 80% of those with type 2 diabetes will have some retinopathy. It seems likely that the genes involved in the development and, particularly, the progression of retinopathy are the same regardless of whether the underlying cause of the elevated glucose levels is type 1 diabetes or type 2 diabetes.

How Are the Genes for Diabetic Retinopathy Going to Be Found?

As discussed above, one of the major reasons that family members seem to have a similar risk of diabetic retinopathy is that they share genes. Can this information be used for finding the genes responsible? What would finding such genes mean for treating, or even preventing, diabetic retinopathy? This brings us back to the human genome—the complete sequence of the genetic material, DNA, that is found in human cells. The single largest scientific project in biology to date has been the project to determine the complete sequence of human DNA and understand how the DNA is organized. The DNA "alphabet" consists of just four letters, A, T, C, and G. Each stands for one of the key building blocks of DNA. These blocks are organized linearly on our chromosomes. Humans have 22 pairs of chromosomes that are found in both men and women. Women also carry two copies of an additional chromosome called the X chromosome, while men carry one copy of the X chromosome and one copy of another chromosome called the Y chromosome. In total then, each individual has 46 chromosomes that together are made up of approximately 3 billion of the A, T, C, and G building blocks.

DNA is organized into genes

These 3 billion building blocks are known as nucleotides. Several years ago, The Human Genome Project announced that the entire sequence of nucleotides had been decoded. This was the result of a monumental effort that now provides much of the raw information necessary to identify the genes involved in human diseases, including those involved in diabetic retinopathy. The human DNA sequence shows that the DNA building blocks are not randomly ordered; they occur in defined clusters of sequences. We call these sequences genes. It is estimated that there are about 30,000 genes in the human body. These genes act in a coordinated fashion to control the processes of growth and development and to allow the body to carry out its normal functions.

Some genes are responsible for hair color or eye color. One gene, the insulin gene, contains the information required to produce the hormone insulin, which is so critical for normal metabolism and is central to the biology of diabetes. Other genes help signal the body to produce insulin after we eat a meal, and regulate its production so that it is not produced when it should not be. Many genes have a variety of functions, and we know at least some of the functions of many genes. Some of these functions relate to how we process and regulate glucose levels, and others control what happens as diabetic retinopathy progresses. As reviewed in the earlier chapter on diabetic retinopathy (chapter 12), the more advanced stages of retinopathy are marked by the growth of new blood vessels that reflect the body's attempt to correct a worsening situation. This new blood vessel growth is "directed" by several genes. As we also learned, the attempt of our bodies in this regard is noble, but the strategy is flawed, and the growth of new blood vessels in the retina may lead to further threats to vision.

Everyone's genes are not the same

All individuals have the same set of 30,000 genes. We may differ, however, in the exact sequence of these genes. It is these differences that give rise to the incredible variation among individuals. For example, consider the ABO blood group. Some individuals have blood type A, while others have B, O, or AB. The differences in what blood type we have result from subtle changes in the sequence of the DNA building blocks. In the several hundred nucleotides that make up the ABO blood group gene, a simple change in sequence of an A to a T at one location may result in our having a different blood type. Similar sequence differences in many genes occur throughout the genome.

We mentioned earlier that the Human Genome Project had sequenced the human genome. This is true, but not everyone has exactly the same sequence. Between any two individuals there are differences at the DNA level every 300 to 500 nucleotides. This means that any two people differ in their DNA sequences at about 10 million positions. These differences give rise to incredible variation such that no two people (except for identical twins) ever have had, or ever will have, exactly the same DNA sequence. This is what makes us so interesting.

So, how is the human genome helpful?

If we were able to look at all the DNA differences between those with retinopathy and those without, we would have to sort through these tens of millions of differences to determine which 1 or 2 or maybe 50 or even 100 differences are the key ones that alter our risk for developing retinopathy. Until this millennium, the task was impossible and largely unimaginable. Technology has changed and is still changing at such a rate that within just a few years it will be possible to do just that. When combined with appropriate methods of statistical analysis, it will be possible to identify those genes and their different forms that are most involved in determining susceptibility to diabetic retinopathy. With this will come understanding of the key biological steps that lead to the development and progression of retinopathy.

Out of this understanding will surely come new strategies for treatment and screening. When these strategies are coupled with existing methods for controlling blood glucose and treating retinopathy (such as with laser treatments), it is anticipated that the impact of retinopathy will be lessened and the chances of those with retinopathy maintaining full visual function will increase. While it is not yet possible to sort through all of the potential genetic differences among individuals, it is possible to measure some of these differences, and many scientists are trying to find ways to use the information we can collect now.

What has been learned so far?

Much is already known about the development of diabetic retinopathy. The condition usually begins with the loss of key cells from the capillary blood vessels in the retina. These cells are lost through a process of cell death called apoptosis. The formation of new blood vessels in the retina comes later in the development of retinopathy and represents an attempt by the body to repair the damage to the retina that has already occurred. Any genes that are involved in these processes become excellent choices for study in the context of retinopathy. By study, we mean looking at these key genes and determining whether there are differences in them between individuals who have retinopathy and those who do not. Not only do these key genes merit detailed study, but so do any other genes that are closely related to them or that interact with them. Studies are now underway in a number of scientific laboratories looking at well over 100 potentially relevant genes to see whether differences in the sequences of any of these genes predict differences in risk for retinopathy.

While these genes are now being examined in great detail, it is possible that many other genes among the 30,000 or so genes in the human genome may also be important. Scientists have used a number of different approaches to find genes that may affect retinopathy. One recent method has been to survey the entire genome using family members and an approach called linkage analysis. To illustrate the approach, recall the notion that pairs of brothers look alike because they share genes. If they both have brown eyes, then they probably have the same form of the gene involved in determining eye color. We may not know exactly where that gene is, but there are strategies for mapping the genome to locate where its genes might be.

In the case of retinopathy, sibling pairs (brother-brother, brother-sister, or sister-sister pairs) are identified in which both members of the pair have diabetic retinopathy. Because each member of the pair has retinopathy, we can presume that they both are likely to share the same forms of the genes that influence retinopathy risk. There are methods for searching the genome for regions that are more similar in siblings who share a trait than you would expect them to be if genes were not involved in determining that trait. In the case of retinopathy, such unexpectedly similar regions may harbor a gene that affects retinopathy, and the siblings may share the same form of that gene. These types of studies have recently been completed for two different populations, and they identify several regions that could contain retinopathy genes. These regions are now the subject of follow-up studies to see whether some genes previously thought to be involved in retinopathy occur in those regions, or whether previously unsuspected retinopathy genes might be present in them.

How else can genes for retinopathy be found?

The linkage studies described above can be thought of as getting investigators into the "ballpark" where retinopathy genes might occur. This is significant because of the enormous size of the human genome—for some conditions, a single change in just one of the three billion or so building blocks in the genome can produce a devastating disease. Narrowing down the region of the genome to just a few places makes the task more manageable and will greatly speed the discovery process. The challenge, however, is that once you are in a ballpark, you still need to find your section, row, and seat. Again, technology is coming to our rescue, and it is now possible to systematically search for every change that occurs in a "ballpark-size" area of the genome to locate differences that might reveal a disease-causing change. It is now possible to thoroughly examine thousands of sites in any given region of the genome, and newer technologies permit every region of the genome to be examined at least partially.

These types of studies were recently completed for an eye disease called age-related macular degeneration, which is the leading cause of blindness in adults over age 50 in the U.S. These studies identified a specific gene playing a major role in risk for this disease. This gene is now under intense investigation to determine exactly how it alters risk for disease and why certain forms of it make people so prone to macular degeneration. It is expected that this knowledge will lead eventually to better treatments for the disease, and possibly even to prevention.

So, If the Genes for Diabetic Retinopathy Are Found, Then What?

As we use technology to take us into a new realm, we sometimes forget why we wanted to go there in the first place. Identifying those genes and their variant forms that lead to retinopathy will hopefully help us to predict who runs the highest risk for retinopathy. It may also suggest new approaches to prevention or treatment, and may reveal disease pathways that can be targeted by new drugs, or possibly even existing ones. These things may reduce your risk and also the risk that your family members have for developing retinopathy.

Real World Gene Research—Phenylketonuria

A simple example of the power of genetics can be seen the next time you pick up a diet soda sweetened with aspartame. If you read the fine print, you will find a warning to individuals with phenylketonuria (PKU). This is a rare inherited genetic disease that is screened for at birth. If untreated, individuals with PKU will develop a series of problems, including mental retardation and behavioral changes. However, individuals who have PKU can be given a special diet that has low levels of the amino acid phenylalanine, which is a major component of aspartame. With such a diet, individuals with PKU can develop normally. PKU thus represents a case in which a genetic disease can have devastating consequences in one environment (i.e., a diet containing phenylalanine), but little effect in another (i.e., a diet without phenylalanine). A basic understanding of the gene involved with PKU allowed the development of strategies to treat the condition. We have reason to hope that the same will be true for genes involved in retinopathy, many of which may exert their harmful effects mainly in the presence of high glucose levels.

While We Are Waiting for Genetic Answers, What Should You Do in the Meantime?

There is so much that we already know about preventing diabetic retinopathy that it would be a mistake for anyone to suppose that any one gene will determine whether they will develop retinopathy and how rapidly it will progress. There are more than likely multiple genes involved. Many of these genes have not yet been identified, and their roles have not been determined precisely. However, we do know that if you have a blood relative with diabetes who develops more severe diabetic retinopathy, and you have diabetes yourself, you may have a higher risk of developing more severe retinopathy. Furthermore, if you develop more severe diabetic retinopathy, your blood relatives will run a higher risk for the condition.

Even though genes can affect the risk of one's developing diabetic retinopathy, particularly in the case of more severe retinopathy, they do not determine the risk by themselves. Better control of blood glucose over the long term can dramatically reduce your risk of both developing retinopathy and having it progress to a more severe form. Even if we find all the genes involved in diabetic retinopathy, this will not change! Furthermore, retinopathy is a diabetes complication that can be readily detected, categorized, and treated. This is why it is so critical to obtain regular eye examinations. Your eye care professional can see when retinopathy develops and when it begins to progress and can also tell when treatments such as laser therapy are appropriate and will be most effective in preventing loss of vision.

As our understanding of the genetics of diabetic retinopathy increases, our present methods for combating retinopathy will be enhanced. We can look forward to the development of new strategies for controlling blood glucose and reducing the risk not only of retinopathy, but of all the complications of diabetes. This will have a remarkable impact on individuals who have diabetes, on their relatives who have diabetes, and on their family members who may not have diabetes, but who nonetheless share in many ways, with little respite, the challenges and trials that attend life with diabetes.

This chapter was written by Craig L. Hanis, PhD, and D. Michael Hallman, PhD.

14

Nerve Damage:
Legs, Feet, and Arms

Case Study

MJ is 52 years old and has had type 2 diabetes for 10 years. Recently her feet began to burn, and she was diagnosed with painful neuropathy in her feet. Her doctor checked the reflexes at her ankles and knees. He also checked her feet with a tuning fork and a thin item called a monofilament and found that MJ had lost some sensation in her feet. This meant that she was at risk of injuring her foot and not realizing it, which could lead to a foot ulcer.

Introduction

Peripheral neuropathy (nerve damage of the legs, feet, and/or arms) is very common long-term complication of diabetes. It affects as many as 75% of all people with diabetes. The symptoms of neuropathy range from unpleasant to severe. On average, the symptoms occur within 10 years after the onset of diabetes. Unfortunately, for many people with type 2 diabetes, the symptoms of neuropathy may be the first sign of something wrong, even though they have actually had diabetes for many years without knowing it. You may develop painful neuropathy soon after you begin treatment for your diabetes. As your blood glucose levels improve, the pain may go away, but the symptoms may last for as long as 6–18 months. Be patient; improving blood sugar makes your whole body healthier.

Peripheral neuropathy is also called sensorimotor neuropathy. It may affect your feet, legs, hands, or arms, although the feet are usually affected first and more commonly than legs, hands, or arms. It usually happens in both lower limbs at once. Table 14-1 outlines the symptoms that can occur.

Table 14-1. Peripheral Neuropathy and Its Symptoms

Syndrome	Symptoms
Small-fiber damage	• Loss of ability to detect temperature • "Pins and needles," tingling or burning sensation • Pain, usually worse at night • Numbness or loss of feeling • Cold extremities • Swelling of feet
Large-fiber damage	• Abnormal or unusual sensations • Loss of balance • Inability to sense position of toes and feet • Charcot's joint (loss of proper fixation of bones in the feet)
Motor nerve damage	• Loss of muscle tone in hands and feet • Misshapen or deformed toes and feet

What Is Peripheral Neuropathy?

Neuropathy is damage to the nerves. Nerves connect your brain to your spinal cord, your organs, and other parts of your body. This is called your nervous system and has several parts—the central nervous system, the peripheral nervous system, and the autonomic nervous system. The central nervous system is made up of the brain and the spinal cord. The peripheral nervous system is made up of the nerves that go farther out to areas such as your feet and toes. Because most nerve damage from diabetes occurs in the peripheral nervous system, it is called peripheral neuropathy. This type of neuropathy affects the sensory nerves, with damage to the longer nerves first. That is why the symptoms begin in the feet, and sometimes the hands, and move up. It is also called "stocking-glove" syndrome because of where the symptoms occur.

The sensorimotor nervous system includes your sensory and motor nerves. The sensory nerves send information about how things feel, from the skin and internal organs to the brain. The motor nerves send information about movement from the brain to the body. For example, if you step on a sharp tack with your bare foot, the sensory nerves send a message to your brain that you are in pain. The brain then sends a message back to the motor nerves telling your foot to move off the tack.

The autonomic nervous system controls involuntary, or automatic, functions, such as heart rate, digestion, and bladder and sexual functions. For example, the autonomic nervous system tells your heart to speed up when you are running and to slow down when you stop. It helps maintain your blood pressure whether you are standing, sitting, or lying down.

What Causes Peripheral Neuropathy?

Neuropathy can occur from a variety of chronic illnesses such as diabetes or lupus, or from exposure to toxins such as alcohol, heavy metals, or chemotherapy drugs. The causes of neuropathy are not completely known, but in diabetes, it is related to high blood glucose levels over a long period. The Diabetes Control and Complications Trial (DCCT) showed that intensive insulin therapy lowered the risk for neuropathy by 60% for participants in that study, who all had type 1 diabetes. The Japanese (Kumamoto) study and the United Kingdom Prospective Diabetes Study (UKPDS) showed the same beneficial effects for keeping blood glucose close to normal among people with type 2 diabetes. In addition, high blood glucose, decreased insulin output by the pancreas, age, obesity, and duration of diabetes have all been linked to neuropathy. It is probably fair to say that neuropathy is caused not only by elevated blood glucose levels but also by a combination of genetic influences and environmental factors.

How Do High Blood Glucose Levels Cause Nerve Damage?

There are several theories about why neuropathy occurs when blood glucose levels are high for a long period. Unlike most cells in the body, nerve cells don't need insulin to pull in glucose from the bloodstream. Therefore, when blood glucose levels are above normal, the glucose level inside the nerve cells is also high. These high glucose levels may be toxic to the nerves.

One theory suggests that changes in the nerve cells function lead to the creation of molecules called free oxygen radicals. Free oxygen radicals are toxic to cells and cause "oxidative stress" that robs sick nerve cells of oxygen and protein molecules, which the cells need to grow. The result is a kind of cell suicide known as apoptosis. Over time, oxidative stress and apoptosis may lead to neuropathy.

Another theory is based on the decreased blood flow that can occur when small blood vessels are damaged from diabetes. Decreased blood flow to the peripheral nerves may damage them over time.

Still another theory points to glycation (sugar coating) of proteins in the nerve cells. When glucose levels are high, glucose molecules stick to the protein molecules that make up new cells. (This is similar to the way glucose builds up on the red blood cells and is measured with an A1C check.) Proteins with glucose coatings may not function normally.

Autoimmunity has also been suggested as a cause of nerve damage. The damaged nerves may be misread as germs, and the antibodies that the body develops are mistakenly directed toward the nerves.

What Are the Symptoms of Neuropathy?

You can have problems with nerve damage without having any symptoms, so you and your doctor may be unaware that you have the condition. The most common symptoms are pain, tingling, or burning in the feet and legs or numbness of the feet. The symptoms depend on the nerves affected and the extent of the damage. Sometimes, numbness is the only sign. Diabetes can cause damage to the autonomic (see chapter 16), sensory, and motor nerves.

How Is Neuropathy Diagnosed?

Neuropathy can be diagnosed by the symptoms or by simple tests (called "signs"). At least once a year, ask your health care provider to test your reflexes and to check your bare feet for their ability to sense heat and cold, vibrations with a tuning fork, and a light touch with a monofilament (plastic line; like a fishing line).

Why Is Neuropathy So Serious?

When sensory nerves are damaged, you may not be able to feel items, objects, heat, cold, or pain. Because there is no pain, you may continue to walk on an injured foot. This can result in an ulcer, which can become infected, leading to gangrene and amputation. Because there is loss of feeling, you need to check your feet every day or have a family member do it for you; this is the best way to find an injury so that it can be treated before it becomes more serious. Ask your provider or nurse educator to show you any places on your feet to which you need to pay special attention, what to look for when you inspect your feet, and how to care for them, including moisture, nail cutting, proper shoes, callus care, etc. If you need help, do not be embarrassed to say so.

Nerves are made up of both small and large fibers. If the small fibers of the nerves are affected, you may have pain and be unable to detect heat and cold, which will increase your risk for burns or frostbite. If large fibers are affected, you lose the ability to sense the position of your feet or to feel a light touch.

If the pain that results from sensorimotor neuropathy lasts for less than 6 months, it is considered acute (recent). Pain that lasts longer than 6 months is considered chronic (long-term). With chronic painful neuropathy, the pain may eventually disappear, and your feet and hands will feel numb or always cold as the nerves become more damaged.

With large-fiber damage, your senses of balance and position may be impaired, which increases your risk for falls. Some people describe this as "not being able to feel where my feet are when I walk." Walking in the dark is especially difficult and risky. Light touch may be involved as well, making it less likely to detect objects and result in mechanical damage to your foot.

When motor nerves are damaged, the muscles in the feet can become weak and eventually atrophy (degenerate). This results in the development of foot and toe deformities, such as hammertoes and claw toes. (See chapter 15.)

What if Your Only Symptom Is Numbness?

Actually, feet that feel numb are more common than painful feet. If you are unable to feel a tuning fork that is vibrating on your toe or a line (monofilament) pressing on the fleshy part of your foot, you have an insensate foot, like MJ in the case study. If you have any foot deformity, you can protect your feet with custom-made orthotics or shoes. These may even save your feet. See chapter 15 for information on shoes and foot care.

What Is the Treatment for Neuropathy?

The treatment for peripheral neuropathy is based on the symptoms you have. There is no cure for neuropathy, so the treatment is mostly aimed at relieving the pain and protecting your feet and hands to prevent injuries. Lowering blood glucose levels as near normal as possible may decrease pain or other symptoms. Other things you can do to care for neuropathy are listed in Table 14-2.

Although people used to be told that the pain was something that they had to live with, there are now medicines that can be used to relieve pain and other symptoms. Vitamins alone usually aren't effective to treat neuropathy caused by diabetes. Pain-relieving medicines that contain narcotics are generally not recommended because of side effects and the risk for addiction. Medicines that your provider may prescribe include medications specifically for the

Table 14-2. Self-Care Practices for Peripheral Neuropathy

- Keep your blood sugar levels as close to normal as is safe for you.

- Protect your feet. You need to do what your nerves used to do for you.

- Give therapies a fair trial before you decide whether they are working. Some medicines take time before they begin to work.

- Talk to your provider about any natural, herbal, or other remedies you are using or hear about. Some may work, but others may actually be harmful.

- Stop cigarette smoking. Ask your provider about smoking-cessation programs or prescription medicines that can help you quit. Nicotine delivery systems (patches, gum) are available without a prescription and may also help.

- Avoid alcohol, because it can increase nerve damage. Ask your provider about programs that can help if you believe alcohol is a problem for you.

- Keep informed and up to date. Take diabetes-education classes to learn the best and latest techniques for protecting your health. Neuropathy is an area of ongoing research. Ask your provider periodically whether there are new medicines or other therapies available. If you are interested in participating in studies of new medications, call the ADA at 1-800-DIABETES, look up diabetes or diabetic neuropathy on the Internet, or contact the diabetes program offered at large medical centers in your area and ask whether there are any studies available.

treatment of painful neuropathy (duloxetine and pregabalin), low doses of antiepileptic agents, and antidepressants. The antiepileptic agents and antidepressants work by interrupting pain transmission. Medicines that can be used for neuropathy are listed in Table 14-3.

Many of these medicines take time to work, so you need to give them a fair trial (4–6 weeks) before you decide whether they are effective. In addition, you may need more than one of these medicines to relieve your symptoms. Like all medicines, they may cause side effects. Most of the time, you will start on a low dose and slowly increase the dose based on relief of your symptoms and any side effects. Common side effects include sleepiness, dry mouth, constipation, nausea, memory problems, and dizziness. Taking your dose at bedtime may help. Tell your provider about these or any

Table 14-3. Medications for Peripheral Neuropathy
(some are used as "off-label" in the treatment of painful diabetic neuropathy)

Antidepressants	Antiepileptic drugs
Duloxetine (Cymbalta)*	Pregabalin (Lyrica)*
Amitriptyline (Elavil, Vanatrip)	Gabapentin (Neurontin)
Nortriptyline (Aventyl, Pamelor)	Carbamazepine (Carbatrol, Epitol,
Desipramine (Tofranil)	Tegretol)
Paroxetine (Paxil)	
Trazadone (Desyrel)	

*approved by the FDA for use in the treatment of painful diabetic neuropathy

other side effects. Your dose may need to be adjusted. You may also find it helpful to see a neurologist.

Therapies used in place of, or along with, medications can also be helpful. Walking or gentle stretching, relaxation exercises, biofeedback, and hypnosis may help relieve your pain. Not drinking alcohol and quitting smoking may help relieve symptoms. Elastic body stockings (available at dance or exercise stores), pantyhose, or foot cradles can help keep clothes and bedcovers away from your sensitive skin. Lamb's wool padding and specially made shoes or orthotic devices can help protect misshapen feet.

Transcutaneous nerve stimulation (TENS) units are battery-operated devices that are about the size of a portable radio. TENS units provide small electrical impulses that block the pain message from getting to your brain. These devices are available only by prescription. There are also clinics in larger medical centers that specialize in pain relief. Ask your provider for a referral if you believe this would be helpful to you. Talk to your physician or nurse educator about any pain remedies you read about in newspapers or magazines; many of these are expensive but not very effective.

Are There Treatments for the Pain of Neuropathy?

Try simple maneuvers first. Painful neuropathy can actually be brought on when you begin to improve your blood glucose levels;

but it usually goes away as you maintain near-normal blood glucose levels. It may take as long as 6–18 months.

Antidepressants

Several studies have shown that tricyclic antidepressants given along with the antiepileptic drugs work for treating painful neuropathy. Duloxetine (Cymbalta) is the medication in this class that is approved for use in painful neuropathy.

Antiepileptics

Pregabalin (Lyrica) is an antiepileptic drug that is approved for treating painful neuropathy. Gabapentin (Neurontin) and other drugs in this class can also be effective.

Lidocaine patches and oral mexiletine

Some people get relief by applying lidocaine patches or cream to the affected areas. Lidocaine is in the same class of drugs as the novocaine your dentist uses. Lidocaine given by slow infusion has provided relief of pain for 3–21 days. This form of therapy may be most useful in self-limited forms of neuropathy. If successful, therapy can be continued with oral mexiletine. These compounds target pain caused by sensitivity of nerve endings near the surface of the skin.

Transcutaneous nerve stimulation

TENS may occasionally be helpful and certainly represents one of the more benign therapies for painful neuropathy. Move the electrodes around to identify sensitive areas and obtain the most relief.

Analgesics

These are rarely of much benefit in the treatment of painful neuropathy, although they may be of some use on a short-term basis.

Biofeedback, exercise, and support

Biofeedback programs, yoga, and exercises such as swimming or stationary bike riding have been shown to help neuropathy. Exercise releases endorphins—which are natural pain relievers—and lowers blood glucose levels. A support team is also an invaluable resource. Find a knowledgeable health care team, which may include

- physicians who are experts in diabetes, endocrinology, and/or neurology,
- nurse educators,
- a dietitian,
- or a psychologist or social worker.

Be sure to let them know if your pain is interfering with your ability to work to take part in activities you usually enjoy, or causing you to feel down or depressed much of the time. Support groups and educational programs are often helpful. There is help available now and hope for the future as research seeks and finds new therapies.

This chapter was written by Aaron Vinik, MD, PhD, FCP, FACP; Martha M. Funnell, MS, RN, CDE; Douglas A. Greene, MD; Eva L. Feldman, MD, PhD; and Martin J. Stevens, MD.

15

Foot Care

Case Study

TJ is 62 years old and has had type 2 diabetes for 10 years. TJ went walking on the beach with his grandchildren and cut his foot on a seashell. He did not feel the cut, nor the ulcer (sore) that developed. By the time he noticed redness and swelling, he had walked on it for weeks, and now it is infected. His doctor has tried dressings and antibiotics, but the ulcer is not healing, even though TJ still has good circulation in his feet. The doctor is afraid the front of his foot will have to be amputated.

Introduction

The foot is a marvelously intricate biomechanical structure composed of 26 bones, 23 joints, and 42 muscles and tendons. When these structures work together normally, your feet feel great. However, when they don't, serious problems can develop.

Foot problems are one of the leading causes of hospitalization for people with diabetes. The good news is that you can prevent most ulcers (and amputations) with daily foot inspections, regular visits to your doctor and podiatrist, wearing proper shoes, and finding problems early. Ovid, the Greek playwright and poet, once wrote, "Stop it at the start, it's late for medicine to be prepared when disease has grown strong through long delays." The "stop it at the start" philosophy is as practical today as it was in Ovid's time, some two thousand years ago.

Is There One Cause for the Foot Problems that Lead to Amputations?

Actually there are four:

1) nerve damage or neuropathy (loss of feeling)
2) poor circulation
3) difficulty fighting infection
4) foot deformity

Add any injury to your "high-risk foot," and you may develop an ulcer that is difficult to heal (Table 15-1).

Table 15-1. Risk Factors for Diabetic Foot Ulcers

Within the Body Factors	Outside Factors
• Neuropathy	• Minor injury
- Loss of feeling	- High plantar pressures: callus buildup
- Muscle weakness	- Shoe pressure: blisters
• Vascular disease	- Injury: cuts, lacerations, etc.
- Poor circulation	• Thermal injury
- Difficulty healing	- Burns from hot soaks, scalds, etc.
• Poor response to infection	- Frostbite
• Foot deformity	• Chemical burns: "corn cures"
• Previous ulcer	• Bathroom surgery on ingrown toenails, calluses, etc.
	• Poor knowledge of diabetes
	• Cigarette smoking

Neuropathy

Nerve damage causes a loss of feeling in feet and legs. You may have numbness or tingling and not be able to feel where your feet are. We rely on pain to protect us from injury. If you buy a pair of new shoes and they rub a blister on your foot, you will stop wearing those shoes. If you can't feel the pain of the blister, you will keep on wearing them and do a lot of damage to your foot.

Neuropathy affects the nerves to the muscles in your feet and causes weakness of those muscles, which can lead to the development of hammertoes, bunions, or other deformities. When we walk, there is pressure on the bottom of our feet. With neuropathy, the bones on the bottom of the forefoot may shift position and increase the pressures on the skin beneath them, but you can't feel it. Continuing to walk on high-pressure points breaks down the skin and causes ulcers.

Poor circulation

People with diabetes often have circulation problems in their feet due to blockage of arteries (arteriosclerosis). Your feet may turn bright red when hanging down and constantly feel cold. Also, the skin may become shiny, thin, and easily damaged, and hair growth may be reduced. Reduced blood flow means your feet don't get enough oxygen or nutrients. When the foot is injured, infected, or ulcerated, healing will be slow or may not happen at all.

Infection

People with diabetes are more likely to have infections, because their immune systems do not fight off infections well. Infections can rapidly worsen and go undetected, especially with nerve damage or poor circulation. The only sign of a developing infection may be unexplained high blood glucose levels.

If you have had a long-lasting (chronic) foot ulcer for several months and suddenly develop a fever and flu-like symptoms, it may not be the flu; it may be spreading of the infection. Such infections must be treated with hospitalization and antibiotics to avoid death of the skin, muscles, and even bone (gangrene). In fact, delaying treatment can make an amputation necessary.

Foot deformities

Foot deformities such as hammertoes and bunions are common for everyone, but they cause more problems for people with diabetes (Figures 15-1 and 15-2). These deformities can cause corns, calluses, blisters, and ulcers when wearing an ill-fitting shoe, a shoe with little support, or no shoes at all. A deformed foot may require a specially molded shoe and/or insert. As Dr. Paul Brand said, "When a person with diabetes complains that his shoes are killing him, he may very well be correct."

What Are Some Common Foot Deformities?

Hammertoe and claw toe

A hammertoe (Figure 15-1) is a buckling of the toe knuckle closest to the ball of the foot, making it look like a swan's neck. A hammertoe of the second toe often occurs with a bunion. If you have diabetic neuropathy, hammertoes are often caused by weak muscles. Claw toes are similar to hammertoes, but with buckling of both toe knuckles (Figure 15-1). Claw toes usually affect those with high

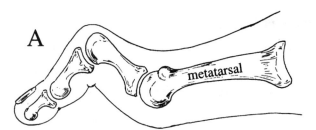

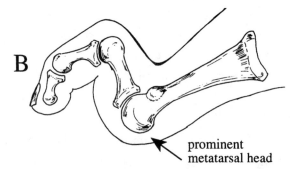

Figure 15-1. A. Hammertoe. B. Claw toe.
Reproduced with permission from Kelikian H: Deformities of the Lesser Toes, in Kelikian H, editor: *Hallux Valgus, Allied Deformities of the Forefoot and Metatarsalgia.* W. B. Saunders, 1965.

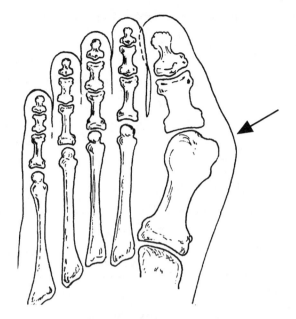

Figure 15-2. A bunion is a significant bone deformity.
Reproduced with permission from Kelikian H: Deformities of the Lesser Toes, in Kelikian H, editor: *Hallux Valgus, Allied Deformities of the Forefoot and Metatarsalgia.* W. B. Saunders, 1965.

arches in their foot, but not always. When the toe knuckles curl into hammertoes or claw toes, they end up sitting on the top of the bones just behind the toes (metatarsal heads) and pushing down. This leads to more pressure at the ball of the foot, which may lead to calluses or ulcers. The increased pressure at the tips and tops of the toes may also lead to calluses or ulcers of the toes.

The metatarsals are the five long bones in the middle of the foot, just behind the toes. The metatarsal heads, which are similar to knuckles in the hand, are located in the ball of the foot and support the body's weight. Normally, these bones share weight evenly. However, if one metatarsal bone is longer or lower than its neighbors, it carries too much weight. When you step on it, the high pressure on this point can cause pain, calluses, ulcers, and sometimes fractures.

Bunions

A bunion is an enlarged bump at the big toe joint. Bunions are most often an inherited characteristic. The big toe angles toward the second toe and may underlap or override the second toe, causing a hammertoe (Figure 15-2). When the foot is forced into a tight shoe, there is pressure over the bunion, which can result in an ulcer. Arthritis may be associated with bunions, leading to pain and stiffness of the joint. Restricted motion in the joint can cause a callus or ulcer beneath the big toe.

Charcot's foot

Charcot's (shar-kos) foot is not a common deformity, but it is very serious. Most people with this deformity go to their doctor because their foot is red and swollen and their shoes won't fit. This redness and swelling is actually caused by severe fractures and dislocations of joints and bones in the foot and ankle (Figure 15-3). When the middle of the foot collapses, it causes a rocker-bottom shape to the foot and increased pressure on the bottom of the foot. This often results in ulcers. The foot can become so deformed that walking is difficult. Special footwear is very important for this condition.

People at high risk for Charcot's foot generally have had diabetes for more than 10 years, have loss of feeling in their feet, and are in their 50s or 60s. People who have complications affecting eyes, kidneys, and nerves appear to be at greatest risk. Injury to the foot can put you at risk, as does smoking, living alone, and not taking good care of your feet.

To treat Charcot's foot you'll need to stop putting weight on the foot. This can be done by bed rest or with a special cast. If you walk on it, you may cause more fractures and deformity.

What Are the Symptoms of Foot Problems?

If you have these warning signs, get prompt treatment:

- Redness, swelling, or increased skin temperature of the foot or ankle
- A change in the size or shape of the foot or ankle
- Pain in the legs at rest or while walking

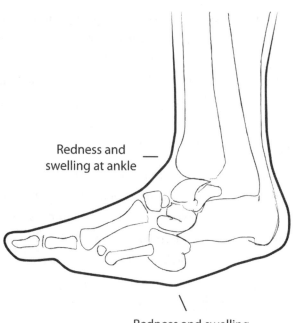

Redness and swelling at ankle

Redness and swelling

Figure 15-3. Charcot's Foot.

- Open sores with or without drainage, no matter how small (ulcers)
- Nonhealing wounds/sores
- Corns or calluses with skin discoloration

Are There Treatments for Foot Deformities?

If you have foot deformities or a loss of feeling, you may need therapeutic footwear (shoes, socks, and shoe inserts). All three can work together to prevent ulcers. There are many types of shoes, socks, and inserts available. Your foot-care specialist can help you choose what is correct for you. In some cases, especially when sores keep coming back, surgery might be an option.

How Do Foot Deformities Cause Ulcers?

It isn't just that your shoes don't fit right. It's more a matter of your bones not being where they're supposed to be. Deformities of the foot and ankle cause increased pressure and irritation of the skin over the bumps and bony areas, causing damage that can lead to ulcers and infection. Your earliest symptoms may be a slight reddening (irritation) or thickening of the skin (corn or callus) beneath the ball of your foot or on your toes. You stress these areas every time you walk, and this may cause open sores and fractures.

What Is an Ulcer?

An ulcer is usually a painless, open sore on the bottom of the foot or top of a toe. It results from pressure from your shoes, a corn or callus that has grown too thick, or an injury such as a splinter or glass. Continued walking on the injury or callus creates even further damage. The open sore frequently becomes infected and may even penetrate to the bone, even though you can only see a small sore on the surface of the skin.

How Can Ulcers Be Treated?

Find it early, see your doctor immediately, and don't walk on it. Your doctor will clean the wound and apply dressings, and may give you antibiotics. All the dead tissue in an ulcer must be removed (debrided), so it will heal. A specimen may be taken from the ulcer to check for bacteria. X-rays may help to determine whether there is a foreign body in your foot, infection in the bone (osteomyelitis), or any gas (air bubbles) or air deep in the tissues (which suggests infection). Sometimes, you need an examination using magnetic resonance imaging (MRI).

Proper wound care is important. There are many treatments for wounds, including saline, healing gels, ointments, and topical disinfectants or antibiotics. There are also many types of dressings to cover your wound, and different ones may be used at different points in the healing process. New products for wound healing include platelet-derived growth factors and tissue-engineered skin substitutes. They are not appropriate for all wounds, but they may help you to heal better than standard saline dressings alone. Both deliver growth factors and live cells to your ulcer to speed up the healing.

Controlling your blood glucose is important because high blood glucose interferes with your white blood cells' ability to fight infection. Signs of the infection getting worse are increased redness around the ulcer or red streaks going up your leg. If you notice increased drainage and the foot has a bad odor, call your physician at once. If you develop pain, or if the foot with an ulcer on the bottom gets red and puffy on the top, call your physician. These are signs of spreading infection. Do not soak your foot.

Most importantly, stay off the foot to avoid further pressure, and do not wear the shoes that might have caused the ulcer. You may use crutches, a wheelchair, or bed rest. Special casts, braces, healing sandals, shoe inserts, or padding may also protect the foot while it heals.

How Can You Get Around While the Ulcer Heals?

The best device for relieving pressure on an ulcer is a below-the-knee total-contact cast or a non-weight-bearing removable cast. Studies have shown that a total-contact cast will heal 90–95% of wounds in an average of 6 weeks. A professional applies the cast, taking care to protect the skin from further injury. The cast protects the wound from the high pressures that caused it. It immobilizes the foot and helps control swelling, and it limits the amount of walking you can do. The cast is fairly heavy, may be hot, and cannot be removed for bathing. It is usually changed every 1–2 weeks. Your other option, a "clam shell" non-weight-bearing cast, can be removed at night and for bathing. However, it is expensive and cannot be adjusted to fit as the swelling goes down.

You might use a walker boot, which has a padded insert and padded uprights to protect the foot from high pressures. The soft insert spreads the pressures over a greater area of the foot. The walker boot can be removed to inspect the wound and for bathing. However, if you take the boot off and do any walking, even in the middle of the night to go to the bathroom, you can undo days of healing.

It is not as heavy as a cast and is easier to put on and take off than a cast, but it may not be as effective in healing an ulcer.

Another choice is a half-shoe. It is lighter than a cast or boot, but it does relieve the pressure on the front part of the foot by forcing weight bearing onto the heel. The sole of the shoe ends before the forefoot, which can make walking difficult. You may need a cane or walker for balance. Healing time is not as fast as with a cast, but it's better than if you wore only therapeutic footwear or no shoes at all.

Should You Use a Cane or Walker When You Have an Ulcer?

A cane, crutches, or a walker can help unload pressure from the foot even further when you use them with casts, boots, or shoes. Any pressure taken by the arms is weight that doesn't have to go through the feet. Use them if you feel more stable; don't if you don't. It's up to you and your doctor.

What Shoes Should You Wear After the Ulcer Is Healed?

After your wound is healed, your foot has a good chance of developing another ulcer. You need to check your feet very carefully every day. Even though the ulcer has healed on the surface, you will wear a walker boot or protective shoe for several weeks or months as the skin gets stronger. Your doctor will refer you to a pedorthist (a person specializing in shoes and inserts) for special shoes to protect your feet.

Why Don't Some Ulcers Heal?

Ulcers can take months to heal. During this time, try to keep your diabetes in good control to encourage healing. When ulcers are slow to heal, or get worse, you have to consider the possible causes. First, some people don't stay off the foot. If walking or weight bearing is the cause of the ulcer, it makes sense that continued walking will prevent it from healing. (You do not cure tennis elbow by continuing to play tennis!) Denial is common, because people with neuropathy can't feel pain. If it doesn't hurt, it is easy to ignore. Walking continues (without a limp since there is no pain), the pressure continues, and the ulcer cannot heal. Also, many people can't take time off from their jobs to heal. Wheelchairs, crutches, or casts can help.

A second reason the ulcer won't heal can be poor circulation, which prevents the blood from delivering nutrients, oxygen, and antibiotics to the ulcer. Without adequate blood flow to the foot, the ulcer will not heal. Your physician can check the blood pressures at your ankles and arms. It should be the same, and if it is not, you may have blocked arteries and will need more tests to determine your situation. When significant blockages exist, you may be referred to a vascular surgeon. Bypass operations in the legs and the feet or other less invasive procedures can restore circulation and promote healing of ulcers (chapter 6).

Deep-seated infection is the third major reason many foot ulcers do not heal. Long-standing (chronic) infections often have no symptoms. Constant draining or a discharge from the ulcer may be a sign of an underlying infection. Wound specimens are taken periodically to check the bacterial growth in the ulcer and to determine which, if any, of the bacteria need to be treated with antibiotics. Keep in mind, however, that sometimes the cultures taken by swabbing may not show the bacteria that are actually causing the infection. Antibiotic treatment based on the incorrect culture results may not help. Tissue taken from the ulcer or a punch biopsy may be sent for analysis instead. If a probe can actually touch bone through the bottom of the ulcer, it strongly suggests bone infection (osteomyelitis) that will require more aggressive treatment. Periodic X-rays will show any bone infection changes. If you have a long-standing ulcer that suddenly gets worse, with fever and elevated blood glucose levels, you need immediate hospitalization.

How Can You Prevent an Ulcer from Developing?

Like with any health problem, you'd rather prevent foot ulcers than treat them. Develop good habits and continue them for your lifetime. Use the "5 Ps" of prevention—professional care, protective footwear, pressure reduction, preventive surgery, and preventive education (Table 15-2).

Table 15-2. The 5 Ps of Prevention

1. Professional care
- Regular visits, examinations, and foot care
- Early detection and aggressive treatment of new ulcers

2. Protective shoes
- Adequate room to protect from injury, well cushioned
- Walking shoes, extra-depth or custom-molded shoes

3. Pressure reduction
- Cushioned insoles, custom orthotics, padded socks
- Pressure measurements, computerized or mat

4. Preventive surgery
- Correct hammertoes, bunions, Charcot's foot, etc.
- Prevent ulcers over or under deformities from reappearing

5. Preventive education
- Patient education: need for daily inspection and early treatment
- Physician education: significance of foot ulcers, importance of regular foot examinations, and current diabetic foot management

---

Professional care

You need regular examinations by a health care professional familiar with diabetic foot care. For example, your diabetes doctor can examine your feet and check for neuropathy, circulation problems, and potential trouble spots. A podiatrist can also check your feet and trim toenails and calluses before they become problems. Studies have shown that such regular care—at least several times each year—is important in preventing foot problems, especially if you have neuropathy.

Protective footwear

Many of the minor injuries leading to foot ulcers are caused by poorly fitting shoes. A professional should assist you in selecting and fitting shoes for the shape of your foot and any deformity you have. Walking or athletic shoes are good for most everyone; but studies have shown that people with a healed ulcer who wore specially designed shoes (with extra depth for the toes and cushioned soles) were much less likely to get another ulcer than were people who continued to wear their regular shoes.

Pressure reduction

You can relieve pressure on the soles of your feet by wearing cushioned shoes, padded socks, and insoles. The most common sign of higher-than-normal pressures on the foot is a callus, which is the skin's normal response to excessive pressure. If you reduce the pressure on this part of the foot, you can reduce the size of the callus and possibly prevent an ulcer from developing under it. Most ulcers occur where there is a callus. If the callus comes back after the ulcer heals, there is a strong likelihood the ulcer will come back, too.

High pressures can be measured by footprint analysis using pressure-sensitive mats or by computerized gait-analysis systems. Potential problem areas or "hot spots" can be detected and treated with inserts for your shoes. In-shoe pressure measurements are useful for seeing how well the insoles work.

Preventive surgery

Occasionally, foot surgery can stop ulcers by correcting a deformity in the foot that would eventually cause an ulcer. Reconstructive surgery is often necessary to heal chronic ulcers that don't respond to other treatments. This does not mean that you need a routine correction of any hammertoe or foot deformity. Most are best managed by special shoes and pressure-reduction therapies. The decision to have surgery must be a joint one made by you, your family, your primary physician, and the surgeon. Avoid unnecessary surgery at all costs. This surgery is done only in people with healthy arteries and requires good post-operative care to be successful.

Preventive education

Many foot ulcers are caused by poor self care or neglect. You need to know what to do. That is why foot-care education from your diabetes educator, nurse specialist, physician, or podiatrist is so valuable. Foot care is seldom accomplished by one health care provider. You usually will have a team, depending on the condition of your feet. Nothing is more important than keeping your feet clean and dry and inspecting them every day. Remove both shoes and socks at every doctor's appointment. Take part in diabetic foot-care courses, and learn to recognize warning signs. That's how you reduce your risk for foot ulcers.

Who Should See Your Feet?

Foot problems may require care from your primary care physician, an endocrinologist or diabetologist, a podiatrist, an orthopedic surgeon, a plastic surgeon, a vascular surgeon, a diabetes educator, a wound-care specialist, or a rehabilitation specialist experienced in the management of people with diabetes. These team members should communicate with each other about your condition and treatment.

What Type of Shoes Should You Wear?

You can buy shoes off the shelf or have them custom made, but in any case, the shoes are meant to protect your feet, not to hurt them. Shoes made of leather easily adapt to the shape of your feet and allow your feet to breathe. Athletic shoes, jogging shoes, and sneakers are excellent choices—as long as they fit well and provide adequate cushioning.

If you can, change your shoes several times a day so that one pair is not worn for more than 4–6 hours. Only wear new shoes a few hours at a time, and then inspect your feet for redness or irritation.

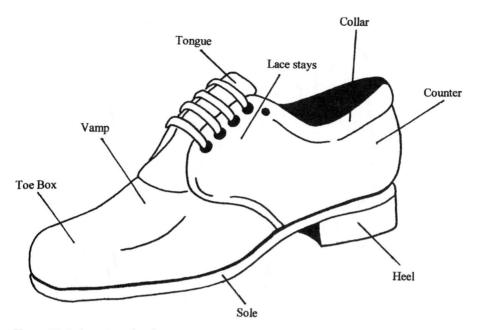

Figure 15-4. Anatomy of a shoe.

Above all, do not walk barefooted indoors or outdoors. Discuss wearing open-toed shoes or sandals with your podiatrist or physician. At the beach or pool, wear water shoes, especially if you have lost feeling in your feet.

What Features Should You Look for in a Shoe?

Make sure the shoes are the kind called "in-depth" or "extra-depth" shoes. In-depth shoes have 1/4–1/2 inch more room from top to bottom in the toe box (area where toes sit) than a regular shoe (Figure 15-4). They usually also have a removable insole that can be taken out for more room, or to make room for a special shoe insert. These shoes are great for accommodating foot deformities or shoe inserts. They can also help prevent deformities, such as hammertoes and bunions.

Steer clear of slip-on shoes, which are generally too tight and often too short. They are designed this way because if they truly fit the shape of your foot, they'd keep falling off. Shoes that tie or have

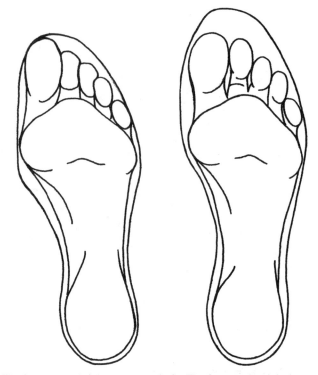

Figure 15-5. The foot on the left is not properly fit. The foot on the right is.

velcro are best. You can loosen them as the day goes on, especially if your feet and ankles swell. Shoes that tie put less pressure on your forefoot and can prevent the development of blisters or calluses.

Look for shoes that come in a variety of widths—narrow, medium, wide, and extra wide. Some shoe manufacturers use letters: "A" means narrow and "E" means wide.

All feet are shaped differently, as are all shoes. The important thing is to get a good match. It's best to find a shoe that resembles the shape of your foot. Try to avoid shoes that have pointed toes, which cramp your toes and bend them into unnatural positions. A shoe with a broad, rounded toe is best (Figure 15-5).

High heels are another thing to avoid. The higher the heel, the more pressure there is on the ball of the foot and toes. High heels are especially bad when they are combined with a pointed toe box, as in cowboy boots and women's shoes.

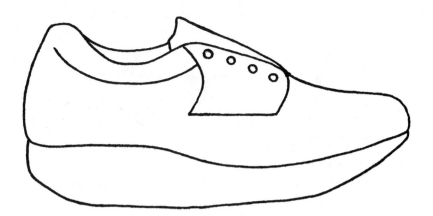

Figure 15-6. Rocker sole shoe.

The soles of your shoes are important to consider. Thick, cushioned wedge soles are appropriate for most people. A wedge sole is flat along the entire bottom of the shoe, with no separate heel. Dense foam rubber soles offer more cushioning than leather soles do. Shoes with built-in rocker soles decrease the pressures under the ball of the foot, helping to prevent ulcers. You can have rocker soles put on most any shoe if you need them (Figure 15-6).

How Do You Know if Your Shoes Fit?

Shoes must always fit comfortably, with adequate length, width, and depth for your toes. If a shoe is hard to put on, don't wear it. It may be too small and cause serious damage, especially if you have neuropathy or poor circulation. Don't "break in" new shoes: If they don't fit when you try them on in the store, don't buy them.

- Have your feet sized every time you buy shoes. Your feet tend to get longer and wider as you grow older. You might be surprised to find what your size is now. And have both feet sized—one may be longer than the other.
- Have your feet measured at the end of the day. Feet often swell during the day, and you want to buy shoes that will fit all day long.

- Keep in mind that sizes vary among different shoe brands and styles. Judge the shoe by how it fits, not by the size marked in the shoe.
- Once the shoes are on, there should be 3/8–1/2 inch of space beyond your longest toe while you're standing; at the same time, the ball of your foot should fit well into the widest part of the shoe. Always try on shoes with the socks you will wear with them.
- Walk in the shoes to make sure they fit well. The heels should not slip very much.

A qualified shoe fitter measures your feet with a special device to get the length from heel to toe, from heel to ball, and width. It is important to be sure that your shoes are not too tight, causing pressure, nor too loose, causing shear.

You should be able to pinch some leather between your fingers across the top of the shoe, or vamp. Properly fitting shoes will tend to slip a little in the heel. No slippage indicates that the shoe is too short. If you have shoe inserts, try them on with your new shoes. They will change the fit.

Will the Shoes Be Ugly?

Most therapeutic shoes nowadays don't look like the orthopedic shoes of the past. They can be walking or running shoes, work boots, or hiking boots. You can even get dress shoes. (The policy for wearing dress shoes, however, is like the one for dessert—not very much and not very often.) The shoes can be very attractive. In fact, unless your feet have severe deformities requiring custom shoes, no one will even know that you are wearing special shoes.

What Kind of Socks Should You Wear?

White socks are preferred so you can see blood or drainage, for example, from a blister. Look for socks made of materials that wick moisture away from the skin, such as CoolMAX or Duraspun. These socks, made of acrylic fibers, are bulkier and provide more cushioning and less friction. There are socks for people with diabetes that don't have seams, wick moisture away, and have special cushioning under the ball of the foot and the heel.

What Will Shoe Inserts Do for Your Feet?

Shoe inserts (also called orthotics or arch supports) cushion and protect your feet. They off-load high pressure in specific areas on the bottoms of your feet by distributing your weight equally over the entire soles of your feet. They are also used to correct the position of your feet or to provide pain relief.

How Do You Obtain Shoe Inserts?

Your physician refers you to a specialist to make molds of your feet for the inserts. A podiatrist or certified pedorthist are the most qualified persons to make foot orthotics. Your doctor may refer you to a certified orthotist, who has had special training in providing braces and supports for the entire body, including the feet. In any case, you will need a prescription. If you have lost feeling in your feet, have diabetes, and have a foot deformity or have had a foot ulcer, Medicare and many health insurance companies will pay for up to 80% of custom footwear.

What Are the Types of Shoe Inserts?

Some inserts are made of soft, lightweight foam. They don't last long, but they offer the best cushioning. They are often bulky, and some people need a larger shoe to use them. Weight-distributing inserts commonly have a soft foam layer on top (next to your foot) and a firmer material, such as cork, underneath. This type of insert offers you cushioning and protection while equalizing pressures on the bottoms of your feet. Sometimes a shock-absorbing material is included. These are full-length inserts. This type of insert routinely wears out after a year or two, but it should be checked by your foot care specialist every six months or so.

A functional shoe insert is made of a thin, rigid plastic that runs from heel to the ball of your foot. If your health care team asks for it, a soft topcover can be applied. The plastic base of this insert lasts for years, but the topcover will need to be replaced periodically.

It's rare, but sometimes, an over-the-counter shoe insert works. Custom-made devices can be costly, and some insurance plans do not pay for them, so an over-the-counter device can be a lower-cost alternative. However, you must have no deformities or nerve damage. And you may need them to be customized for you.

Where Can You Buy Therapeutic Shoes?

Specialty shoe stores or comfort shoe stores are better equipped to help you than a large discount shoe store or a department store. Some stores specialize in walking shoes and therapeutic shoes and may have a certified pedorthist on staff. Certified pedorthists are trained in foot anatomy and the construction of shoes, shoe modifications, and foot orthotics (inserts). Like a pharmacist, a pedorthist fills the prescription for therapeutic shoes that was written for you. Check out the store thoroughly, because this is likely to be a long-term relationship. There may also be pedorthic facilities near you. They have pedorthists on staff and stock a more specialized inventory of shoes.

About 85% of people can be fitted with off-the-shelf shoes. Off-the-shelf shoes may need some adjustment to fit your needs. The uppers may need to be stretched for prominent toes, wedges and flares can be added to the soles for better stability, and rocker soles or metatarsal bars can be added to reduce pressure on certain areas of the foot. Shoes with laces can be converted to Velcro closure if needed. Lifts are added to the inside or outside of the shoes if your legs are different lengths. If your feet can't fit into standard footwear, the pedorthist can fit you for custom-made shoes. These take 3–6 weeks to make.

What Sort of Follow-Up Do You Have with Special Shoes?

Your shoes and shoe inserts should be checked by your foot care specialist every 6 months. When you get shoes and inserts, your practitioner will tell you how long it will take to break them in. There will be a few scheduled follow-up appointments during the first month or two, but then you are on your own. Most facilities send you a reminder about setting up a visit every 6 months, but it is your responsibility to make sure your shoes and inserts are working properly. If you develop any red spots, blisters, calluses or other pain, make an appointment to see your health care team, pedorthist, or orthotist immediately.

Will Your Insurance Pay for Therapeutic Shoes?

In 1995, legislation called the Therapeutic Shoe Bill (TSB) was passed. The TSB provides a special exception for people with diabetes to get coverage for their shoes and inserts, because Medicare does not normally pay for shoes and/or inserts. There are several points that you will need to know regarding the TSB.

Only people with diabetes are eligible for the benefits under the TSB. You also need to have another qualifying complication, such as an ulcer or a thick callus, a history of ulcers, deformity in your feet, loss of feeling, or poor circulation. The physician managing your diabetes must certify that you have diabetes and have foot complications. There is a standard form for your physician to fill out before you can get your shoes and inserts, and a prescription is required as well.

A facility that is either a registered Medicare provider or a registered Medicare supplier must be used. A Medicare provider performs the service and then bills Medicare directly. A Medicare supplier has you pay up front, and then submits a claim to Medicare, so you are reimbursed for the amount that Medicare allows for the services provided.

The TSB covers in-depth shoes and shoe inserts. The shoes can be either off-the-shelf or custom made, but the inserts must be specifically designed for your feet, not just ones purchased over-the-counter.

One pair of shoes per calendar year and up to three pairs of inserts are covered. Modifications to shoes, such as rocker soles, can be substituted for inserts. Medicare covers 80% of the allowable costs for these goods. If you have supplemental insurance, it will often cover the other 20%.

Call your insurance plan's customer service center and verify whether they cover therapeutic footwear. Unfortunately, many private health insurance carriers do not recognize how important therapeutic footwear is and will not pay for these services.

How Should I Care for My Foot After an Amputation?

An amputation can "create" a foot deformity and put unusual pressure on the remaining bones in the foot. Although the surgery may be necessary to save the foot, it increases the risk for future ulcers and amputation. You will need padding in your shoe and well-fitting therapeutic shoes.

If you ever have an amputation, give yourself time to adjust. Physical therapy can help with strength and mobility. You may be surprised, however, by the emotions you feel. Talking with a counselor or a support group can help you regain your emotional balance, too.

What Are the Guidelines for Good Foot Care?

- At each doctor's visit, remove your shoes and stockings, and have your feet examined.
- Don't walk barefoot.
- Look inside your shoes for sharp tacks, rough linings, or foreign objects before you put them on.
- Wear sensible shoes that are properly fitted and change them several times each day if possible.
- Inspect your feet daily for blisters, bleeding, and sores between toes. Make this part of your ritual.

- Use a long-handled mirror to see the bottom of your foot and heel. Ask a family member for help if you can't see well.
- Do not soak your feet.
- Avoid hot water bottles, heating pads, or electric blankets on your feet. Test bath water with your elbow to avoid unnoticed burns.
- Wash feet daily with warm, soapy water and dry them well, especially between the toes. Put on clean socks.
- Use moisturizing lotion (whose first ingredient is not alcohol) daily but not between the toes.
- Do not use acids or chemical corn removers.
- Do not perform "bathroom surgery" on corns, calluses, or ingrown toenails.
- Trim your nails, leaving them long and following the curve of the toes. If necessary, file them gently. Have a podiatrist do this if you have difficulty doing it, and especially if you have neuropathy.
- Call your doctor immediately if your foot becomes swollen, red, or painful. Stay off the foot.
- Don't smoke.
- Learn all you can about diabetes and foot care.
- Have regular foot examinations by your physician or podiatrist.

This chapter was written by Robert G. Frykberg, DPM, MPH; Beth Noe, DPM; Lee J. Sanders, DPM; Erick Janisse, CPed, BOCO; Michael Mueller, PT, PhD; and David R. Sinacore, PT, PhD.

16

Nerve Damage: Internal Organs and Localized Damage

Introduction

Autonomic nerves help with the activities of your body that you don't have to think about—heartbeat, breathing, food digestion, breathing, as well as bladder and sexual functions. Neuropathy can be further classified as either diffuse or focal—diffuse meaning scattered and focal meaning only one or a few nerves are involved. Diffuse neuropathies develop slowly over time, but focal nerve damage can occur suddenly if it is due to a single nerve involvement or more slowly if due to an entrapment such as carpal tunnel syndrome. Damage to the autonomic nerves can affect major systems in your body, such as the heart, the stomach and intestines, or the sexual organs. This chapter deals with autonomic neuropathy in nerves affecting the bladder, eye, heart, and sweat glands, as well as those involved with the awareness of hypoglycemia and the ability to recover spontaneously from a blood glucose low (hypoglycemia responsiveness).

What Are the Possible Causes of Neuropathy?

There can be many causes of neuropathy—diabetes is not the only one. To rule out the other possible causes, your provider must consider:

- Your family history of neuropathy
- Vitamin B12 and folate deficiency

- Syphilis
- Lyme disease
- Leprosy
- Chaga's disease if you have traveled in South America
- Amyloid if you have a family history of neuropathy and are of Mediterranean origin
- Autoimmune diseases
- Toxic causes of neuropathy including alcoholism, arsenic, and a variety of drugs

Tests to confirm or rule out these other conditions will need to be done. The condition causing your neuropathy must be treated along with the neuropathy if you are to get well.

How Is Neuropathy Diagnosed?

To diagnose neuropathy, your health care provider may gather information from five different categories. First, of course, are your symptoms (Table 16-1). For autonomic neuropathy, it is necessary to check your body's responses to stimuli, for example, in the heart or gastrointestinal wall. There is a series of simple, noninvasive tests for detecting cardiovascular autonomic neuropathy. These tests are based on detection of heart rate and blood pressure response to a series of physical movements. Specific tests are used to evaluate gastrointestinal, genitourinary, and sweating functions and peripheral skin blood flow, all of which can be affected by diabetic autonomic neuropathy.

How Does Autonomic Neuropathy Affect Your Bladder?

The genitourinary system includes your bladder and sex organs. The kidneys filter your blood and make urine to take away waste products. The urine goes from the kidney, through the ureter, into the bladder. The bladder is an elastic bag and can expand and contract. After about 1 1/2 cups (10 oz) of urine collects in your bladder, you feel the urge to go to the bathroom. Bladder function is controlled by three different types of nerves. One transmits the signal to your

Table 16-1. Symptoms of Diabetic Autonomic Neuropathy

Genitourinary
Bladder
Urinating less often
Frequent urinary tract infections
Difficulty emptying bladder completely
Weak urinary stream
Difficulty starting to urinate and dribbling afterwards; incontinence

Sexual function

In males:	*In females:*
Impotence	Diminished vaginal lubrication
	Decreased frequency of orgasm

Gastrointestinal
Stomach
Difficulty swallowing
Feeling full just after beginning to eat
Bloating and abdominal pain
Brittle diabetes hyper and hypoglycemia after meals
Nausea without vomiting
Vomiting food that was eaten many hours before
Intestinal
Diarrhea, especially at night
Constipation

Cardiovascular
Severe dizziness on standing with a drop in blood pressure
Fixed heart rate
Exercise intolerance
Cold dry feet with poor blood flow

Hypoglycemia Counterregulation
Loss of early warning symptoms of hypoglycemia
Failure of counter-regulation and recovery from hypoglycemia without intervention

Sweating
Dry hands and feet
Increased sweating on upper body
Sweating while eating certain foods

Pupils
Delayed or absent response of pupils to darkness/light
Decreased pupil size

brain when your bladder is full. Another causes your bladder to contract so you can pass urine. A third maintains the tone of the sphincter that opens for you to urinate and closes when you are finished. Diabetes can cause damage to all three types of nerves.

What Are the Symptoms of Neuropathy of the Bladder?

When people first begin to have this type of damage, they may urinate less often. Some people will have the desire to urinate frequently, but will pass only small amounts of urine each time. This is because the bladder does not empty completely each time. Tests for bladder function might include blood tests of your kidney function, measurement of the amount of urine left in your bladder after you urinate, or an ultrasound test of your bladder when it is full.

One of the concerns is that urine remaining in your bladder provides an excellent place for bacteria to grow, especially if there is also glucose in the urine. This can cause a bladder or urinary tract infection (UTI). If untreated, these infections can cause kidney damage. Symptoms of a bladder infection are frequent urination of small amounts, pain or burning when you urinate, and being unable to urinate even though you feel the urge. UTIs usually go away quickly with antibiotics. You need to call your provider at the first signs of an infection. If you have more than two bladder infections each year, it may be an early sign of nerve damage to your bladder. Talk to your provider about the need for tests of your bladder function.

What Is the Treatment for Bladder Neuropathy?

The treatment for bladder dysfunction includes both self-care activities and drug therapies. Patients with neurogenic bladder may not feel when their bladders are full. You'll have to think for your bladder. Drink plenty of fluids, and go to the bathroom every 2 hours. You may need to press on your bladder to determine when it is full, and if necessary, push on it to start the flow of urine. Medicines to improve bladder function are available and may be effective. Drugs such as bethanechol are sometimes helpful, but they often do not help you fully empty your bladder. The sphincter can be relaxed with terazosin or doxazosin. Self-catheterization can be useful in the case of a contracted sphincter, with generally a low risk of infection. Bladder neck surgery may help to relieve spasm of the internal sphincter. Because the external sphincter remains intact, urine will not leak out.

How Does Autonomic Neuropathy Affect Your Eyes?

The pupils in your eyes react to light and darkness by becoming smaller in very bright light and larger when it is dark. The response of the pupils is controlled by autonomic nerves. If these nerves are damaged, the pupils respond more slowly to darkness, so it can take longer for your eyes to adjust when you enter a dark room. More importantly, they do not constrict in response to light. You may have more difficulty driving at night because your eyes don't respond as quickly to the lights of an oncoming car or when going from a well-lit to a darker area. You need to take precautions to ensure your safety in these situations.

How Does Autonomic Neuropathy Affect Your Cardiovascular System?

Autonomic nerves control your heart rate and blood pressure, which normally change slightly throughout the day in response to position (lying, sitting, and standing), stress, exercise, breathing patterns, and sleep. If the nerves to the heart and blood vessels are damaged by diabetes, the blood pressure and heart rate may respond more slowly to these factors. If the nerves that regulate your blood pressure are damaged, blood pressure can drop quickly when you stand up and not return to a normal level as quickly as it did before the nerves were damaged. You may feel lightheaded or dizzy, see black spots, or even pass out. This is called orthostatic hypotension. This results from blood pooling in the feet, which can lead to swelling or edema. Orthostatic hypotension is often a late development of autonomic neuropathy in patients with diabetes.

How Is Orthostatic Hypotension Diagnosed?

Because it is not unusual to feel lightheaded when you stand up too quickly, your provider needs to take your blood pressure and heart rate when you are lying and standing to diagnose orthostatic hypotension. This should be done at least once a year. If you have concerns, ask your provider to do these simple tests again.

The situation can be complicated by the fact that people with advanced diabetes may have complications involving the kidney, eyes, and blood vessels, making it difficult to determine which condition is responsible for the person's symptoms. There is also "meal-induced hypotension," in which people become dizzy soon after breakfast, occasionally after lunch, but not at all with dinner. It is difficult to relieve the morning or breakfast-related low blood pressure without making the afternoon or evening blood pressure high. Loss of the daily rhythm of blood pressure control is the hallmark of autonomic neuropathy—blood pressure tends to rise at night and fall during the day. There is a risk of stroke. Low blood pressure medications are discussed below.

What Is the Treatment for Orthostatic Hypotension?

Treating orthostatic hypotension requires a delicate balancing act— trying to elevate blood pressure in the standing position without elevating it too high in the lying position. Treatment for orthostatic or postural hypotension includes better blood glucose control, an adequate salt intake to be sure that you have a large enough volume of plasma in your bloodstream, avoidance of medications such as diuretics, and safety measures to prevent falls. Raising the head of your bed on blocks (to a 30-degree angle) is helpful, and putting on waist-high elastic stockings before you get up may help prevent your blood pressure from dropping. You should put them on while lying down and not remove them until you have returned to lying down. Clearly, they can be uncomfortable, especially in hot weather, which means that people don't like to use them. In severe cases, you may need a total body stocking or an Air Force antigravity suit. Get out of bed slowly, and stand at your bedside until your head clears before you move off. Avoid very hot showers or baths, as the hot water relaxes your peripheral blood vessels and can worsen the drop in blood pressure.

Medications such as fludrocortisone (Florinef) may help to expand plasma volume. You must be on the alert for edema (swelling), because there is a risk of developing hypertension and congestive heart failure. Other drugs (for example, phenylephrine, ephedrine, Neo-Synephrine nasal spray, beta-blockers, clonidine, octreotide, and Epogen) that work more directly on the blood vessels are used to treat orthostatic hypotension. A few patients may be helped with propranolol (Inderal). Postural hypotension that occurs after eating may respond to therapy with octreotide (Sandostatin).

It is particularly important for you to discuss with your health-care team all of the medications you are taking. Drugs commonly used in people with diabetes, such as diuretics and blood pressure agents, may be the cause of these symptoms, and their doses should be modified. Other drugs, such as those used to treat pain, may also lower blood pressure.

Interestingly, it has been recently recognized that the symptoms of orthostasis may not be due to a fall in blood pressure but rather to either an inappropriate rise in heart rate, called postural orthostatic tachycardia syndrome (POTS), or a fall in heart rate, called postural orthostatic bradycardia syndrome (POBS). Thus, when doing the test for your symptoms, your doctor should measure you blood pressure as well as your heart rate when you stand from a lying position. POTS is easily treated with a beta-blocker such as propranolol or an inhibitor of acetylcholine breakdown, pyridostigmine. Bradycardia syndrome can be treated with an anticholinergic drug such as propantheline.

Can Autonomic Neuropathy Affect Your Heart Rate in Other Ways?

Yes, it can. If the nerves that control heart rate are affected, the heart rate tends to be fast and does not change very much in response to breathing patterns, exercise, stress, or sleep.

How Is the Effect of Neuropathy on Your Heart Diagnosed?

It can be diagnosed through measuring the changes in your pulse rate as you breathe deeply, during a Valsalva maneuver (done by bearing down as hard as you can or simply blowing into a sphygmo-manometer cuff like you would if you were blowing up a balloon), or before and after standing. An electrocardiogram (ECG) and specialized computer programs may be used to do this. This effect on the heart is a serious complication because it may increase your risk for irregular heartbeat and prevent you from feeling the pain or warning symptoms of a heart attack (see box). The computer programs are now sophisticated enough to be able to tell which part of the autonomic nervous system is involved, which is vital to making the right choice of drug with which to treat you.

Sometimes the nerve damage prevents you from getting the usual cardiovascular benefits from aerobic exercise. If this is the case, ask your provider what kind of exercise you can do.

If there is any question as to whether you may have heart disease, whether there is pain or not, you should have cardiac stress testing. This is especially true if you have two or more risk factors for coronary artery disease (see chapter 10) or if you are considering starting an exercise program.

Silent Heart Attack?

One problem with autonomic neuropathy and the loss of the nerve supply to the heart is the fact that a heart attack may be "silent," as in there may be no pain whatsoever. However, there may still be symptoms. A heart attack in someone with autonomic neuropathy that affects the heart may feature:

- No pain
- Unexplained persistent coughing
- Nausea and vomiting
- Shortness of breath
- Excessive tiredness
- Electrocardiographic changes found upon doing an ECG

If you experience these symptoms and have autonomic neuropathy, seek medical attention immediately. Pain is not the only indication that something is wrong.

How Are Changes in the Daily Pattern of Blood Pressures Connected with the Risk of Sudden Death?

Normally, blood pressure declines at night. It has been shown that people with type 1 and type 2 diabetes and albuminuria (protein in the urine) have blunted blood pressure cycles and that their hearts may be at full throttle all the time, which may help explain why heart-related events are so common at night for those with this cluster of conditions. Damage to the vagus nerve, which supplies the lungs and heart and regulates blood pressure, may be an important factor in sudden cardiovascular death and silent heart attacks. These findings help explain the mortality risk for people with autonomic neuropathy. When you are taking blood pressure medication and you have blunted or reversed blood pressure patterns, your doctor must be careful to consider the effects of that medication on your overnight blood pressure. There is also evidence that nerve damage in the heart isn't distributed evenly and that a rapid irregular heart beat is most common. Fortunately, there are now tests that can show this pattern of nerve supply damage, and this sudden arrhythmia often can be prevented with a beta-blocker.

Can Neuropathy Cause Unusual Sweating?

Yes. Sweating is one way your body regulates your temperature. The sudomotor nerves control where and how much you sweat. If these nerves are damaged, you may sweat less on your hands and feet and more on your face and trunk. One explanation for this situation is that the body needs to get rid of heat by increasing blood flow and sweating in the upper body to compensate for the loss of peripheral autonomic nerves in the lower body. In addition, you may sweat while eating, particularly spicy foods, cheese, chocolate, red sausages, red wines, and some soft drinks. (Even people with a normally functioning autonomic nervous system may have head and face sweating when eating spicy foods.)

When your sweating response is damaged, your body can't adjust its temperature. This increases your risk for heat stroke. The skin on your feet and hands can get too dry and, as part of the damage process, may not be getting the essential nutrients usually delivered by the blood vessels. Your feet may feel cold. Your skin may also thicken in response to decreased sweating and lubrication. The thickened skin can crack open and provide a site for bacteria and infections to start. Most importantly, many of the new devices developed to recognize hypoglycemia rely on sweating as a symptom. These may prove useless if you have autonomic neuropathy—a little-recognized fact.

How Is Sweat Gland (Sudomotor)Nerve Damage Diagnosed?

Obviously, the symptoms lead to the diagnosis. Your provider can dust you with a special starch powder that turns purple when it gets wet or check your ability to feel warmth in your feet and hands. There are also more sophisticated tests using electrical stimulation of these nerves and laser Doppler blood flow studies that can help make the diagnosis.

What Is the Treatment for Sweat Gland (Sudomotor) Neuropathy?

The important thing is to keep your feet and hands healthy and to use lubricating creams and oils after you bathe to keep in the moisture. You should also avoid intense heat and humidity because your body cannot regulate extreme temperatures well. Medications (propantheline hydrobromide, scopolamine patches) may help relieve unusual sweating if it is severe. Your provider may also prescribe a cholinergic blocker to decrease upper-body sweating. High doses of these medications are usually required, and therapy is usually limited by the side effects, such as dry mouth, urinary retention, and constipation. Glycopyrrolate is an option for those who sweat while eating. An injection of botulinum toxin type A may also be used to treat this disorder.

Does Autonomic Neuropathy Affect Your Body's Response to Hypoglycemia?

Yes. Autonomic nerves orchestrate your body's symptoms of, and response to, hypoglycemia. When there is severe autonomic damage, both the capacity to respond to hypoglycemia and the ability to counteract it are seriously limited. This can be life-threatening. To counteract low blood glucose, your body should release gluca-gon (a hormone that causes you to release glucose from your liver), adrenalin (epinephrine), growth hormone, cortisol, and glucose from the liver (chapter 5). If it does not, you probably won't experi-ence symptoms of low blood glucose, a condition known as hypo-glycemia unawareness. The autonomic symptoms of hypoglycemia usually are heart palpitations, irregular heartbeat, anxiety, tingling around the mouth, and sweating. When you have autonomic neu-ropathy, your symptoms—when you have any—are more likely due to the shortage of blood glucose in the brain: irritability, tiredness, confusion, forgetfulness, and loss of consciousness.

Furthermore, the epinephrine response is important to counteract hypoglycemia. When you have autonomic neuropathy and repeated episodes of hypoglycemia, this no longer happens. More and more people practice intensive blood glucose control, which has led to a threefold increase in hypoglycemic episodes requiring the assistance of another person. Although tight control may delay autonomic neuropathy, it also puts you more at risk for hypoglycemia, and you may be unaware of it happening. If your hypoglycemia becomes life-threatening, it may be necessary for you to relax your blood glucose goals. Sometimes this will restore your body's responses.

You should also be aware that the symptoms of hypoglycemia will fade over time. The longer you have had diabetes, the more likely you will have at least some degree of hypoglycemia unaware-ness. To catch hypoglycemia before it goes too low, check your blood glucose level often, especially before you drive.

What Is Focal Neuropathy?

Focal neuropathy is damage to a single nerve (mononeuropathy), to nerve clusters (mononeuropathy multiplex), to nerves in the chest or abdomen (plexopathy), or to nerve roots (radiculopathy), which often mimics the pain of heart attack or appendicitis. Mononeuropathy that affects nerves to the head is called cranial neuropathy and can cause, for example, severe headache, drooping of one side of the face, or double vision. Mononeuropathies in areas where nerves can be trapped or compressed, such as in the wrist and palm, upper arm, elbow, and thigh, are called entrapment neuropathies. Carpal tunnel syndrome is an example of an entrapment neuropathy and is fairly common in people with diabetes.

Mononeuropathies

Mononeuropathies are lesions in a single nerve that spontaneously heal. Common mononeuropathies involve cranial, thoracic (in the chest), and peripheral nerves. Their onset is sudden and associated with pain, and they generally go away over 6–8 weeks. They must

---

Hypoglycemia Awareness Training

If you feel you may have hypoglycemia unawareness, check your blood glucose often and try to determine what your symptoms of hypoglycemia are. This is called hypoglycemia awareness training. If you do not have symptoms, such as sweating or tingling around the mouth, try to recognize the earliest symptoms of a drop in glucose supply to your brain—it may simply be irritability. In addition, you and your family members and friends should know the symptoms, causes, and treatments of hypoglycemia. You need to have a source of carbohydrate with you always and an up-to-date glucagon kit handy. The kit can be prescribed by your provider, and your family and friends need to be taught how to use it. To prevent hypoglycemia from surprising you, check your blood glucose levels often. You may also want to wear identification jewelry stating that you have diabetes in case hypoglycemia happens when you are away from home or work. In general, if you have bona fide hypoglycemia unawareness, your targets will probably be higher-than-normal glucose and A1C levels, which will help you avoid life-threatening situations. Often, an insulin pump will help you avoid hypoglycemia. Rapid-acting insulin may help also.

---

be distinguished from entrapment syndromes, which start slowly, progress, and do not go away without intervention, because the treatment for each is quite different. One example is the condition called femoral neuropathy, which involves damage to motor and sensory nerves in the thigh. The symptoms include pain that is sometimes worse at night in the thigh and calf. Muscle weakness can be disabling and can limit hip and knee movements. To distinguish it from sciatica, your provider may have you straighten your leg and raise it. This will be very painful if you have sciatica, but not if you have femoral neuropathy. You should recover completely, but it may last for several years before muscle strength returns to normal.

Entrapment neuropathy

Entrapment neuropathies are common in people with diabetes and should be checked in every person with symptoms of neuropathy. Common entrapments involve the median nerve in the wrist with impaired sensation in the first three fingers (carpal tunnel syndrome). Ulnar nerve entrapment in the elbow decreases sensation in the little and ring fingers. Damage to the radial nerve (in the upper arm) can cause weakness, loss of sensation on the back of the hand, and dropping of the wrist when extended. Damage to the lateral cutaneous nerve of the thigh causes thigh pain. Damage to the peroneal nerve in the knee causes foot drop. In your foot, medial and lateral plantar nerve entrapments decrease sensation on the inside and outside of the foot, respectively. Finally, tarsal tunnel syndrome may cause numbness and tingling in the foot.

Carpal tunnel syndrome and other entrapment neuropathies
Carpal tunnel syndrome occurs twice as frequently in people with diabetes. This may be related to repeated trauma (from simple things such as using a weed whacker or even a Blackberry), metabolic changes, or accumulation of fluid within the confined space of the carpal tunnel. The diagnosis can be confirmed by electrophysiological study, and therapy may require surgery. The symptoms may

spread to the whole hand and arm in carpal tunnel, and the signs may extend beyond those caused by the trapped nerve. They often involve the thumb, index finger, and one side of the middle finger. Other nerves that are frequently trapped include the peroneal nerve, which causes pain on the outside of the lower leg and inability to raise the foot or the big toe; the ulnar nerve that causes pain in the ring and little fingers; and the medial plantar nerve with pain on the inside of the foot. The problem is often that the true nature of your trouble goes unrecognized, and an opportunity for successful therapy is missed.

To treat carpal tunnel (and avoid surgery), you can change how you use the wrist, do special exercises, wear a wrist splint, or take anti-inflammatory medications. Surgical treatment consists of sectioning the volar carpal ligament and releasing the entrapped nerve. The rest of the entrapment neuropathies can be treated the same way—rest, splinting, diuretics, and if there is weakness, surgical decompression. One should not, however, resort to surgery for common neuropathy. This has become the vogue in certain surgically oriented centers, despite the fact that there is as yet no proven evidence of value.

Radiculopathy

Radiculopathy is damage to a nerve or nerves in the trunk of the body. The primary symptom is pain in the chest (and sometimes the abdomen) that comes on suddenly and is worse at night. The pain does not seem to get worse with exertion. Pain in the chest leads your provider to look first for heart or lung problems. Once these are ruled out, other conditions that can cause similar pain are spinal disk problems, pneumonia, gastrointestinal disease, ulcers, or appendicitis. Ruling out these conditions requires several different diagnostic procedures. Radiculopathy generally goes away within 6 months to 2 years.

Are There Self-Care Activities for Living with Neuropathy?

Yes. As is repeated throughout this book, maintaining near-normal blood glucose levels is most important, but there are other simple things you can do each day to help yourself live better with the effects of neuropathy. (See Table 16-2.)

Table 16-2. Self-Care Activities for Diabetic Autonomic Neuropathies

Genitourinary
Bladder dysfunction
Empty bladder every 2–3 hours whether you feel the urge or not.
Call your provider at the first sign of a urinary tract infection.
Sexual dysfunction
Talk with your health care provider about your symptoms.

Gastrointestinal
Gastroparesis
Eat 4–6 small, mostly liquid meals each day.
Eat foods low in fat and fiber.
Take medications before eating, as recommended.
Monitor blood glucose levels often.
Give medications a fair trial.
Avoid some of the newer medications, such as exenatide or pramlintide, that slow the rate of gastric emptying.
Intestinal
Constipation
Increase fiber in your diet.
Increase fluid intake.
Increase activity.
Use laxatives with caution.
Diarrhea
Increase fluid intake to prevent dehydration.
Use antidiarrhea medications with caution.
Take antibiotics to counteract bacterial overgrowth.
Talk to your doctor about medications such as questran, viokase, creon, or san dostatin.

Cardiovascular dysfunction
Rise slowly after sitting or lying. After sleeping, sit on the side of the bed and let your feet dangle off the side until you adjust.
Elevate the head of your bed 30 degrees.
Use elastic stockings as recommended.
Avoid strenuous and aerobic exercise or activity.
Avoid straining or lifting heavy objects.
Stop smoking.
Have a cardiovascular evaluation before starting an exercise program.
Learn to use rate of perceived exertion when exercising and do not rely on heart rate or use a heart rate monitor.

Impaired hypoglycemia counter-regulation

Test your blood glucose often, especially before and on breaks during driving on long trips.

Wear diabetes identification.

Teach family, friends, and co-workers how to recognize and treat hypoglycemia.

Keep an up-to-date glucagon kit on hand, and be sure someone around you knows how to use it.

Impaired sweating

Avoid foods that can lead to sweating.

Use lotion on dry skin.

Use caution when the weather is very hot or humid.

Impaired pupil

Turn on the light when entering a dark room.

Use nightlights in dark hallways and bathroom.

Use caution when driving at night.

This chapter was written by Aaron Vinik, MD, PhD, FCP, MACP; Martha M. Funnell, MS, RN, CDE; Douglas A. Greene, MD; Eva L. Feldman, MD, PhD; and Martin J. Stevens, MD.

17

Diabetic Kidney Disease

Case Study

A 37-year-old woman who has had type 1 diabetes since age 10 noticed ankle swelling and increasing girth over a 6-month period. Over the years, her blood glucose had not been well controlled, ranging from 140 to 300mg/dL. She had high blood pressure (145/90 to 185/110). Albuminuria (increasing amount of albumin, a protein, in her urine) had been showing in her lab tests for the last 2 years. She recently needed laser therapy for proliferative diabetic retinopathy. Her serum creatinine was 2.1 mg/dL (normal is less than 1.2 mg/dL). When the kidneys start to fail, the blood creatinine begins to rise. Her physician diagnosed nephrotic syndrome, a condition characterized by urinary protein loss, water retention, and high cholesterol. He prescribed an ACE inhibitor, a medicine that lowers blood pressure and helps preserve kidney function by blocking an enzyme (angiotensin-converting enzyme), and a diuretic, a drug that increases salt and water excretion in urine. A statin drug was included to reduce LDL cholesterol to less than 100. He sent her to a registered dietician for help in following a reduced-fat, limited protein, low-sodium and low-potassium diet.

Case Study

After 15 years of type 2 diabetes, a 54-year-old man with poor health care coverage and high blood pressure (180/110 mmHg) complained of being unable to concentrate and of constantly feeling cold. Weakness, nausea, a 12-pound weight loss, and itchy skin were also problems that were affecting his quality of life. Physical examination and lab tests indicated that he had advanced renal failure with a serum creatinine of 14.5 mg/dL. (Normal is less than 1.5 mg/dL, since men have a higher "normal" level than women.) The diagnosis of diabetic renal disease is supported by the presence of diabetic retinopathy, for which he recently underwent laser treatment. His primary care physician referred him to a nephrologist (kidney specialist) to discuss options in renal replacement therapy, including various types of dialysis and kidney transplantation. At the end of the evaluation, he opted for a kidney transplant. Subsequently, a very good friend and his wife offered to donate a kidney.

Introduction

In most industrialized nations, diabetes is the leading cause of kidney (renal) failure, accounting for 25–50% of all new cases. This epidemic, now termed a pandemic, can be explained by a slightly paradoxical situation—there are more people taking better care of their diabetes. The more successful patients and health care professionals are at handling diabetes, the longer and healthier the life of people with diabetes should be. A longer life span, however, can give some people with diabetes enough time to develop late complications of diabetes, including renal failure. African Americans, Latinos, and Native Americans (especially the Pima tribe) are three to five times more likely to have both diabetes and kidney complications.

Of people with type 1 diabetes, 30–50% are likely to develop diabetic nephropathy after having diabetes for more than 20 years. In patients with type 2 diabetes, diabetic renal disease is a bit of a mystery. Damage to their kidneys also means that they are at risk for a stroke or heart attack.

Ongoing research and improvement in the management of diabetes and its complications have progressively enhanced the quality of life of people afflicted with severe kidney disease. Over the past decade, dialysis and kidney transplant have steadily improved the survival rate of kidney failure for those with diabetes.

What Do Normal or Healthy Kidneys Do?

Most people have two kidneys located in the back of the abdomen on either side of the spine (Figure 17-1). Each is about the size of an Idaho potato weighing approximately 1/2 pound, and together they process about one-quarter of the blood pumped by the heart. One kidney can do the work of two in terms of permitting an otherwise normal life, which is why people born with only one kidney or who lose a kidney by trauma or disease, or as a transplant donor have a normal life expectancy. Blood flow through the kidneys amounts to about 1 quart every minute. The kidneys maintain a

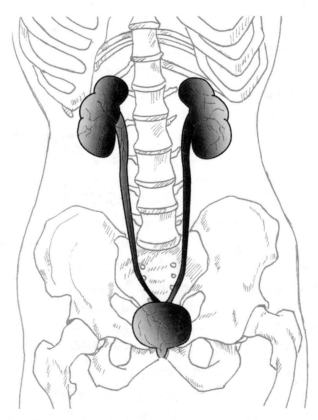

Figure 17-1. The kidneys and urinary system.

balance of sodium and potassium and remove nitrogen-rich end products of protein digestion as well as water. Kidneys also produce hormones (chemicals that work throughout the body) that stimulate the bone marrow to make red blood cells and regulate calcium absorption from the intestines. Like other vital organ systems, renal function has a large reserve capacity.

Each kidney is made up of between 600,000 and nearly 1.5 million subunits called nephrons. Specialists in internal medicine who work primarily with diseases of the kidneys are called nephrologists. Individual nephrons begin with a complex of tiny blood vessel loops called a glomeulus, through which blood from the heart is filtered. The blood is delivered by an arteriole, a small artery. Blood, minus what was filtered, leaves through another arteriole to return through to the heart. The filtrate enters a long channel in the nephron called a tubule, where it is changed into urine and discharged into the bladder via the ureters, tubes connecting the kidneys to the bladder (Figures 17-1 and 17-2).

Disease of the kidney (renal disease) is called nephropathy, and people with diabetic kidney disease have diabetic nephropathy. Sometimes confusingly, people with diabetes may have kidney disease not related to diabetes. For instance, an individual may inherit a kidney disorder, have a tumor or enlargement of the prostate gland that obstructs urine flow and puts backup pressure on the kidneys, or have an infectious disease that affects the kidneys. Many beneficial drugs can injure kidney function. That is why it can be difficult to determine whether kidney disease is related to diabetes or caused by something else.

Who Is at Risk for Developing Diabetic Nephropathy?

The longer you have diabetes, the more at risk you are for developing diabetic nephropathy. However, after 40 years of diabetes, only 30–50% of people with type 1 diabetes develop kidney disease. Individuals whose blood glucose control has not been good are at higher risk for developing the disease. Some people have a genetic tendency to develop diabetic renal disease, as signaled by relatives with kidney disorders. Subjects with high blood pressure appear to be more likely to have diabetic nephropathy than those with normal blood pressure. On the other hand, renal disease may make high blood pressure worse. Other risk factors for kidney disease include high cholesterol levels and smoking.

What Are the Symptoms of Diabetic Kidney Disease?

Unfortunately, diabetic nephropathy is silent, meaning it has no symptoms, until it is pretty far advanced. Therefore, laboratory tests, especially urine protein measurement, need to be done at regular intervals to tell you and your doctor how your kidneys are doing before serious symptoms occur.

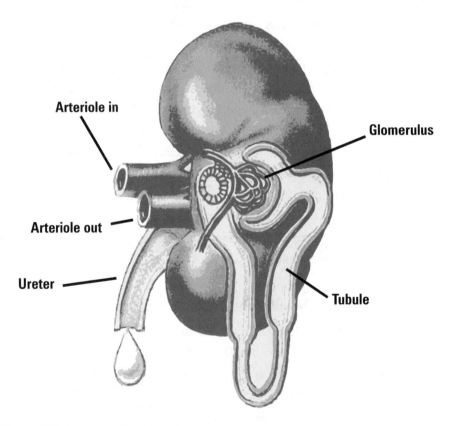

Figure 17-2. A cross section of a kidney.

What Are the Stages of Diabetic Nephropathy?

The stages of diabetic nephropathy have been divided into hyperfiltration, microalbuminuria, nephrotic syndrome, renal insufficiency or chronic kidney disease, and end-stage renal disease. (See Table 17-1.) However, not all stages are seen in every subject.

Hyperfiltration

The first stage of diabetic kidney disease has no symptoms and is called hyperfiltration. Early in the course of diabetes, in as many as 70% of those with type 1 diabetes and about 33% of those with type 2 diabetes, an above-normal amount of blood passes through the filtering glomeruli in their kidneys. This phenomenon has been linked to long-standing high blood glucose levels. You kidneys will enlarge in early the course of diabetic nephropathy, but blood glucose control can correct hyperfiltration and reduce your kidney size to normal. A kidney test named "clearance" may show that you are experiencing hyperfiltration, but that does not mean your kidneys are getting worse. Fewer than 50% of people who have diabetes and hyperfiltration will advance to the later stages of nephropathy.

Microalbuminuria

Microalbuminuria is a condition characterized by the presence of small amounts of a protein called albumin in your urine. Each day, healthy people pass less than 25 mg of albumin in their urine. Microalbuminuria (30–300 mg/day) occurs in 4–15% of adults with diabetes, usually in those who have had diabetes for at least 5 years. Hyperfiltration may not be present with microalbuminuria. It is important to detect microalbuminuria because people with type 1 diabetes who have it are most likely to progress to later stages of diabetic nephropathy. Subjects with type 2 diabetes who have microalbuminuria are more likely to have a stroke or a heart attack. Strenuous exercise, hypertension, sudden illness with fever, urinary tract infection, or congestive heart failure can temporarily increase microalbuminuria. Albumin excretion can also vary from day to day.

Table 17-1. Stages of Diabetic Nephropathy and Treatment Targets

Stages	Glomerular Filtration Rate* (GFR) (mL/minute)	Clinical Assessment and Treatment Targets
Hyperfiltration	Increased (GFR >125)	• Strive for normal blood glucose (BG). A1C less than 7%. • Lifestyle modification (weight reduction, smoking cessation).
Microalbuminuria	Normal or increased (GFR ≥ 90)	• Strive for normal BG. A1C less than 7%. • Treat high blood pressure. BP below 130/80. • Reduce serum lipid levels. LDL cholesterol below 100 mg/dL. • Lifestyle modification. • Your doctor will assess and treat other diabetic complications.
Nephrotic Syndrome and Chronic Kidney Disease (CKD) Stage 1	Normal or increased (GFR ≥ 90)	• Strive for normal BG. A1C less than 7%. • Extract edema. Your doctor will give diuretics. • Blood pressure below 125/75. Your doctor will use ACE inhibitor and/or A2 receptor blocker + one or two other BP-lowering drugs. • Protein restriction (0.8 to 1 gram/kg of body weight). • Lipid reduction. LDL cholesterol less than 100 mg/dL. • A dietitian can help with dietary requirements.
CKD Stage 2	Mildly decreased (GFR 60–89)	• Same recommendations as in CKD stage 1. • Your doctor will refer you to a nephrologist. • He will estimate the progression of your renal disease.
CKD Stage 3	Moderately decreased (GFR 30–59)	• Same recommendations as in CKD stage 1. • Your doctor will search for and treat complications associated with CKD (high serum potassium, phosphorus, and low serum calcium levels and anemia. • He or she will continue to treat other diabetic complications. • Your kidney doctor will educate you and your family about the different types of renal replacement therapy. • Save blood vessels for access creation.
CKD Stage 4	Severely decreased (GFR 15–29)	• Get ready for uremia therapy. • Access creation for hemodialysis or peritoneal dialysis. • Look for potential kidney donors. • Monitor psychosocial adjustment.
CKD Stage 5	End Stage Renal Disease/Kidney failure (GFR < 15)	• Initiate replacement therapy (dialysis or transplant).

*The GFR is the rate of filtered fluid through your kidney, and in general, a measure of your overall kidney health. Your doctor will determine this rate using various factors, including creatinine tests, age, gender, and other variables.

Therefore, two or three urine specimens should show elevated levels of albumin (30–300 mg/day) before a diagnosis of microalbuminuria is made.

Although microalbuminuria has no signs or symptoms, we know there are changes in the small blood vessels of the kidneys that are unique to diabetes and blood pressure increases in the filters (glomeruli) of both kidneys. Microalbuminuria signals the need for treatment with ACE inhibitors or a class of drugs called A2 receptor blockers. Both ACE inhibitors and A2 receptor blockers lower the blood pressure within the glomerulus so that less albumin leaks from the blood into the urine. Many doctors advise an ACE inhibitor or A2 receptor blocker for every person with diabetes. About 10% of people treated with an ACE inhibitor may develop a dry cough or other side effect and have to stop taking the drug. If you are a woman of childbearing age, both ACE inhibitors and A2 receptor blockers should be used cautiously and stopped immediately if you become pregnant.

Nephrotic syndrome

Nephrotic syndrome is a condition characterized by large amount of albumin in the urine, low levels of albumin in the blood, high levels of cholesterol and fats in the blood, and water in the feet and other areas of the body. When the injury to the blood filters in the kidneys gets worse, albumin loss in the urine rises to 3,500 mg per day or more. Because of the loss of albumin in the urine, the concentration of albumin in the blood decreases to less than the normal range of about 3.9–4.6 mg/dL. This diminishes the ability of the blood to hold plasma water inside tiny blood vessels. Water then accumulates in the tissues as edema in the chest (pleural effusion), around the heart (pericardial effusion), and in the abdomen (ascites). These are the areas where you may notice symptoms if the disease has progressed this far. The liver also produces more cholesterol and fats (hyperlipidemia), which can cause other health problems.

In the nephrotic syndrome, fluid is retained in the body, and water weight may reach 50 pounds. Carrying this much extra water causes fatigue and shortness of breath. People with nephrotic syndrome often note that their shoes do not fit and dresses and pants will not button because of the water weight, and even routine activities are difficult and tiring to complete.

Renal insufficiency or chronic kidney disease

This stage is called renal insuffeciency, or chronic kidney disease (CKD). At this stage, the damaged kidney is no longer able to filter all the toxins from the blood or prevent protein from leaking into the urine. Often, physicians monitor the condition of the kidneys by measuring serum creatinine. The preferred method of measuring kidney function is the glomerular filtration rate (GFR), which is reported in mL per minute. Your GFR estimates the amount of fluid filtered by your kidneys, with decreasing levels indicating a worsening of kidney disease. GFR can be determined using your serum creatinine levels, urine clearance test results, age, and other factors, though your doctor may use a variety of formulas to determine your rate. Estimation of GFR is extremely important and clarifies the staging of chronic diabetic kidney disease. In addition, studies have indicated that significant GFR reduction may be seen in adults with type 1 and type 2 diabetes in the absence of increased urine albumin excretion.

If your GFR falls to 60 mL/minute or less, you should be referred to a nephrologist right away. Once your GFR drops below 50, renal function continues to deteriorate, though you may not have many symptoms until your GFR hits 30 or lower. At this point, loss of appetite, nausea, feeling cold, being unable to concentrate, and itching are common complaints. Anemia is also common. Once GFR declines to less than about 15, most people begin to experience the symptoms of kidney failure such as intermittent vomiting, abnormal or metallic taste, weight loss, fatigue during the day and insomnia at night, restless legs, and lethargy. At this stage, progressive reductions in insulin and oral diabetes medications are necessary to prevent hypoglycemia because less insulin is eliminated by the kidneys.

End-stage renal disease (ESRD)

After months to years of renal insufficiency or chronic kidney disease, kidney function decreases to the point where life is no longer possible without renal replacement therapy. Untreated ESRD may induce major swelling of the abdomen and fluid collection into the sac surrounding the heart, thereby limiting its ability to pump blood. Muscle cramps and even death may occur when blood potassium rises because potassium cannot be excreted in the urine. High blood potassium levels affect heart function. Patients may have convulsions. Uremia, Greek for "urine in the blood," is the term applied to ESRD in its last stages. Dialysis and kidney transplant can reverse all the signs of uremia.

What Happens When Your Kidneys Do Not Work as They Should?

When kidney function in both kidneys falls below about 25% of normal for age, sex, and body size, you develop uremia. Nitrogen-containing compounds build up in your blood and tissues. Subsequently, edema (excess fluid in your tissues) can be seen and felt in your legs, beneath the skin, and around your eyes. Edema occurs because you are not excreting as much water as you should in your urine. This causes your blood pressure to go up. Hypertension (high blood pressure) is very common in people with diabetes or uremia.

What Can We Do to Slow or Prevent Diabetic Nephropathy?

Several studies done in England, Japan, and the United States found that kidney injury can be prevented or slowed by controlling high blood pressure and maintaining near-normal blood glucose levels. Eating a balanced diet that is lower in fats, cholesterol, and protein will also help. There is evidence that cigarette smoking increases the pace of diabetic kidney disease.

Controlling hypertension

Hypertension (high blood pressure) significantly escalates the progression of diabetic nephropathy and other complications. Early detection and effective treatment of hypertension decrease protein leakage into urine and help slow the rate of deterioration of renal function. Your target blood pressure should be lower than 130/80 mm Hg. If you have urine protein loss higher than 1 gram a day, your blood pressure levels should be lower than 125/75 mm Hg. In fact, anyone with diabetes who also has microalbuminuria or proteinuria should be treated with certain blood pressure–lowering drugs, particularly an ACE inhibitor or A2 receptor blocker or both, even when they do not have hypertension. At every stage of diabetic nephropathy, having normal blood pressure not only is advisable, but is the mainstay of successful therapy.

Improved diet

Eating less protein may help. Current guidelines suggest limiting daily protein intake to 0.8–1 gram per kilogram of body weight. It is also important to have a diet low in saturated fats and cholesterol. You may want to change your diet to unsaturated fats and to take blood cholesterol–lowering medication. A dietician can help you with dietary requirements.

Blood glucose control

Lessons learned over the past 25 years demonstrate that keeping blood glucose levels normal helps prevent or slow the progression of kidney complications for people with type 1 and 2 diabetes. Shoot for an A1C level below 7.0 as advised by the American Diabetes Association.

What Else Can Harm Your Kidneys?

Over-the-counter drugs such as ibuprofen and naproxen may injure your kidneys when taken in excess. Some antibiotic, cancer, and psychiatric drugs prescribed by your doctors can also harm your kidneys. When your renal function is already reduced, the risk of damage from those drugs is greater. Always remember to ask your physician and pharmacist whether a drug you are going to take could possibly damage your kidneys. You and your doctors must weigh the potential harm against the potential benefit of every drug you take. Frequently, there are safer substitutes for most of these medicines.

When the dye used for X-ray studies—angiograms, angio-plasties, or CT scans—is injected into your vein or artery, it carries a risk of acute kidney failure starting within one day. Although this condition is usually reversible, sometimes it requires a period of dialysis. If dyes must be urgently used, you can be given intravenous fluids before and after the procedure to decrease the likelihood of acute renal failure.

Several clinicians report that metformin may create a dangerous condition called lactic acidosis (increased blood level of a chemical called lactic acid) in people with acute or chronic kidney disease. Consequently, you should avoid metformin if you are on dialysis or have less-than-normal kidney function, or have your regimen suspended if you are scheduled to receive dye for X-ray studies.

Finally, it should be noted that your own bladder can harm your kidneys. Some people with diabetes may develop a condition called neurogenic bladder. It means diabetes has damaged nerves to your bladder, preventing urine from emptying normally and causing urine to back up to the kidneys, producing damage. Infection of the urine is common in people with neurogenic bladder. The symptoms may be burning when urinating and, in severe cases, fever.

What Should You Do if ESRD Happens to You?

Until its later stages, diabetic nephropathy is silent, meaning it has no symptoms. Other parts of the body harmed by diabetic complications as kidney function declines may divert your attention from the presence of ESRD. You may become sleepless, apprehensive, and depressed when you realize that you are faced with what seems to an unending maze of doctors, procedures, and problems with other major organs. Medical expenses and lost wages often impose a huge financial stress on family members. At this point, a medical team captain serving as patient advocate, physician coordinator, and friendly advisor can make the difference for you. Your kidney doctor will help you decide when you need to start renal replacement therapy (Table 17-1). This decision is based on your medical condition and nutritional health, and on how much renal function you have left.

What Is the Treatment for ESRD?

ESRD is treated by repeated dialysis or a kidney transplant (Table 17-2).

What Is Dialysis?

There are two types of dialysis used to treat kidney failure—hemodialysis and peritoneal dialysis. Hemodialysis is a process that uses a machine (an artificial kidney) to remove the waste products and fluids that have accumulated in your body. There must be a connection to a blood vessel, usually in your forearm or arm, permitting blood to flow to and from the artificial kidney. Typically, hemodialysis is performed three times a week for 4 or 5 hours each time. Hemodialysis can be performed in hospitals, in dedicated dialysis centers, or at home. With home dialysis, you and a partner are trained in all the steps of the procedure. Home dialysis provides the freedom to plan treatments to fit your own schedule. Recently, a new schedule of dialysis has been introduced—daily hemodialysis. The plan calls for six treatments a week, each for 2 or 3 hours. Another schedule calls for dialysis at night while sleeping. This "nocturnal dialysis" is done at home for 6 to 8 hours. Several reports indicate that anemia is less frequent and blood pressure lower in people receiving daily or nocturnal dialysis. Unfortunately, daily dialysis is not yet widely available.

Table 17-2. Choices for Uremic Patients with Diabetes

Variable	Peritoneal Dialysis	Hemodialysis	Kidney Transplant
Other serious disease	No limitation	No limitation	Not for patients with cardio-vascular disease
Geriatric patient	No limitation	No limitation	Determined by program
Complete rehabilitation	Unlikely, persistent problems	Unlikely	Common as long as transplant functions
Death rate	Higher than for nondia-betic patients	Higher than for nondiabetic patients	About the same as nondiabetic patients
First-year survival	About 80%	About 80%	Greater than 90%
Survival to second decade	Undetermined	Increasing but rare	About 1 in 5
Progression of complications	Continuing attention to other conditions is essential	Persistent problems	Probably reduced in type 1 diabetes by functioning pancreas and kidney; fewer complications than in dialy-sis patients
Special advantage	Can be self-performed; avoids swings in solute and intravascular volume level	Can be self-per-formed; efficient in removing water and solutes in hours	Cures uremia; freedom to travel
Disadvantage	Peritonitis; long hours of treatment; increased hospitalization rate-	Access complica-tions	Cosmetic disfigurement, hypertension, induced malignancy
Patient acceptance	Variable, usual compli-ance with passive toler-ance for regimen	Variable, noncompli-ance with diet and medicines	Enthusiastic during periods of good allograft function; exalted when pancreas proffers euglycemia
Relative cost	Has been used to cir-cumvent initial outlay for dialysis equipment required by hemodialysis; expense of dialysate is about the same as a kid-ney transplant	Less expensive than kidney transplant in first year; subse-quent years most expensive due to professional fees and cost of supplies	Pancreas + kidney engraft-ment most; after first year, kidney transplant alone is lowest cost option

Peritoneal dialysis, a technique based on cycling a rinsing fluid (dialysate) into the abdomen several times a day, removes wastes from the blood in small blood vessels located in the membrane lin-ing your abdominal cavity. After your physician inserts a catheter in the abdominal cavity, dialysis fluid or dialysate can be put into and drained from the abdomen at regular intervals. Continuous ambulatory peritoneal dialysis (CAPD) is the most common form of peritoneal dialysis. During CAPD, approximately 2 liters of dialysate are infused and drained every 4–6 hours by the patient. Some patients prefer continuous cyclic peritoneal dialysis (CCPD), in which dialysate infusion and drainage are carried out by a machine while patients are sleeping. Both CAPD and CCPD can be performed at home.

Motivated and well-trained individuals are very successful with peritoneal dialysis. The advantages of CAPD are freedom from a machine, rapid training, minimal cardiovascular stress, and no need for an anti-clotting drug called heparin. The main drawback of peritoneal dialysis is the need to pay constant attention to fluid exchange in order to lower the risk of peritonitis (infection of the lining of the abdomen). Recurring infection can seriously damage the lining of the abdomen and decrease the effectiveness of peritoneal dialysis.

Maintenance hemodialysis is the most widely used ESRD treatment in America. About 76% of people with diabetes and ESRD receiving uremia therapy are treated with hemodialysis, but only 5% are on peritoneal dialysis. The remaining 18% have a functioning kidney transplant. Although home hemodialysis is, by consensus, preferred to dialysis at a medical facilitiy, a very small number of people with diabetes select this form of treatment.

Dialysis generally does not have the excellent outcomes one can get from a kidney transplant. Current statistics show that about half of the people with diabetes who start on hemodialysis die within 4 years, often from a heart attack. By contrast, more than half of those who receive a live donor kidney transplant are alive after a decade. The good news is that both the rate of ESRD in persons with diabetes and the death rate in those with diabetes and ESRD are continuously falling.

This chapter was written by Eli Friedman, MD.

Other Complications

18

Gastrointestinal Complications

Case Study

Mr. T is a 67-year-old man who has had diabetes for over 30 years. He currently takes long-acting NPH insulin in the morning and at bedtime, and rapid-acting insulin aspart 5–10 minutes before meals. He has some diabetic complications, including mild retinopathy and peripheral neuropathy. His diabetes is poorly controlled, and he has many high and low glucose readings. Sometimes he wakes up with high glucose for no reason (at other times his blood glucose is in the target range of 80–130 mg/dL). He also has noted that his glucose sometimes drops very low 1–2 hours after giving himself insulin and eating a meal.

At a clinic visit, his doctor looks at his glucose readings and asks him if he has any nausea, vomiting, or abdominal pain. Mr. T replies, "No, but I do have a little bloating sometimes." His doctor wonders if he might have a stomach problem called gastroparesis, which slows the rate at which food is emptied from the stomach to the intestines. She tells him that he needs more tests.

Case Study

Mr. RZ is a 59-year-old man with type 2 diabetes who has had diarrhea for the last 3 to 4 years. Sometimes he has loose, watery stools with no trace of blood. He does not have stomach pain or cramps.

The diarrhea does not seem to be related to any particular food. He is not taking a medication that causes diarrhea. Occasionally, he does not feel a bowel movement coming and soils his underwear. His primary care provider tells him that he may have a problem called diabetic diarrhea and needs further testing.

What Is Gastroparesis?

When a person chews and swallows food, it travels from the mouth to the food tube (esophagus) to the stomach. The muscles of the stomach grind food into small particles and push it into the intestines (gut). There, muscles also squeeze, moving partially digested material along. Chemicals from the pancreas help to break food down further so that it can be absorbed into the bloodstream. The body then stores it or uses it for energy.

There are nerves that control the muscles described above. In poorly-controlled diabetes, high blood glucose levels damage these nerves and slow the rate at which food is emptied from the stomach into the gut. When this problem is severe, it is called diabetic gastroparesis. There are other causes of slowed gastric (stomach) emptying besides diabetes. Many pain medications, low potassium levels, thyroid disease, and some diseases of the nerves can all lead to gastroparesis. How common is gastroparesis in people with diabetes? Some studies suggest that 30–50% of people with long-standing diabetes may have it.

How Do You Know if You Have Gastroparesis?

Some people with gastroparesis have no symptoms at all. Others have frequent nausea and bloating after they eat. They may complain of feeling full after a few bites of food. Sometimes, they also vomit. Lots of high and low blood glucose levels may be a sign of gastroparesis. Since it takes longer for food to move along the gut and be absorbed into the bloodstream, blood glucose levels rise many hours after meals. People with gastroparesis may have low blood glucose levels a few hours after taking rapid-acting insulin because the insulin is absorbed by the body faster than food.

Besides gastroparesis, there are other medical conditions (like a stomach ulcer or acid reflux) that cause stomach pain, nausea, and vomiting. If your provider suspects that you have gastroparesis but wants to make sure that you do not have other problems, he or she may send you for a barium swallow or an endoscopy. In the first test, you swallow barium contrast material, and X-rays show abnormal areas in your esophagus or stomach. An endoscopy is a special test where a doctor gives you a medication to make you sleepy and then inserts a small tube with a camera down your throat to your stomach. It is a way of looking directly at the lining of your esophagus and stomach to see if it is inflamed or has an ulcer.

There are special tests that can be used to look at the way the stomach empties food. In one standard test, you eat a meal (usually scrambled eggs) that has been labeled with a small amount of radioactive tracer chemical. The amount of radiation used in this test is the same as that in a plain X-ray of the stomach. The level of radioactivity in the stomach is then measured at different times. The test tells your health care provider how much of the meal is emptied by your stomach after a given amount of time. In a second type of test, you eat food labeled with a tracer called carbon 13. The labeled food is emptied from the stomach, absorbed from the intestine, and processed by the liver, and a small remaining part is transported to the lungs. Carbon 13 is then measured in your breath as you exhale.

How Do You Treat Gastroparesis?

If you have gastroparesis, you should work with your healthcare team to control your blood glucose levels. You should try to eat small, frequent low-fat meals and avoid foods that are difficult to digest, such as legumes, lentils, and citrus fruits. There are some medications that increase the rate of gastric emptying. Metoclopramide (Reglan) is taken one-half hour before meals and also treats nausea. Its main side effects are dizziness and, less commonly, abnormal movements or muscle tone. Erythromycin is often prescribed as an antibiotic but it can also be used for gastroparesis. It is given three times a day, and its main side effect is stomach cramps. However, it can also cause changes in the conduction of the heart electrical system. Check with your doctor before taking erythromycin. Tegaserod (Zelnorm) speeds up gastric emptying and the movement of food through the small intestines. It can cause diarrhea. There are a few similar medicines available in other countries outside of the United States.

It is often helpful to take a medicine that treats nausea specifically, such as promethazine (Phenergan), prochlorperazine (Compazine), or ondansetron (Zofran). People with severe nausea and vomiting may benefit from electrical stimulation of the stomach (gastric pacemaker). In a few severe cases, medicines, diet, and other treatments do not help, and the patient with gastroparesis may be malnourished and lose weight. He or she may then need to have a feeding tube placed. A J-tube (the "J" is for jejunostomy) is a more permanent tube that goes through the skin to the small intestine and is used for feeding. If you have type 1 diabetes and severe gastroparesis with nausea and vomiting, and become dehydrated, you are at risk for a life-threatening condition called diabetic ketoacidosis. It is important to check your glucose frequently and to seek medical attention immediately.

What Are Some Other Common Problems that Cause Stomach Pain in People with Diabetes?

People with diabetes may be at increased risk of forming gallstones, which can cause right upper abdominal pain after meals. Poor circulation in the gut can also lead to abdominal pain and is a concern as people grow older and develop blockages in other blood vessels (of the heart, neck, and legs). One type of diabetes-related nerve damage (diabetic neuropathy) can affect the nerves in the chest or abdominal wall. This can cause pain that seems to wrap around the abdomen from front to back.

Heartburn may be more common in people with diabetes compared to those without diabetes. A ring-like muscle (the LES, or lower esophageal sphincter) separates the esophagus and stomach. When food reaches the stomach, it closes and stops food and acid from backing up into the esophagus. When the muscle is weak, there is a backup of food and acid that is called gastroesophageal reflux (GERD). GERD can lead to a burning feeling in the throat and chest after eating or when lying down. It can also leave a sour taste in your mouth all the time.

How Do You Treat Acid Reflux?

If you have the symptoms described above, your healthcare provider may diagnose you with GERD and may suggest that you change your diet and lifestyle in the following ways.

- Stop drinking alcohol, coffee, soda, and other caffeine-containing beverages.
- Avoid foods that increase acid, like chocolate, tomatoes, and spicy meals.
- Do not lie down less than 2 hours after a meal.
- Raise your head on two pillows when you do lie down.

GERD can also be treated with medications. If you have heartburn only occasionally, you may feel better with antacids and lifestyle changes. If heartburn bothers you several times a week, then your provider may recommend an H2 blocker, which decreases stomach acid production, or a proton pump inhibitor, which is a very strong acid blocker.

If You Have Heartburn, When Do You Need More Tests?

In GERD, acid can irritate the lining of the throat and voice box (larynx), causing a sore throat and/or hoarse voice. If these problems do not get better when you treat your heartburn, your health care provider may refer you to a head and neck specialist. If you have difficulty swallowing, you may need a test to look for a blockage in your esophagus. If you have burning or aching in the upper part of your stomach on a regular basis, you may need an endoscopy to look for an ulcer.

What Are Some Causes of Diarrhea in People with Diabetes?

Studies have show that 4–22% of people with diabetes have diarrhea. People with diabetic diarrhea (diarrhea caused by diabetes) may have loose watery stools some times, and normal stools or constipation at other times. They do not have much stomach pain.

Diabetes can cause diarrhea by damaging the nerves to the gut and possibly by increasing the growth of bacteria in the gut. Metformin, a diabetes medication, is a common cause of diarrhea. Large amounts of sorbitol, an artificial sweetener used in diet drinks, can also cause loose stools. Other causes of diarrhea in people with and without diabetes include medications, lactose intolerance, infections, thyroid disease, diseases in which there is inflammation of the gut (ulcerative colitis or Crohn's disease), diseases of the pancreas, and celiac sprue. Type 1 diabetes increases the chance of developing celiac sprue, a disease in which the body's own immune system reacts to foods that contain gluten, such as wheat, barley, and rye.

Blood tests and stool tests may be necessary in order to find the cause of diarrhea. It is also important to review your diet and medications (including those sold over the counter) with your provider. In some cases, a healthcare provider may recommend a test called a colonoscopy, in which the patient is made sleepy with a medication and a tube with a camera at the end is inserted into the anus in order to look at the lining of the colon.

How Do You Treat Diabetic Diarrhea?

Antibiotics may be used to treat the growth of bacteria in the gut. Other medications that treat diarrhea include loperamide (Imodium), codeine, and diphenoxylate (Lomotil). If these do not work, clonidine (Catapres), which is sometimes used to treat high blood pressure, can be used to decrease the number of stools. The side effects of clonidine are dry mouth and dizziness. If other treatments do not work, octreotide (Sandostatin, a special injectable medication) may be helpful. When people with diabetes start octreotide, they need to watch for changes in their glucose. If there is another medical condition (besides diabetes) causing diarrhea, then it should be treated. If a medication is causing it, the medication can be stopped. People with lactose intolerance can avoid dairy products or take an enzyme called Lactaid. The treatment of celiac sprue is a gluten-free diet (avoiding foods that contain wheat, barley, and rye).

What Is Fecal Incontinence?

People with diabetic diarrhea may not only have loose stools but also may not feel any warning when a bowel movement is coming. As a result, they may leak stool and soil their underwear. Diabetes may affect the nerves that control the muscles of the rectum (the last part of the intestines) and the anus (the ring of muscle at the end of the rectum). When these nerves are damaged, the muscles may lose tone, and it may not be possible to control a bowel movement. This is called fecal incontinence. On rectal exam, the anus may have reduced muscle tone, and there may be loss of the anal wink reflex (the anus normally squeezes when you stroke the skin around it). There are more complicated tests to examine this problem, such as anorectal manometry, in which a balloon is inflated in the rectum, and the body's ability to feel and squeeze are tested. There are ways of treating fecal incontinence by improving feeling in the rectum and retraining the muscles of the anus.

What Is Constipation?

Constipation affects many people with and without diabetes. People use "constipation" to describe many problems with bowel movements: straining, lumpy or hard stools, feeling "blocked" in the rectum, fewer than three bowel movements a week, needing laxatives to have a bowel movement, among others. In general, food moves more slowly through the large intestine, or colon, when you are constipated. The main causes of constipation are diseases affecting nerves (diabetes, Parkinson's disease, multiple sclerosis, spinal cord injury), thyroid disease, low potassium levels, and drugs (pain medications, some antidepressants, iron, some blood pressure medications).

How Do You Treat Constipation?

The treatment of constipation involves fluids, dietary changes, and medications. Drinking lots of water, exercising, and sitting on the toilet 30 minutes after meals may help. Dietary fiber speeds up the rate at which food travels in the gut and is found in food such as bran, prunes, apricots, many vegetables (spinach, cabbage), and many beans. Laxatives such as psyllium (Konsyl, Metamucil) and methylcellulose (Citrucel) absorb water and increase the "bulk" of bowel movements; the usual adult dose is 1 tablespoon in water or juice two to three times a day, and the main side effects are gas and bloating. Docusate (Colace) is a stool softener that can be taken once or twice daily. Bisacodyl (Dulcolax) and senna (Senna, senokot) change the way that salts are transported by the gut lining and increase the movement of food through the gut. When overused, they can cause low potassium levels. Castor oil has long been used to treat constipation but is not recommended because it can cause problems with the body's fluid and salt contents.

Many laxatives can be obtained over the counter. Lactulose requires a prescription and works by dragging water, salts, and stool out with undigested glucose. Sorbitol acts in a similar way and is less expensive. Both medications can cause bloating and can raise blood glucose in people with diabetes. Polyethylene glycol solutions can also improve the texture and frequency of bowel movements. Rectal suppositories (bisacodyl or glycerin) and enemas (mineral oil or Fleet's phospho soda) may be effective in treating severe constipation. Phosphate-containing enemas (such as Fleet's) should be avoided if you have severe kidney disease. Some people with severe constipation may require manual disimpaction, in which a trained medical provider inserts his or her finger into the rectum and gently breaks down very hard stool. Tegaserod (Zelnorm) is one of the newest medications approved for the treatment of irritable bowel syndrome and constipation. A few people with very severe constipation may require surgery.

When Do You Need More Tests for Constipation?

If you have constipation that does not respond to lifestyle changes and first-line medications, your health care provider may order one of several tests to look at your intestines. A plain X-ray of the abdomen can show whether you have stool in the intestines. A barium enema is a test in which X-rays are taken after you have been given an enema containing a chemical called barium. A proctosigmoidoscopy is a short test in which a doctor uses a flexible tube with a light to look at your rectum and the last part of your intestines. Colonoscopy, rectal exam, and anorectal manometry are also options. In a "colonic transit" study, you swallow markers, and X-rays are taken as they move through the intestine.

What Is Fatty Liver Disease?

Nonalcoholic fatty liver disease (NAFLD) is found in most patients with diabetes and obesity (see chapter 19). Most people with NAFLD do not have symptoms. Other people may feel slightly full in the right upper abdomen. Often, elevated liver enzymes on routine blood tests are the first clue that someone has NAFLD, usually prompting more blood tests. A liver ultrasound may also show a fatty liver. NAFLD is common in people with diabetes because it is related to insulin resistance, one of the problems in type 2 diabetes. When you have insulin resistance, your body (especially the liver, muscle, and fat) does not respond normally to insulin.

The treatment of NAFLD is gradual weight loss, approximately 1–2 pounds a week. There are some diabetes medications that may help to decrease liver enzymes and decrease fat in the liver. Gradual weight loss is important, as rapid weight loss may actually worsen the disease.

Conclusion

People with diabetes can develop problems with the stomach and intestines that may or may not be related to the disease itself. Uncontrolled diabetes may damage the nerves that control the muscles of the gastrointestinal tract and thus can affect the rate at which food moves from the mouth to the anus. Common problems are gastroparesis, diabetic diarrhea, fecal incontinence, or constipation. It is important to tell your health care provider about stomach pain, nausea, bloating, diarrhea, and constipation, so that he or she can decide whether you need further testing to look for causes other than diabetes. In most cases, these problems can be treated by changing your lifestyle or by adding and/or stopping medications. In many cases, working to control your diabetes can also make a difference.

This chapter was written by Nalini Singh, MD.

19

Fatty Liver and NASH

What Are Fatty Liver and NASH?

Fatty liver disease is a condition where there is an excess accumulation of fat within the liver (more than 5–10% of a liver's weight). There are two main forms of fatty liver:

1. Fatty liver where there is only excessive fat deposition in the liver
2. Steatohepatitis, where there is injury to the liver along with fat accumulation, which can lead to further damage or cirrhosis of the liver

Both fatty liver and steatohepatitis can be caused by excessive alcohol consumption. In all other cases, it is called nonalcoholic fatty liver (NAFL) or nonalcoholic steatohepatitis (NASH). Both conditions are described under the umbrella term nonalcoholic fatty liver disease (NAFLD).

NASH is associated with liver-damaging inflammation and sometimes, the formation of fibrous tissue. An inflamed liver may become scarred and hardened over time and progress to either irreversible liver scarring known as liver cirrhosis, or to liver cancer. While NAFL itself rarely causes cirrhosis of the liver, the presence of excess fat in the liver increases the risk of developing diabetes, high blood pressure, and hardening of the arteries.

How Common Are Fatty Liver and NASH?

Fatty liver is the most common liver disease in the United States, and NASH is one of the leading causes of liver cirrhosis in America. Overall, NAFLD occurs in nearly 1/3 of those living in the United States, and 1 out of every 20 to 30 Americans has NASH. For those who are overweight or obese, the rate is even higher.

Who Is at Risk?

NAFLD can occur in all age and ethnic groups. However, those of Hispanic origin have the highest risk. On the other hand, African Americans have a low risk of getting NAFLD. People tend to have a higher risk of developing NAFLD if they have certain conditions such as:

- Obesity
- Diabetes
- High cholesterol and triglycerides
- Rapid weight loss, especially in those who were obese beforehand
- Malnutrition
- Use of certain drugs (see box)

Some Common Drugs Associated with Fatty Liver

• Estrogen	• Tamoxifen
• Methotrexate	• Corticosteroids
• Amiodarone	• Diltiazem
• Isoniazid	• Coumadin
• Valproic acid	• Nifedipine

Several of these conditions often occur together, especially obesity, diabetes, and high blood fats (cholesterol and triglycerides).

However, some people may develop fatty liver even without obesity and diabetes. In Western countries, fatty liver has become a growing problem, though one that is not often discussed. Some studies have shown that close to 20–40% of people who are overweight will develop NASH.

What Is Insulin Resistance and How Is It Related to Fatty Liver?

Insulin resistance is caused most commonly by obesity. However, genetics and immune processes in your body are also possible causes. This condition occurs when your body becomes resistant to the effects of insulin and is therefore unable to utilize insulin properly, resulting in high blood glucose levels and an increased metabolism of stored body fat. Insulin resistance is often measured from a fasting blood sample by the levels of glucose and insulin. Insulin resistance leads to changes in the liver that affect the regulation of fat production, degradation, and secretion, which all contributes to the progression of fatty liver.

What Are the Symptoms of Fatty Liver and NASH?

Most people have no symptoms. When symptoms do occur, they usually include fatigue, malaise, weakness, or pain and discomfort in their abdomen, especially in the upper right side. This pain is very often described as dull and aching, without a predictable pattern. It is not an intense, sudden, and severe pain, as might occur with, for example, gallstones. The abdominal pain in NAFLD and NASH is thought to be due to the stretching of the liver covering (capsule) when the liver enlarges and/or when there is inflammation in the liver.

When liver cirrhosis occurs, a person may experience yellow eyes and skin (jaundice) or itchiness (pruritis). Some symptoms of chronic liver disease may also start appearing, such as abdominal swelling, enlarged liver/spleen, and mental changes. These are usually signs of very advanced disease and occur late in the course of the disease.

What Are the Complications of Fatty Liver and NASH and Why Should You Worry?

NASH may progress to fibrosis (an excess growth of connective tissue in the liver) and lead to end-stage liver disease, a complete failure of the liver that can only be treated by a liver transplant. Cirrhosis develops in 20% of cases, which can also lead to end-stage liver disease and is associated with an increased risk of liver cancer.

How Are Fatty Liver and NASH Diagnosed?

Most people are diagnosed with fatty liver when they receive abnormal liver-test results that have been done for unrelated issues. Sometimes, the liver is found to be slightly enlarged during a routine physical check-up. To rule out another type of liver disease, more blood tests, an ultrasound, a computed tomography (CT) scan, or a magnetic resonance imaging (MRI) test may be indicated. A liver ultrasound may suggest the presence of a fatty liver, but it cannot rule out inflammation and fibrosis scarring. CT scan and MRI are better suited to evaluating the degree of fat infiltration, but these tests are more expensive, and neither CT scan nor MRI can distinguish NAFL from NASH. The only definite way to find out for certain is to get a liver biopsy, a procedure in which a needle is inserted through the skin to remove a small piece of the liver.

A diagnosis of NAFLD and NASH is made based on two conditions:

1. Evidence that the condition is not caused by alcohol abuse
2. A liver biopsy demonstrating fatty infiltration with or without presence of inflammation, cell injury, and scar tissue

The liver biopsy is the essential piece of the diagnosis. Without a liver biopsy, your doctor can presume that you have NAFLD, but cannot prove it.

What Can a Liver Biopsy Show and When Should It Be Done?

In order to precisely diagnose fatty liver and NASH and determine just how severe the condition is, there is still no substitute for performing a liver biopsy. Only by examining the liver tissue under a microscope and noting fat along with inflammation and damaged liver cells can one determine whether the condition is NASH (without the damage and inflammation, it's fatty liver).

Severe NASH would indicate that the risk of developing cirrhosis later on is high. A biopsy is also the only way to assess how much scar tissue there is before the development of cirrhosis. Therefore, a liver biopsy can provide important information about outcome. At the same time, it can exclude the presence of other liver diseases.

A liver biopsy involves identifying the exact location of the liver, often by ultrasound or by percussion. The site is then cleaned, and a local anesthetic is applied. A needle is then inserted into the liver, and a small core of tissue is removed. The procedure takes about ten minutes, and most patients are sent home the same day. It is a relatively safe procedure, with discomfort at the site of needle insertion and shoulder discomfort the most common complications. Rarely, there can be bleeding from the liver that can be severe and require blood transfusion or surgery (the risk for this is about one in one thousand).

At this time, there are no specific drug treatments available for NAFLD or NASH. In other words, if you are obese and/or have diabetes, you will be encouraged to lose weight by diet and exercise, regardless of your biopsy result. However, weight-loss surgery (bariatric surgery) has recently been shown to improve liver tests in severely obese individuals and improve NASH. Also, several drugs are currently in clinical trials for NASH.

In general, the decision to perform a biopsy usually requires your doctor to assess your specific circumstances. Knowing the state and severity of your condition can significantly affect your treatment and prognosis.

How Are Fatty Liver and NASH Treated?

Since there is no established drug therapy of NAFLD/NASH, treatment generally focuses on controlling the risk factors (obesity, insulin resistance, diabetes) associated with the condition. Fatty liver is not irreversible. Weight loss through exercise and diet, along with good diabetes control, will help reverse fatty infiltration of the liver and improve your condition.

Weight loss and exercise

Weight loss has been widely studied and has been shown to improve not only biochemical results but also liver biopsy findings. Those who are overweight and have fatty liver should aim for a target weight loss of 10% of their current weight at a rate of 1–2 pounds per week. In general, high- to moderate-intensity exercise, such as 30-minute walks three to five times a week, is recommended. You should also try to incorporate moderate activity into your everyday life (for example, climb the stairs instead of taking the elevator, walk instead of driving your car). It is important to consult your physician before starting on an exercise program to ensure that your heart and overall medical condition are stable enough to handle a given degree of physical activity.

Weight loss surgery

For those who are significantly obese and have not been able to lose weight through dieting and lifestyle modifications, weight loss surgery (bariatric surgery) is an option. Surgery has been shown to reduce fat in the liver and improve diabetes and related complications. Bariatric surgery is suggested for those who have a body mass index (BMI, see page 371) greater than 40 or for those with a BMI greater than 35 and obesity-related complications.

Diet

To lose weight and improve NAFLD/NASH, you will more than likely need to lower the number of calories, fats, and saturated fats you eat. Working with a registered dietitian (RD) to craft a weight-loss meal plan can be extremely helpful.

Medications

Studies on lipid-lowering drugs and antioxidants have been some-what promising, though no obvious improvement in liver biopsy findings has been seen. Diabetes medications that improve insulin resistance, such as metformin and piaglitazone, may help fatty liver by improving one of the factors that leads to fatty liver. However, no long-term study has shown this definitively, and more research is needed. At this time, there are no medications specifically designed to treat NAFLD or NASH.

Conclusions

NAFLD and NASH affect millions of Americans and are strongly associated with obesity and insulin resistance. These are serious diseases with serious consequences and it is very important to detect NAFLD and NASH early, especially if you have diabetes, are overweight, or both. Speak with your health care team about screening for liver conditions. Early detection is the absolute best way to ensure you avoid serious and life-threatening complications later on.

This chapter was written by Arun Sanyal, MD, and Onpan Cheung, MD, MPH.

20

Men's Sexual Health

Diabetes can affect blood flow and nerve function throughout the body, so it's no surprise that the penis is just as prone to problems as the feet and internal organs. In fact, a common complication of diabetes in men is erectile dysfunction (ED), the consistent inability to attain and maintain an erection for satisfactory sexual intercourse (an occasional problem is not necessarily ED). As many as 80% of men with diabetes develop ED, compared with 25% of similarly aged men who do not have diabetes. Indeed, men who have had diabetes for more than 10 years have a more than 50% chance of having ED. It also affects those with diabetes at a younger age. While most non-diabetes-related ED affects men over the age of 60, those with diabetes often begin to note ED in their 30s.

What Are the Symptoms of ED?

There are many symptoms of ED, and some men may have more than one symptom simultaneously. Symptoms of ED can include:

- A less rigid penis
- Short-duration erections
- Premature ejaculation
- Retrograde ejaculation, where sperm is redirected into the bladder instead of out through the urethra

What Is Normal Erectile Function?

The penis is composed of two erectile cylinders called corpora cavernosa that run the entire length of the penis. The corpora cavernosa are contained within a thick, fibrous tissue called the tunica albuginea. Within this tunica albuginea, the erectile bodies are made up of spongy tissue composed of smooth muscle fibrous tissue vascular spaces called lacunar spaces, veins, and arteries. The urinary channel, or urethra, through which ejaculation occurs courses beneath the corpora cavernosa and is surrounded by spongy tissue termed the corpus spongiosum.

For an erection to occur, stimulation from the central nervous sytem, whether psychological or physical, trigger local nerves causing the smooth muscles of the corpus cavernosa to relax. When these muscles relax, there is an increase in blood flow to the penis and a decrease in outflow of blood from the penis, causing pressure within the penis to produce an erection. When stimulation is diminished, the smooth muscle relaxation reverses, and blood flows out, producing a flaccid penis.

Erectile dysfunction is caused by any interruption of the events leading to normal erectile response. This can include nervous system problems, such as psychological difficulties, depression, head trauma, strokes, and medications. More commonly, however, the problem is a vascular one. Diabetes, arthrosclerosis, hypercholesterolemia, hypertension, and other vascular risk factors can be responsible for decreasing erectile function. Lifestyle issues such as smoking, obesity, and sleep apnea can cause problems. Hormonal factors, such as decreased testosterone or thyroid dysfunction, can also lead to ED. In fact, as many as 40% of those with diabetes who complain of ED may have decreased testosterone levels.

Surgical procedures can also produce ED by injuring the nerves and arteries supplying the penis. These surgical procedures, including radical prostatectomy, radical surgery for bladder cancer, and radical surgery for colon cancer, can interfere with erectile response after surgery. Radiation therapy for these same conditions can likewise produce ED.

Medications can lead to ED as well. The most common culprits are antidepressants, antihypertensives, antihistamines, and tranquilizers. Speak with your doctor about your medications. Choosing blood pressure medications such as hydrochlorothiazide may worsen ED, while alpha-blockers, ACE inhibitors, calcium channel blockers, and A2R inhibitors can preserve or even improve erectile function.

How Do You Diagnose ED?

Patient history is the most important part of the diagnosis of ED. It is important for your doctor to ask specific questions regarding ED, including when it started, descriptions of what's happening, predisposing factors and medications, associated diseases, relationship issues, and any psychological problems. It is important to know if you have erections in the morning, while you sleep, or during masturbation. Your doctor may also ask about premature ejaculation, as it is often mistaken for ED or may occur with ED. Abnormal penile curvature, such as that associated with Peyronie's disease, should also be investigated.

Your doctor should also conduct an examination of your testicles, penis, prostate, secondary sexual characteristics, and vascular supply. A prostate problem is often associated with ED in younger men and a thorough prostatic examination is critical.

Lab work is also helpful. This should include blood glucose, A1C, blood lipids, creatinine, liver enzymes, and testosterone evaluation. While low testosterone is often associated with decreased libido, low libido is not necessarily a sign of low testosterone, and despite a history of normal libido, testosterone screening is important if you have ED.

Other studies can be performed to further evaluate patients with ED. Nocturnal penile tumescence monitoring (NPT), which measures erections while you sleep, may be helpful in ruling out some psychological causes of ED. Similarly, Doppler penile ultrasound may help identify decreased penile blood flow abnormalities. If you have a strong history of sleep apnea, sleep studies may be helpful. Treating sleep apnea may improve testosterone, improve depression, and thus improve erectile function.

How Do You Treat ED?

There are a number of options available to treat ED, including medications, injection therapy, urethral suppositories, vacuum devices, hormone therapy, and surgery.

Oral medications

The treatment of ED was revolutionized by the introduction of sildenafil citrate (Viagra) in 1998. After more than 10 years of use, this medication and its successors have been proven effective and safe. Viagra, vardenafil (Levitra), and tadalafil (Cialis) are all in a class of drugs called phosphodiesterase type 5 (PDE5) inhibitors. PDE5 inhibitors are oral medications that enhance the smooth muscle relaxation in the penis, thus improving erectile function. Sildenafil and vardenafil can improve erectile function for up to 8 hours, while tadalafil can be effective for as long as 36 hours. PDE5 inhibitors may be taken daily. However, if you have a severe heart condition that requires nitroglycerine or nitroglycerine-type drug, you shouldn't take a PDE5 inhibitor. Other side effects common to the three PDE5 inhibitors include headache, facial flushing, nasal congestion, acid reflux, muscle pain, and back pain.

Injection therapy and urethral suppositories

Medications don't always work, however. If you have severe vascular or anatomic disease, you may need to consider other options, including injection therapy or urethral suppositories. Urethral suppositories are small tablets you place approximately 2 centimeters into your urethra with an applicator and activate by massaging your penis. While the oral ED medication requires sexual stimulation for activity, injection therapy and suppository therapy produce erections without sexual stimulation. Erections begin 10–15 minutes after applying these therapies and usually subside within 45–60 minutes. Side effects include penile aching, prolonged erections, and penile scarring, the last two effects being quite rare. However, you can use these therapies if you are taking nitroglycerine, making them attractive options for those who can't use oral medications for ED.

Vacuum erection devices

Using a vacuum erection device (VED) is also an effective ED treatment if you do not respond to, or cannot take, oral medications. These devices are placed on the penis and resemble a syringe barrel. They provide an erection by creating a vacuum. Blood is drawn into the penis, causing engorgement and expansion of the venous channels. To maintain the erection, you will slide a tight elastic ring from the base of the vacuum cylinder onto the base of your penis, maintaining the blood within your penis during erection and intercourse. While these devices may be useful for some patients, the constriction ring is often uncomfortable and inhibits normal ejaculation.

Hormone therapy

Testosterone deficiency is common in men with diabetes and, if you're suffering from ED, your testosterone levels should be evaluated. Getting testosterone into the normal range should improve your response to oral ED medications. If you have testosterone levels of less than 300 ng/dl and symptoms of ED, low libido, low energy, and low strength, you should consider testosterone therapy. Testosterone can be returned to normal with testosterone gel (the most commonly used treatment alternative), injections, long-term injections (available only in Europe), or testosterone patches. There are very few side effects to getting your testosterone into normal ranges. Effects on your prostate can be a concern, however, testosterone replacement therapy has not been shown to cause problems.

Surgery

If the more direct forms of ED therapy are not effect, surgical intervention can produce excellent results. Penile prostheses have been available for the treatment of ED since the mid 1970s, and these devices that have enjoyed great success and high satisfaction rates. The most common device is an inflatable penile prothesis that consists of a pair of cylinders that are inserted surgically along the length of your penis. An incision either above or below the penis can be used to insert the entire device. The two hollow cylinders are connected to a small pump device placed in your scrotal sac. To activate the device, you compress the pump until the two cylinders inflate with a saline solution and provide a rigid, normally functioning erect penis. The erection will be maintained as long as you like and then deflated by pressing the release valve on the pump. The penis then returns to a normal flaccid appearance, allowing you to comfortably wear any kind of clothing and shower in public. This surgery does not affect sensation or ejaculation. Older procedures ran a small risk of infection—a particular problem for men with diabetes—but an antibiotic coating has reduced infection risk to fewer than 1% of patients.

While other surgical procedures have been performed, they are rarely appropriate for those with diabetes. Arterial reconstruction is used in young men who have suffered traumatic blockage of an artery responsible for erections, but because men with diabetes run a much higher risk of cardiovascular problems, these surgical procedures are not recommended. Other surgery options simply do not produce effective, long-term results.

What Is the Future of ED Therapy?

Newer medications and surgeries continue to improve the treatment of ED. However, the future of ED treatment may arrive in the form of gene therapy. A decade of gene therapy research has yielded promising results in animal models and in some early human studies. Advanced human studies are ongoing, and this therapy, which consists of injecting gene therapy into the penis, looks to reinforce those early findings. By restoring vascular damage in the diabetic penis, gene therapy may eventually restore normal erectile function.

Conclusion

If you suffer from ED, it not only affects your own quality of life, but that of your partner and family as well. ED should be taken seriously and treated appropriately. The diagnosis of ED requires careful history, a physical examination, and laboratory studies that include a hormone profile. Once the diagnosis has been established and refined, treatment alternatives available in the 21st century can restore most men to normal erectile function. These treatment alternatives include the three PDE5 inhibitors currently available, urethral suppositories, VEDs, and finally, penile prostheses in those who have not responded to less invasive alternatives. By identifying and evaluating ED, an important part of your life can be restored safely and effectively.

This chapter was written by Culley C. Carson, MD.

21

Women's Sexual Health

Case Study

LO, a 46-year-old woman diagnosed with type 2 diabetes 5 years ago, has always tried to maintain good glucose control. She and her husband have been married 20 years and have three children. Through most of their marriage, they have enjoyed an active sex life. Lately, however, LO no longer initiates sex and finds ways to avoid it. Even when she feels emotionally aroused, she takes a long time to feel physically aroused and then experiences discomfort during intercourse. As a first step, the doctor suggests an over-the-counter vaginal lubricant and that she talk to her husband about what she has been experiencing.

Case Study

BN, a 36-year-old woman who has had type 1 diabetes for 27 years, came to her physician to plan a pregnancy. She had high blood pressure, protein in her urine, high blood glucose levels, and an A1C level of 9.8% (normal range is 6% or less). Her insulin therapy consisted of two insulin injections a day.

BN's blood pressure and glucose levels needed to come down before she became pregnant, and the protein in her urine was too high. Her physician was also concerned about her retinopathy. She was referred to an ophthalmologist for laser therapy. After the treatment stabilized her retinal status she was given the "green light" to plan her pregnancy. For six months, her health care team also helped her with a program of diet, exercise, and medication to bring her blood glucose levels close to normal. A nephrologist also placed BN on an ACE-inhibitor and birth control pills during this period; her blood pressure normalized and proteinuria decreased dramatically. The nephrologist then switched her to methyldopa and hyralazine, a combination of antihypertensive medications that have been proven safe in pregnancy.

After 6 months, her A1C was in the normal range, and her blood pressure was less than 130/80 mmHg. BN was given the "go-ahead" to become pregnant and was told she could stop taking her birth control pills. During the pregnancy, her blood pressure, blood glucose levels, and health status all remained good. She delivered a healthy, 7-pound baby boy.

Introduction

Some women define sexuality as the ability to bear children. This definition tends to devalue the whole woman. Sexuality is as important to a woman in her 60s as it is to a woman in her 30s. Women with diabetes can have a healthy and sexually fulfilling life.

Which Sexual Problems Can Happen to Any Woman?

It may help to divide sexual problems into two categories: sexual difficulties and sexual dysfunction.

Sexual difficulties

Sexual difficulties are problems in the communication between two people that impact their sexual activity. Generally, these difficulties are a result of lack of knowledge of each other's sexual needs and preferences. They do not, or cannot, tell each other what they want. A woman will complain that her partner wants sex too often or not often enough, that he does not engage in enough foreplay, or that there is no affectionate closeness after intercourse. She may not feel attracted to her partner, may dislike his habits or sexual practices, or may be unable to relax with him in sexual play.

Sexual dysfunctions

Sexual dysfunctions are physical problems. Human sexual response normally consists of four sequential phases: desire, arousal, orgasm, and satisfaction. Different physiological processes are involved in each phase, so you may have difficulty in one phase but not the others.

Desire is defined for both sexes as the motivation or wish to have a sexual experience. It frequently is a response to an external cue such as an erotic picture or genital pressure. This is an activity that begins in the brain and depends on a certain blood level of hormones. Degree of desire, however, is not dependent on levels of hormones, although a complete lack of any hormones can inhibit desire.

Arousal is the emotional and physical response to mental or tactile erotic stimulation and is expressed both as a feeling of excitement and as an accumulation of blood in the genital area. In women, it is demonstrated by vaginal lubrication. Vaginal lubrication and engorgement is an important component to achieving orgasm and satisfaction. Without lubrication, the irritation of intercourse is distracting and often painful, and thus diminishes your desire.

Orgasm, primarily orchestrated by the nervous system, is characterized by a series of rhythmic contractions of the muscles of the internal reproductive structures and vagina. Some women may have several consecutive orgasms before experiencing relaxation and pleasure, and some may be unable to reach orgasm at all.

Dyspareunia is genital pain that occurs during or after intercourse. Pain occurs when there is not enough lubrication and/or the vagina is inflamed by infection. Vaginismus is the involuntary contraction of the vaginal muscles that interferes with vaginal penetration by the penis or fingers.

The most common problem that women report is low sexual desire, with 30–50% of women seeing sex or marital therapists complaining of desire problems. Essentially, if the head is not happy, neither is the tail.

What Causes Sexual Dysfunctions?

Sexual dysfunctions can be caused by any disease or medication that interferes with the hormones, brain, and nerve involvement; blood circulation; or muscles involved in sexual response. Additionally, pain or disability can interfere. Just as important are psychological factors. Physical and emotional factors can interact to cause problems.

What Are the Symptoms of Sexual Problems in Women with Diabetes?

Some women with type 1 diabetes have difficulty becoming physically aroused. They may have less vaginal thickening and lubrication. Both penile erection and vaginal lubrication depend on the increase of blood flow to the genital area. Along with vaginal dryness, an inadequate accumulation of blood in the genital area can cause irritation or pain with sexual activity. Many of these women report improvement when they use lubricants. Women with type 2 are even more likely to have these problems. Even though their frequency of intercourse and masturbation are the same as women without diabetes, women with type 2 have reported being much less satisfied with almost every aspect of their sexual relationship. Fear of rejection, lack of self-esteem about body image and/or depression or the negative consequences of future complications also affect many women.

What Puts You at Risk for Developing Sexual Problems?

The damage that high levels of blood glucose in diabetes can do to the blood vessels and nerves affects both circulation and sensation. Clearly, this damage may affect what one can feel and how one responds.

Persistent high blood glucose levels can increase the chance of vaginitis (inflammation of the vagina) or yeast infections. If you have problems with unusual discharge from the vagina, itching, or yeast infections, the best advice is to consult with your doctor to determine the best treatment for correcting the problem and improving your blood glucose control and treatment for the vaginal infection. High blood glucose can also sap your energy and sense of vitality. Feeling sluggish and tired can interfere with how attracted and receptive you are to engaging in sexual activity.

Being able to enjoy the wide range of physical and emotional feelings associated with sexual contact is linked to your emotional state. This can have as powerful an effect on sexual dysfunction as a physical problem.

Women who have multiple health problems may be taking medications that interfere with their ability to have fulfilling sexual contact. Some medications can interfere with one's desire to have sex (libido). Others cause drying of the vaginal tissue, which leads to painful intercourse. Ask your doctor about the effects of your medications on your sexual health.

Should You Be Concerned About Diabetes During Sex?

If you take insulin or certain diabetes pills (sulfonylureas or meglitinides), the physical exertion of sex might result in low blood glucose. You could reduce the dose of insulin before having sex, or eat something beforehand. If blood glucose goes low, you may find that you are unable to perform as usual and cannot enjoy the experience. Discuss with your partner the potential for low blood glucose, the symptoms, and the treatment, and how to help you.

Do Your Monthly Cycles Affect Diabetes Control?

You may have noticed your blood glucose levels are higher around or during your period. Blood glucose is affected by the natural release of hormones that cause your body to be more resistant to its own insulin or to insulin that you inject. Normally, blood glucose remains high for 3–5 days and gradually returns to the level it was before your period.

During PMS, menstruation, and menopause, you might have less energy and not want to exercise. If you stop exercising, your blood glucose may rise even higher. Your ability to control food cravings and to continue with your exercise program will help you balance your blood glucose (and your emotions). Chart your responses during your cycle. Also note the effect of caffeine and alcohol on blood glucose levels at these times. Women with uncontrolled blood glucose may have irregular monthly cycles and acne.

What Do Your Provider and Diabetes Educator Need to Know?

Women are often reluctant to raise the subject of sexual health, believing that their concerns are embarrassing, trivial, or inappropriate unless the provider brings up the topic. It may not be easy to communicate your concerns to your partner or to your provider. Yet, if you want to honor yourself as a woman and this is an issue for you, take the risk. Let your provider know if you have noticed any changes in your sex life. Do you have:

- A decrease in sexual desire or interest?
- Vaginal dryness or tightness with intercourse?
- Pain or discomfort with intercourse?
- Soreness and irritation after sexual activity?
- More difficulty reaching an orgasm than in the past?
- Less satisfaction with your sexual relationship now than you had before?

To assess the possible emotional causes of your sexual dysfunction, your provider needs to know the following:

1. What were your levels of sexual activity and responsiveness (how often, how varied, who initiates it) before diabetes?

2. What are the sexual needs and expectations of you and your partner?
3. What other or underlying difficulties are the two of you having?
4. How do you feel about having diabetes? To what extent does it interfere with your life and relationship?
5. What effect do you feel diabetes has had on your relationship in general and your sexual relationship in particular?

Why Is It Helpful to Know When the Problem Began?

Knowing when the sexual problem began can help determine the cause and whether it is related to diabetes complications or psychosocial adjustment. It is also helpful to know whether the problem is generalized (occurs in every sexual situation or with different partners) or situational (occurs only during specific sexual activities).

Does Your Spouse or Partner Need to Speak with Your Provider?

Of course. Your spouse or sexual partner plays the other important role in the situation. Your partner's viewpoint on any sexual problems or any changes in your sexual relationship might help you find and treat the cause—and improve communication between you. Chronic illness can place stress and strain even on strong relationships. It is important to assess how your partner is affected by the illness, because this can impact your sexual relationship, too.

What Can You Expect from Treatment?

If your sexual problem is mild, began recently, or has a strong diabetes-related cause, some practical and brief interventions by your health care team may be effective.

If your sexual problems are long standing or complicated, you probably need to work with both your physician for treatment of your diabetes and a counselor or therapist in sexual, marital, or individual counseling. You may need accurate sexual education about normal sexual behaviors—there are many excellent books on the subject. It helps many women to realize that their concerns, thoughts, fantasies, and experiences are normal and shared by many other women.

What Part Do Hormones Play in the Treatment of Sexual Dysfunction?

A woman who has lost ovarian function or has gone through menopause may experience less desire for sex because of a hormonal deficiency. Estrogen replacement can improve vaginal elasticity and lubrication, but additional supplementation with male sex hormones (androgens) is more likely to directly increase sexual desire. Although androgen therapy has been helpful to women who undergo surgical menopause, it has no documented benefit for premenopausal women with low sexual desire.

The arousal-phase problem of poor vaginal lubrication is often easy to treat. A woman who has low estrogen levels can use replacement estrogen as a pill, patch, or vaginal cream. The estrogen can actually reverse vaginal atrophy within a few months. For premenopausal diabetic women or for those postmenopausal women who don't take estrogen, vaginal lubricants are quite helpful.

Are There Any Exercises that Help with Sexual Difficulties?

To minimize pain during intercourse, you can learn to relax the pubococcygeal muscles. You can identify these muscles by contracting them during urination and noticing that the flow stops. You can put a finger inside of the vagina before squeezing the muscles and feel the slight vaginal contraction. Once you have found the muscles, you can practice squeezing them for a count of 3 and then releasing them, 10 times in a row. If vaginal penetration for intercourse feels tight and painful, you can tense and relax the muscles before and during the process. If you have pain on penetration or with deep thrusting, you should use positions that give you more control. These include sitting or kneeling over your partner or both partners lying on your sides facing each other.

Is Difficulty Reaching Orgasm a Separate Problem for Women with Diabetes?

No. Rather, it is often a product of lessened desire and arousal, or physical discomfort during sex. Before assuming the trouble is related to neuropathy, your physician may ask if you are orgasmic with clitoral stimulation (by your hand, with a vibrator, or from a partner). Many healthy women have a difficult time reaching orgasm from penile-vaginal thrusting alone, and the woman with orgasmic difficulty may simply require more adequate clitoral stimulation to reach orgasm.

When Might You Be Referred to a Specialist?

A referral to a specialist in sexual problems may be appropriate when:

- The sexual problem is severe or has been present for several years
- The problem does not respond to primary care provider's treatment
- The woman is poorly adjusted psychologically or has a highly conflicted close relationship
- The problem does not appear to be related to diabetes

For most, the referral of choice is to a mental health professional who has special training in treating sexual dysfunctions. The most common causes of sexual problems in women with diabetes are psychological—depression, anxiety about attractiveness, poor sexual communication, relationship conflict, or a history of a traumatic sexual experience. The specialist is likely to be a qualified social worker, psychiatrist, or psychologist who has specialty training at the postgraduate level. These professionals can be located on the faculty of a local psychology department or medical school.

County or state mental health organizations can also provide referrals. Professional organizations, such as the Society for Sex Therapy and Research, are also sources of reliable referrals.

Can Depression Cause Sexual Difficulties?

Loss of desire for sex is most often related to depression. If you also have trouble sleeping, a change in appetite for food, depressed mood, chronic fatigue, physical symptoms without clear cause, and trouble with concentration or memory, you probably could benefit from treatment for depression. Antidepressant drugs and brief, symptom-focused psychotherapy are both effective. Keep in mind, however, that antidepressant drugs may also cause loss of libido all by themselves. Also, any problem with the couple that decreases communication or increases anger may negatively affect sexual desire.

When Might You Be Referred to a Gynecologist?

A gynecologist is especially helpful with dysfunctions related to menopause or to genital pain. The examination should assess tenderness around the vagina, the condition of Bartholin's glands (which secrete vaginal lubrication), the mucous membranes of the vagina, and the presence of pain deep in the vagina or pelvis with pressure or movement of the cervix and uterus. Women who have vulvar (external genitalia) tenderness, burning, and pain with sexual stimulation sometimes have a syndrome known as vulvar vestibulitis. Inflammation of numerous glands around the vaginal opening can be diagnosed with colposcopy. Common causes of pain that occur only on deep thrusting include endometriosis, pelvic adhesions, abnormalities of the uterine ligaments, or ovarian cysts. Only ovarian cysts have been associated with diabetes.

High insulin levels are irritating to the ovarian outer wall. The wall becomes thickened and thus prevents the normal ovulation of an egg that needs to move from the ovary into the fallopian tubes. When an egg is not released, the egg's sack (corpus luteum) swells, and the sack becomes a cyst. The overproduction of insulin in pre-diabetes or undetected type 2 diabetes affects the ovaries and causes polycystic ovary syndrome (PCOS), which is usually diagnosed before type 2 diabetes. However, many women with type 1 diabetes can also be predisposed to ovarian cyst formation because of the high blood levels of insulin that circulate when insulin is injected under the skin, as opposed to released naturally from the pancreas.

Does Diabetes Affect Your Choice of Contraception?

Options range from abstinence to the pill. In the past, a woman with diabetes was advised against taking the pill for two reasons. First, taking oral contraceptives could worsen her blood glucose control. Even today, a woman may find that this is true. Second, she may be at risk of developing problems with circulation and clotting, such as heart attack or stroke. Because the doses of estrogen and progestin have been decreased in newer pills, so has the risk for these problems. A newly developed progestin counteracts androgen (the male hormone that produces acne in women) and prevents it from stimulating hair growth and oiliness. This progestin is not associated with premenstrual symptoms either—a real plus.

Women on the pill who smoke are at greater risk for circulation problems. Smoking causes the blood vessels to narrow, the walls of the vessels to thicken, and the blood to clot. That's why it is important for a woman to quit smoking. High A1C levels (indicating poor blood glucose control) or dehydration may also increase your chances of having blood clotting problems.

A class of pills for type 2 diabetes, the "glitazones," can decrease the effectiveness of estrogen by 30%. If you take rosiglitazone or pioglitazone while you are on a low-dose birth control pill, you may have breakthrough bleeding (bleeding between periods) or may even become pregnant. If you are on the pill and taking these drugs, ask your physician whether your birth control pill needs to be changed. Also, use a backup method of birth control the first couple of months that you are taking a 'glitazone.

It is important for a woman on the pill to have her blood fats and blood pressure checked regularly. If you have untreated high blood pressure or high blood fats, you may need to use a different method of contraception. However, once the blood pressure is normalized with adequate therapy, low-dose contraceptives are safe. Taking the pill when you have high blood pressure can increase the chance that eye or kidney disease will get worse. The pill can also cause a rise in blood cholesterol, LDL, and triglyceride levels. Barrier methods, such as the diaphragm or condoms, have no effect on blood glucose or blood fats. Speak with your provider about the best options for you.

How Does Diabetes Affect Pregnancy?

Women with diabetes need to establish near-normal blood glucose levels before getting pregnant. A baby's organs (heart, brain, lungs, and kidneys, etc.) are formed in the first 8 weeks of pregnancy, often before you know you are pregnant. Good blood glucose control helps protect your baby from birth defects and keeps you healthy during pregnancy, too. If you maintain normal blood glucose and see your health care team regularly, you and the child should be fine. If you already have complications, especially retinopathy, CAD, or nephropathy, they may get worse, and you and your baby could run a higher risk of problems. With your spouse and doctor, weigh the risks before you get pregnant.

You cannot take diabetes pills during pregnancy, so you'll switch to insulin. Taking three or more insulin injections a day or using an insulin pump provides you the best chance for normal blood glucose levels. You will need to check your blood glucose more often (six to ten times a day) and, most importantly, the checks need to be after eating. Other medications used in diabetes, such as cholesterol-lowering drugs and ACE-inhibitors, are also not recommended during pregnancy.

During pregnancy you have an increased risk of headaches, DKA, urinary infections, and preeclampsia.

As soon as you deliver the baby, your insulin needs return to your normal level, or you can return to your diabetes pill. However, if you choose to breastfeed, diabetes pills are not an option. Insulin therapy must be sustained during lactation to keep the sugar content of your milk normal. The insulin doses need to be appropriately changed for lactation, since lactating causes your body to convert some blood glucose into lactose, or milk sugar. Therefore, if you breastfeed, you may have more severe low blood glucose reactions that occur more often than before you were pregnant. See a dietitian before and during pregnancy to be sure you're getting the calories you need. Snacking, along with a decrease in the basal or overnight insulin doses, is important to cover bedtime and middle-of-the-night feedings.

How Might Your Diabetes Affect Your Baby?

If you have near-normal blood glucose levels throughout pregnancy, from conception through delivery, your child will have the same low risk of birth defects as any other child. The infant of a mother with diabetes usually weighs more than normal, which can lead to birth injuries, such as a broken collarbone. The baby may have jaundice after birth because his or her liver is not mature. If your blood glucose is high during labor, he or she may have hypoglycemia once the cord is cut. This may occur 1–3 hours after birth and should be checked for the first 2 days of life. Some babies may have breathing difficulties and need oxygen at birth because their lungs have not matured as quickly as they have grown. If you have type 1 diabetes, your child is a little more likely to develop diabetes (1–4%). However, if your husband has type 1 diabetes, this risk may be up to 6%. If you have type 2, your child's risk is one in seven. Your child is more likely to be obese after puberty, so give him or her a healthy lifestyle of well-balanced meals and plenty of exercise.

How Can Pregnancy Cause a Woman to Get Diabetes?

Babies in the womb need a different mix of oxygen, sugar, fats, and proteins than their mothers, so hormones are released in the mother's body to get the right mix to the baby. However, these pregnancy hormones make the mother's body resistant to insulin, which causes high blood glucose. The mother's pancreas produces more insulin, but sometimes she can't make enough, and her blood levels of glucose, fats, and protein increase. The baby's pancreas reacts to this high glucose mixture by producing more insulin, which causes the baby to grow faster than it should.

Women who develop diabetes only during pregnancy, called gestational diabetes, do not have the same risks as a woman with diabetes before she gets pregnant. You don't have complications of diabetes, and your baby's organs are formed before the diabetes develops. To keep the baby from being too large, you should follow a meal plan and check your blood glucose levels after eating to ensure that they are normal. If they are high despite an adequate diet, you may need insulin to keep your blood glucose normal. Big babies are harder to deliver, and you may need a cesarean section (C-section). Your blood glucose should return to normal soon after the birth, but you are more likely to develop type 2 diabetes later on in life.

How Are Menopause and Diabetes Connected?

Each woman experiences menopause differently. Your experience will be influenced by your body, your attitudes and fears about menopause, and the thoughts and beliefs of your friends. It is a natural process, but it is a time of unpredictable swings in hormones and emotions. Swings in hormones can cause difficulty sleeping, mood swings, and foggy thinking. They can also affect your blood glucose control.

The symptoms experienced during menopause can often be confused with the symptoms of low and even high blood glucose. Hot flashes, moodiness, and short-term memory loss can be mistaken as low blood glucose, when in fact they are related to shifts in hormone levels. It is important for you to check your blood glucose level before assuming that it is low and eating unnecessary calories.

During menopause, dropping hormone levels can cause insulin requirements to drop. Thus, appropriate adjustments to the insulin doses need to be made. If menopause leads to weight gain, insulin needs may rise. Menopause is a time when a woman needs to make frequent blood glucose checks and change her insulin regimen as needed. Many women often report low blood glucose levels that are stronger and more frequent, especially during the middle of the night. Sleep is often disrupted. Controlling your diabetes can be difficult—as it is for teenagers, who also experience wide swings in hormone levels. Dealing with the unpredictability of blood glucose and hot flashes can leave you feeling frustrated and sad. Hormonal replacement therapy (HRT) is sometimes recommended to treat theses symptoms, but because HRT may carry other risks this is something that needs to be discussed with your health care provider.

Keep your diabetes regimen going, get adequate sleep and exercise, and try relaxation techniques to help balance the effects of emotional and physical stress. Nap when you need to, and learn to breathe deeply. You might try a yoga class to calm yourself and feel more comfortable in your body. It is important for you to realize that the demands of your diabetes regimen, when added to the challenge of hormonal changes and feeling older, can change your personality. Try to choose a positive outlook each day, and be kind to those around you.

As the levels of the hormones estrogen and progesterone decrease, your body will be less resistant to insulin. Some women experience more hypoglycemia. You may find that you need to decrease the dose of your insulin or diabetes pills during or after menopause. Another body change that you may see during and after menopause is vaginal dryness, resulting in painful intercourse and increased risk for urinary tract infections. Persistent high blood glucose levels can make this condition worse. Cream and gel lubricants can be used during sexual activity. Prompt treatment of vaginal and urinary tract infections is important. Good nutrition, weight training, aerobic exercise, and sleep are the foundation for a healthy transition during menopause. You may want to consider yoga, tai chi, meditation, and other stress-reduction techniques to help relieve the symptoms and enhance your overall feeling of well-being.

An RD can help review your needs for calcium supplements and make changes to your meal plan. Some women report that calcium-magnesium supplements help to reduce headaches, irritability, depression, and insomnia. Calcium can be found in high amounts in dairy products; green, leafy vegetables; cauliflower; pinto beans and soybeans; and nuts. The daily requirement for calcium before menopause is 1,000 mg/day. Postmenopausal women need 1,000 mg if they are on HRT and 1,500 mg if they are not. Calcium replacement will also help prevent osteoporosis. Some women report success using a higher soy diet and supplementing with bioflavinoids. If you choose to supplement with herbs, be aware that herbs are like medicines and must be taken under the supervision of someone trained in this area.

How Does Menopause Affect Your Heart?

Estrogen provides a certain degree of protection against heart disease. Estrogen, released from the ovaries, helps to increase the production of HDL cholesterol, the good cholesterol, and to break down LDL cholesterol, the bad cholesterol. It also relaxes the smooth muscle of the blood vessels. Once a woman experiences menopause, the production of estrogen goes down.

As a woman with diabetes, you are already at risk for developing heart disease earlier. Diabetes negates the protective effects of estrogen and puts you at risk for heart disease and a life-threatening heart attack. If you have heart disease, try to avoid hypoglycemia because of the increased chance of having a heart attack (chapter 6).

Does Diabetes Put You More at Risk for Osteoporosis?

As a woman ages, her bones tend to become weaker, putting her at risk for osteoporosis. Yet, there are things you can do today to protect your bones.

Osteoporosis, which means "porous bone," is a condition in which bone mass is lost as a result of losing minerals and protein. Bones become very fragile and fracture easily. Estrogen, calcium, vitamin D, and weight-bearing exercise are important to the health and strength of your bones. Even though all humans lose a little bone mass, not all women are at risk for osteoporosis. Men can develop it, too.

You are more at risk for osteoporosis if you are a smoker, thin, or fair skinned, or if you have experienced menopause early, have been on steroid therapy, or have had prolonged high blood glucose levels. In addition, if you do not take in enough calories or calcium, or you have a history of anorexia or bulimia, your bones have not received the nutrients they need to stay strong. If you have been caught up in quick weight–loss diet fads or have a diet low in calcium, high in alcohol, or very low in fat, your bones have probably been weakened. Your body needs a little bit of dietary fat to make estrogen, which is needed for building bone and preventing bone loss.

Because most women with type 2 diabetes are overweight, they are less likely to develop osteoporosis. However, this is not true if their blood glucose levels are always high.

How Is Osteoporosis Prevented and Treated?

No matter what age you are, you should consider the suggestions below.

- Engage in weight-bearing exercise, which is the best way to increase muscle mass and protect your bones. Your body will respond nicely to exercise that involves repetition and muscle strengthening of the large muscle groups. Even lifting 1 or 2 pounds helps increase bone mass and muscle strength

- Stop smoking! Smoking interferes with calcium absorption and leaves the bones fragile and thin. Smoking is also a risk because smokers tend to eat a high-fat diet, drink excess alcohol, and exercise less—all risk factors for developing osteoporosis.
- Eat a balanced meal plan that has enough calcium, phosphorus, and vitamin D. Ask a dietitian how you can increase these minerals in your diet.
- Get your diabetes under control!
- Consider HRT or other medications (Calcitonin, Fosamax), especially if you are at high risk or if you are postmenopausal. Explore this option and its side effects with your provider.

This chapter was written by Lois Jovanovič, MD.

Skin Complications

Introduction

The skin is the largest organ of the body and there are specific and non-specific skin changes related to diabetes. The skin has two layers—an outer covering called the epidermis and an inner collagen layer called the dermis. It is often difficult to determine whether diabetes is directly related to many skin conditions, but there are some conditions that are more common in people with diabetes. The skin problems of diabetes are usually not serious, but some conditions can lead to concerning complications. It is important to check your skin for:

- Dryness
- Abnormal moisture (maceration)
- White, wet keratin between the toe webs
- Blisters
- Hemorrhage
- Breaks in the skin called erosions (loss of epidermis)
- Ulcers (loss of dermis and possibly deeper tissues).

As the years with diabetes pass, you are more likely to have waxy, thick skin, especially on the hands, feet, arms, and legs. You need to know what other potential effects diabetes could have on your skin.

In this section, you will see the common and some uncommon skin conditions associated with diabetes and options for prevention and treatment. Treatment of the skin requires the treatment of the whole person, including the management of the common factors that can increase the complications of diabetes (see box, The ABCDEs of Diabetes Management).

The ABCDEs of Diabetes Management

- A1C Control
- Blood pressure control
- Cholesterol control
- Diet
- Exercise
- Smoking cessation

Following these ABCDEs and taking care of your whole body can be the best preventative and treatment for many skin conditions associated with diabetes.

Why Does Diabetes Cause Thick Skin?

People with diabetes commonly have thick skin, where the skin often has a yellow, waxy appearance and loses some of its surface flexibility. It may relate to abnormal glucose metabolism, accelerated aging, or fraying of the elastic tissue. Thick skin is most obvious on the upper back, affecting over 10% of adults with diabetes. Thick skin of the finger tendons may decrease the joint mobility and limit finger extension (though usually without pain). This change is more common when blood glucose control is poor. You can check for this condition by trying to put your hand flat on the tabletop with the palm down or by putting your hands together in a praying position. If you cannot straighten your fingers out completely, you may have this condition.

Improving blood glucose control has been shown to make the skin less thick. Otherwise, there is no known effective treatment.

Joint Mobility Problems and Diabetes

People with diabetes are also more at risk for developing Dupuytren's contracture, scleredema, or a joint mobility problem, often in the form of "frozen shoulder" (adhesive capsulitis). If you have difficulty or pain raising your arm or using your shoulder, see your health care provider. The condition is easier to treat with physical therapy in the early stages.

Dupuytren's contracture

When the tendons attached to your fingers become contracted, your fingers gradually become permanently bent, and you are unable to extend them. This bending is more severe than what you would see with thick skin. In some cases, surgery is necessary to release the tendons.

Scleredema

Scleredema is a rare disorder characterized by thickening of the skin on the back, shoulders, and neck and restricted movement of the surrounding muscles. This is different from the serious disorder scleroderma, which has a similar-sounding name. You may not be able to see all the areas involved, but the surface skin may look like the skin of an orange.

Scleredema sometimes affects children and, in this form, will generally clear up on its own. In people with diabetes, scleredema diabeticorum is a bit different, and it often does not go away on its own accord. You may have decreased sensation to pain or light touch in these areas, and it may be accompanied by redness of the skin. The only possible treatment for this form of scleredema is improved blood glucose control.

Are Yellow Skin and Nails Associated with Diabetes?

People with diabetes may have a yellowish tint to their skin and fingernails, and toenails may also become yellow. The cause is thought to be due to large glucose residues that accumulate on collagen, referred to as glycosylation. It was previously thought to be due to increased carotene deposits in the skin, but more recent studies have worked to disprove this.

Some people with diabetes, especially the elderly, develop yellow nails because of peripheral arterial disease (PAD) or a fungal infection. However, about half of the cases of yellow nails in people with diabetes have no other known cause. The first sign may be a brown or yellow color on the nail. Eventually, all the nails can turn bright yellow. This color change is generally harmless and does not require treatment.

Why Does Diabetes Cause Your Skin to Be Dry and Itchy?

You may feel that your skin is always dry or even itchy. Also, your heels may have peeling skin or cracks. When your blood glucose is high, your body makes more urine, which can lead to dehydration. This dehydration may be responsible for keeping your skin dry. Also, peripheral neuropathy can inhibit the sweat glands in your hands and feet, which leads to further drying (Figure S-1). Unfortunately, this drying and cracking leaves your skin prone to different infections. You should keep your skin moisturized, because every crack on skin can be a source of penetration for bacterial germs!

While some itching may be due to high blood sugar or nerve changes due to chronic diabetes, much itching is due to another problem. Yeast infections and eczema (dry skin) are also very common causes of itching. Early symptoms of poor circulation may include itching legs.

If your skin becomes dry, use mild neutral soaps, such as Dove or Basis, and apply a moisturizer cream to the skin while it is still wet. There are two types of moisturizer. One binds water to the surface of the skin and contains urea or lactic acid. The other is an oil-based moisturizer called emollient cream that may contain silicone or dimethicone. These prevent evaporation of water from the skin surface. Choose a moisturizer cream without fragrance and other allergic components. While you want the skin to still be wet when you apply these creams, you should dry off excess moisture before applying. The moist areas such as the toe webs, groin, and under the arms and breasts should be kept dry because they are very prone to yeast or fungal infection. Avoid very hot baths or showers because not only can you easily burn due to a decrease in skin sensation, but hot water also dries your skin by washing off the normal moisture-retaining components on the surface of the skin. (See the box for more tips on skin care.)

Important Tips for Skin Care

- Inspect your feet daily.

- A blister indicates movement in the shoes, and a callus the presence of too much pressure. If either appears, see your foot care specialist.

- If you notice your feet have become abnormally cold, new black areas appear (especially on the toes), or a break in the skin develops, see your doctor or foot care specialist immediately.

- Avoid foot soaks.

- Avoid baths or showers that are too hot.

- Use mild soap and a moisturizer cream after bathing while the skin is still damp.

- After bathing, gently dry off your skin, especially in the skin folds between the toes, in the groin, and under the arms or breasts.

- Apply talc or an antifungal powder (undecyclic acid) on any fold where skin touches other skin.

- Treat cuts right away. Wash minor cuts with soap and water. Do not use Mercurochrome antiseptic, alcohol, or iodine to clean skin, because they are too harsh. Only use an antibiotic cream or ointment. Cover minor cuts with sterile gauze. See a doctor right away if you get a major cut, burn, or infection.

Why Should You Avoid Scratching if You Have Diabetes?

About one third of those with diabetes will experience itching, burning, stinging, shooting, or stabbing pain in their legs and feet. When this happens, it may be very bothersome and cause you to scratch a great deal. This is a problem because scratching can damage your skin, especially if you are elderly. Our skin becomes thinner as we age and we are more susceptible to environmental drying influences. This may include the drying effects of low relative humidity in the winter months or the dehydrating effects of bathing, especially if we take long warm baths or showers with lots of water pressure.

Treating your itch will make it easier to avoid scratching. Itching may be due to neuropathy. Itchy skin may be one of the symptoms of kidney complications (chapter XX). Uremia, or elevated levels of urea in the blood with kidney disease, can also cause itching. Maintaining close-to-normal blood glucose levels, following the ABCDEs above, and improving your kidney function may help. If your itch is interfering with sleep, sedating oral antihistamines, such as hydroxyzine or diphenhydramine, may be required. Because these are sedating, you should take either a full dose right before bed or smaller doses through the day and larger dose at night.

Why Does Diabetes Cause Skin Infections?

High blood glucose levels provide a rich environment for microorganisms. They thrive on the skin surface, where your sweat also has a high glucose content. At the same time, your white blood cells do not fight infection as well when glucose levels are high—they become sticky. When you combine these factors with increased skin injuries that happen when you can't tell your skin is being damaged, as seen in sensory neuropathy, you have a recipe for more infections. People with a history of cellulitis, leg swelling, peripheral arterial disease, hardening of the arteries, or superficial fungal infections are also more likely to have serious skin infections.

What Are Some of the Common Skin Infections Associated with Diabetes?

People with higher levels of glucose in their blood are more likely to have skin infections. High levels of glucose in the skin promote the growth of yeast (especially candida), other fungal infections, and bacterial infections, which are all discussed below.

Yeast (candida) infections

Candida is yeast that will grow on moist areas of the skin or mucous membranes, commonly inside the mouth, at the corners of the lips, under the arms, the groin and vaginal region, or the area surrounding the rectum. Candida infections appear differently in various regions of the body. Inside the mouth, a white, curd-like growth appears on the tongue or inner surface of the cheeks. When these white areas are removed, the surface often bleeds. At the corner of the mouth, yeast infections are often red and moist with a red line, called perleche, appearing at both corners of the mouth. The body folds where skin touches skin (under the arms, the breasts, on the sides of the groin, and around the anus) also provide warmth and moisture that attracts candida growth. In these locations, smaller dotted satellite spots that may have central yellow pustules often surround a bright red spot. In the vagina, candida infections are similar to those in the mouth, with a white, curd-like appearance that bleeds when removed. Involvement in the vagina and other areas of the body is often extremely itchy.

The treatment of yeast infections is aided by good blood glucose control. In the mouth, nystatin solution (an anti-yeast antifungal agent) may be used in a swish-and-spit technique three or four times a day for 5–7 days. Clotrimazole (another antifungal agent) oral lozenges can be used daily until the condition clears up. Sometimes, candida in the mouth is resistant to topical treatment, or the problem may extend down the throat into the esophagus. In these cases, oral fluconazole or another similar oral antifungal drug may be used. At the corners of the mouth, topical antifungal drugs—

Nystatin, terbinafine, clotrimazole, miconazole, ketoconazole, or econazole—may be useful. They are generally applied once or twice a day at first and then once or twice a week after the rash has resolved to prevent further outbreaks.

Keep the corners of your mouth clean and dry. Eat fruits and vegetables with a fork, and drink juices with a straw to prevent moisture from accumulating at the corners of your mouth.

In the body folds, it is important to control yeast infections because they can lead to secondary bacterial infections and surface breakdown of the skin. Keep these areas clean using a mild soap. After cleansing, these areas should be thoroughly patted dry, and an antifungal topical cream should be applied.

In the vaginal area, internal yeast infections are treated with over-the-counter or prescription vaginal creams or vaginal suppositories. These infections often cause a disturbing itch and may be accompanied by a vaginal discharge. Difficult cases may require oral anti-yeast therapy.

In the rectal area, it is necessary to cleanse the affected area with water to remove any residual fecal material before using a topical antifungal agent. If you have liquid or loose stools, you should eat more fiber (bran, bran buds, fruits, and vegetables) or add bulk-forming agents to your diet (Metamucil).

Candidal infections often come back, so your physician may suggest a preventative program of using antifungal and/or talc powders or periodic application of topical antifungal creams to prevent the infection from returning.

Tips for Treating and Preventing Candida Infections

- Control your blood glucose levels.

- Keep all body folds clean and dry.

- Use topical antifungal treatments, such as nystatin or clotrimazole, as necessary.

- For resistant yeast problems, see a health care professional about oral medications (itraconazole, fluconazole, or ketoconazole).

- Check your skin, especially the body folds, regularly for recurrence of infection, and use talc or antifungal powders (Undecyclic acid) for prevention.

Other fungal infections

Fungal infections are usually caused by one of two types of fungi— true fungi (dermatophytes) or yeasts, such as candida. True fungal infections cause redness, scaling, itching, and sometimes skin breakdown. They are easily treated with antifungal creams and can be improved by keeping the areas clean and dry and by controlling blood glucose levels.

The risk of toenail fungal infection is three times higher if you have diabetes (Figure S-2). Because of the potential for skin barrier breakdown and a subsequent entry for bacterial infection, treating and diagnosing a fungal infection early is very important. Fungal infections may appear between your toes, around your groin, under breasts or armpits, on the bottoms of your feet, on the palms of your hands, or in your nails.

Fungal infections usually start between the fourth and fifth toes, where the skin between the toes is most tightly compacted. White and softened skin (maceration) is the first sign of infection and it gradually spreads to the other toe web spaces. It can be treated with topical, over-the-counter antifungal creams (clotrimazole, miconazole) twice a day. It is important to gently dry the skin between your toes after bathing and then apply the topical antifungal agent. When the infection clears, use an antifungal powder daily to keep the toe webs dry.

Infections of this type of fungus in the groin is more common in men (yeast infections are more common in women). The fungal infection involves the inner thighs, with a red active scaly area and central clearing. It usually spares the scrotum. Use topical antifungal creams once or twice a day for an active infection, and antifungal powder to help prevent it from coming back. Boxer shorts can help keep the area dry, while tight-fitting clothing, being overweight, sweating, and local friction can aggravate the situation.

Another fungal infection involves the soles of your feet and palms of your hands. The fungus on the bottom of the feet has a dry, powdery scale that often starts on one foot or hand in a small, asymmetric area and gradually spreads to the entire sole or palmar surface. The dry skin often spreads around the sides of the feet, which is referred to as "moccasin-type" changes. If topical antifungal cream is not successful, you may need a short course of oral antifungal agents especially if your nails become involved.

The most cosmetically disturbing fungal infection involves your fingernails and toenails. The nails become thick and yellow. This infection is most common in the large toenails but can spread to the other nails of the feet or hands.

Tips for Treating and Preventing Fungal Infections

- Control your blood glucose.

- Keep the folds of your skin (toe webs, under the arms, under the breast, and groin) dry and clean.

- Use a topical antifungal cream.

- For more resistant infections or if the nails are involved, use an oral antifungal medication such as terbinafine or itraconazole.

Bacterial infections

There are number of bacterial infections that regularly affect people with diabetes, both on the outer layer of the skin (epidermis) and the deeper inner tissue (dermis). Some of the more serious and common infections are impetigo, erythrasma, erysipelas, folliculitis, cellulitus, necrotizing fasciitis, and abscesses.

Impetigo. Impetigo is a yellow, honeycomb-crusted spot on a red base that is often seen on the face or hands. It may sometimes be associated with blisters. This infection involves the epidermis. The bacteria *staphylococcus aureus, streptococcus,* or both have been known to cause impetigo.

Localized impetigo is often successfully treated with topical antibacterial agents. If multiple spots are present, oral antibiotics are often necessary. People with bacterial infections (as well as their close personal contacts) may be carrying organisms in their nostrils, groin, or other parts of the body not involved with the skin rash. Your doctor may want to sample these areas and test them in a lab to see whether further treatment is necessary.

Erythrasma. This bacterial infection that affects the outer layer of the skin appears as brownish, itchy patches in moist skin folds, particularly in the genital, underarm, and moist bottom of the foot (plantar) areas (Figure S-3). Erythrasma resembles fungal skin infections, but the spots have indistinct borders that are not elevated, there are no satellite lesions, and fungal elements do not show up under a microscope. Using an ultraviolet light, often referred to as a black light or Woods light, can make diagnosis easier—the patches emit a characteristic coral-red glow. The condition often has no symptoms, but it may cause itching or even breakdown of the skin. If treatment is required, the topical use of imidazole agents will often successfully treat this bacterium. The oral antibiotic erythromycin is usually effective as well.

Erysipelas. Erysipelas is an infection in the deeper, second layer of the skin. Erysipelas usually appears as a hot, hive-like change, often on one side of the face. It may spread quickly and will often make you feel ill, with general flu-like illness and fever. Prompt attention is important, and an emergency visit to your doctor or the nearest hospital is advised. Treatment usually requires intravenous antibiotics for the first 24–48 hours and then a switch to oral agents for the remainder of the therapeutic course.

Folliculitis. Diabetes may increase your likelihood of developing several common bacterial infections, usually caused by *staphylococci.* If these infections involve the superficial part of your hair follicle, they are called folliculitis. Larger and deeper infections are called furuncles or boils. If the boils progress to involve adjacent hair follicles, they are then called carbuncles. These infections most often occur on the back of the neck, groin, armpit, or legs. They cause red, warm, tender, or boil-type swellings of your skin. Once the central pus forms, they require drainage, either spontaneously or by surgical incision. Mild infections may respond to drainage or local treatment with topical antibiotic therapy alone, but more extensive lesions require surgical drainage and systemic anti-microbial medications, especially if there is extensive deep tissue infection.

Cellulitis. Another type of skin infection that may be more frequent or severe in people with diabetes is cellulitis (Figure S-4). This infection involves the surface and deep parts of the dermis and causes a red and tender swelling with an advancing red border, often on the feet or legs but occasionally elsewhere. Like impetigo, cellulitis may be caused by *staphylococcus aureus* or *streptococcus* bacteria. This infection often responds promptly (within 36–48 hours) to antibiotic therapy, usually initially by the intravenous route. Clinicians will draw a line with ink or skin marker around the advancing margin to be sure the infection starts to shrink, although it may worsen in the first 24 hours. If the infection does not improve, it is important to reevaluate and consider the possibility of bacteria resistant to the antibiotic you are taking, or a more serious infection, such as a necrotizing fasciitis.

Necrotizing fasciitis. People with diabetes are more susceptible to this potentially life-threatening, subcutaneous (below the skin) soft-tissue infection. The skin has many layers—epidermis, superficial and deep dermis, subcutaneous fat, and fascia. "Fasciitis" means involvement of the skin down to the fascia, the tissue that covers the muscle, and "necrotizing fasciitis" means an infection that causes death to this soft tissue. Necrotizing fasciitis often involves the muscle as well. Gangrene may also develop, and it usually causes gas in tissues.

Necrotizing infections appear and spread rapidly, destroying tissue. Symptoms include severe pain, with the development of hemorrhaging and blisters on a warm, red, tender skin surface, like you would see with cellulitis. Your blood glucose level may be higher than normal. Fortunately, this infection is uncommon. Fasciitis is more likely to affect those with impaired circulation after trauma, and as part of deeper infections, especially of the lower extremities, genital, or rectal areas. Treatment for these infections must include immediate, aggressive removal of the dead tissue and broad-spectrum intravenous antibiotics.

Abscesses. An abscess is a confined area containing microorganisms (usually bacteria) and white blood cells (pus). In people with diabetes, abscesses may occur at insulin injection sites and are often associated with contaminated needles, syringes, or multiple-dose insulin vials. To help prevent this problem, you should carefully clean both your injection site and the tops of any multiuse vials with alcohol or other topical antiseptic.

What Do You Need to Know About Leg and Foot Ulcers?

This issue warrants its own chapter in this book (chapter 15). In a nutshell, four keys are required to heal an ulcer: good blood flow, good nutrition, elimination of infection and inflammation, and reduction of swelling (edema). Diabetic ulcers (Figure S-5) usually appear when an unnoticed injury goes untreated, generally because sensation in the lower extremities has been dulled by diabetes complications. Twice-daily foot exams are absolutely critical. *Know your feet, keep your feet.*

What Is Intertrigo?

Intertrigo is inflammation of your skin due to recent skin-on-skin frictional contact. The areas most frequently involved are the groin, under the breasts, and underarms. High heat and humidity in these areas predispose all people to intertrigo and certain infections in these areas, but even more so in those who are overweight or obese. People with diabetes are more likely to develop intertrigo when they have high blood glucose levels, urinary or fecal incontinence, decreased sensation of skin damage (usually from neuropathy), and increased sweating (due to nerve changes).

The most common infectious agents complicating intertrigo are bacterial and fungal, but intertrigo does not require infection. Sweat, heat, and friction are all that are needed to produce macerated skin-on-skin rashes. However, infection needs to be treated when present.

Good glucose control, loose clothing, minimized skin-on-skin rubbing, and keeping high-risk areas dry and clean can help prevent an outbreak of intertrigo.

What Causes Skin Tags?

Skin tags (Figure S-6) are most often caused by long-term skin-on-skin friction. These growths are harmless and often run in families. Frequent locations for skin tags are around the neck, under the breasts, and under the arms—very common areas for friction. Friction is more likely in overweight people, so weight control can help reduce skin tags. Though they don't cause any medical problems, skin tags may be treated by snipping or freezing.

What Is Diabetic Dermopathy?

Diabetic dermopathy (Figure S-7) refers to small, round, flesh- to brown-colored spots on the lower legs, usually on the shins. These spots are more common in older men with diabetes and, in some studies, have been documented in 70% of men with diabetes over 60 years of age. They are the most common skin-related sign of diabetes, but on occasion may appear on people who do not have diabetes. They are also completely harmless.

Diabetic dermopathy starts as small, pink spots that gradually turn brown. They are approximately the size of a pencil eraser, and the skin may be thinned with tiny scales on top. Although the cause is unknown, they may be caused by trauma, especially if you have neuropathy. It is believed that the brown color is caused by the effect of high glucose levels on collagen or the small blood vessels in the skin. The spots will disappear spontaneously; however, new individual or clusters of spots often appear nearby. No treatment is necessary.

What Is Necrobiosis Lipoidica Diabeticorum?

Necrobiosis lipoidica diabeticorum (NLD) is the name of the red-yellow spots that may appear on the lower legs of people with diabetes (Figures S-8 and S-9). The condition is rare, affecting only about 3 in 1000 people with diabetes, often women, but NLD appears almost exclusively in those with diabetes. One-third of the people who develop NLD may develop an area of skin breakdown or ulceration within a lesion.

NLD starts with red bumps that gradually join together and enlarge, often with a raised active purple margin. The spots then develop a thin, yellow center, the skin becomes shiny and transparent, and you can see tiny blood vessels under the surface. The most common location of NLD is the shin (in 90% of patients), but lesions can occur on the scalp, face, arms, and body. If the lesion ulcerates, you should seek advice from your health care provider.

The cause of NLD is not known. Changes in small blood vessels, an immune system response, or an injury to the skin may all play contributing roles in this condition. These spots are chronic, but they disappear spontaneously in 10–20% of cases. It is common for them to return.

If you do not have an ulcer, you may only need to protect the area from being bumped by other people or objects. Shin pads are often recommended, as is turning on the light before you get up at night to walk around. Your doctor may have you apply a steroid cream or inject steroids under the surface of the skin on the red or purple active margin. The topical steroid should not be used on the thinned central region where a moisturizer alone should suffice.

It is not clear whether improved blood glucose control can help. Low-dose aspirin and the anti-platelet drug dipyridamole may improve NLD, but further studies are necessary to show whether routine use of these drugs is beneficial. Ulcers, of course, require prompt treatment.

Cosmetic treatment is often important, especially for young women. Seek expert cosmetologist advice on applying a waterproof cosmetic cover-up for swimming and other athletic activities (for example, a green-based cosmetic cream may cover areas of red discoloration).

Things to Remember if You Have NLD

- Protect your legs from trauma, and see your physician immediately if you develop an ulcer.

- Your physician may recommend topical creams or injections, depending on the severity of the spots.

- Oral medication, such as aspirin and dipyridamole, may also be prescribed.

- Stop smoking; one study has suggested this is a risk factor.

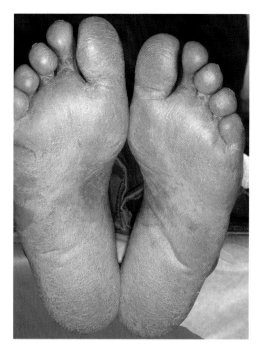

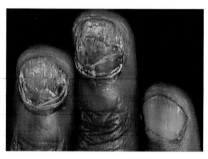

Figure S-1. The dry skin on the plantar surface of the foot, as illustrated in the picture, may be due to either a loss of protective sensation (autonomic neuropathy) or a fungal infection (see section on fungal infections).

Figure S-2. Tinea of the nails is a common fungal infection in people with diabetes.

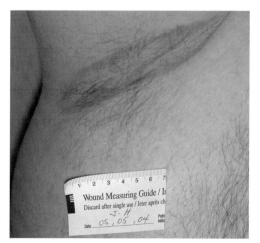

Figure S-3. Erythrasma is a bacterial infection that commonly affects areas where skin touches skin (folds).

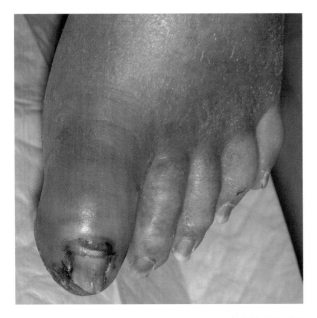

Figure S-4. This image shows a patient with an abscess at the base of the large toe with surrounding cellulitis. This infection is limb-threatening and requires excision and drainage of the abscess, possible removal of the toenail to check for infection or abscess below the nail, and the use of intravenous antibiotics to control the cellulitis.

Figure S-5. Diabetic foot ulcers like this are typically seen on pressure points on the feet. Calluses often surround the ulcer. The ulcers are usually painless and may or may not be infected. Most are caused by small trauma to a "numb" foot (caused by neuropathy), but some are caused by poor blood supply or both a "numb" foot and poor blood supply.

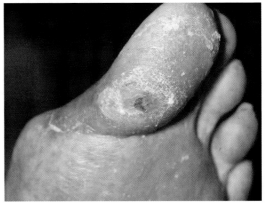

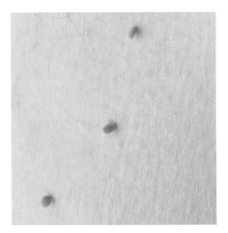

Figure S-6. Skin tags often appear like little "out pouchings" in the soft parts of our skin (such as the underarm area).

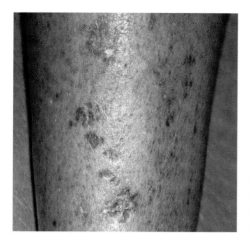

Figure S-7. Diabetic dermopathy is also called diabetic "brown spots." These are a harmless skin pigmentation often occurring on the shin of the leg. These may be easily traumatized, so be careful.

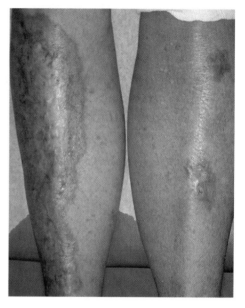

Figure S-8. Necrobiosis Lipoidica Diabeticorum (NLD) is rare, but appears most often in women with diabetes. One leg has a large longstanding lesion with a peripheral active border, central atrophy, and early ulcer formation. On the other leg, smaller evolving lesions are forming the characteristic components of NLD.

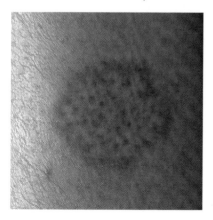

Figure S-9. Another example of an early lesion of NLD.

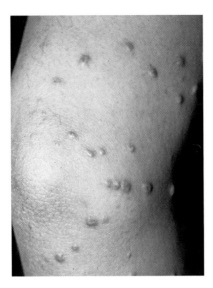

Figure S-10. Eruptive xanthomas are caused by high levels of lipids (fats) in your bloodstream. The best treatment is to control your blood lipid levels.

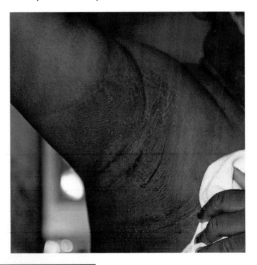

Figure S-11. Acanthosis nigricans may occur in any ethnic group. It is a dark discoloring of the skin that is not due to dirt but an excessive growth of cells that changes the color of the skin.

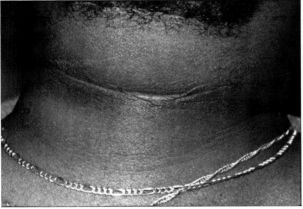

Figure S-12. Acanthosis nigricans commonly occurs on the neck, underarms, and groin areas. However, it may also be seen in joints of the hands, fingers, elbows, and knees.

What Is Generalized Granuloma Annulare?

Granuloma annulare is an inflammatory skin disease characterized by ring-shaped rows of small, raised, bead-like bumps without any surface scale. The flesh-colored, red, or red-brown bumps often surround an oval central spot that may be flesh colored or light brown. The most common form of this condition appears on the hands or feet of children and young adults. There are no other symptoms, and generally, the condition is self-limiting.

The disorder may take other forms. If it spreads to extensive areas on the arms, neck, and trunk, it is called generalized granuloma annulare. Unlike NLD, it is not associated with thinning of the skin or skin sores (ulcers). Also, while NLD is strongly associated with diabetes, the relation between granuloma annulare and diabetes is not clear. Granuloma annulare may appear in a number of ways, and a skin biopsy is sometimes necessary to confirm the diagnosis. Treatment of granuloma annulare is similar to that for NLD, with common first-line treatment including topical and injected steroids. However, this condition may disappear spontaneously without any treatment.

Can You Get a Blister Without an Injury to Your Skin?

Yes. The official name is bullosis diabeticorum, and although it is uncommon, people with diabetes sometimes do develop blisters without any apparent cause. This condition mostly affects those with renal failure. The blisters are clear and appear spontaneously on your forearms, fingers, feet, or toes. They arise from normal skin, have a wide range in size, are painless, and usually go away in 2–4 weeks. They may become dark or black from associated local bleeding. They are common in people who have loss of nerve sensation (neuropathy) and in those with long-standing diabetes. Other than local care, there is no specific treatment needed. You should let the blisters dry up by themselves, but notify your physician if you experience frequent recurrences.

What Are Xanthomas?

Xanthomas (Figure S-10) are firm, non-tender, yellowish, flat or elevated skin spots that can accompany poorly controlled blood glucose levels and high blood fat levels (triglycerides and cholesterol). In fact, xanthomas can be considered a warning sign that blood fats have gotten out of control. They most often appear on the elbows, knees, buttocks, or the site of an injury. Eruptive xanthomas can appear suddenly, and the small lesions are usually 4–6 millimeters in diameter with a yellow or red base.

Diagnosing and treating the cause of xanthomas, high lipid levels, will not only help reduce xanthomas, but will also help prevent arthrosclerosis and the other complications of high triglycerides and cholesterol. In the presence of high serum lipids, diet and lipid-lowering agents are effective. Improving blood glucose control and lowering blood fat levels makes xanthomas disappear.

Lipid collections around the eyelids are called xanthelasma palpebrarum. This is the most common type of xanthoma. They may be caused by high blood fats (high cholesterol) and are a sign to your health care provider to check your cholesterol level. The spots begin as small, yellow-orange bumps, then grow, thicken, and can eventually cover the entire eyelid. They are more likely to occur in women than in men.

Things to Consider if You Have Xanthomas

- Lowering the amount of fat and refined carbohydrates you eat can help lower your blood glucose and blood fats, which can then help xanthomas caused by lipids.

- Surgery or locally destructive therapy may be used to treat xanthomas that are not related to blood lipids.

- Controlling blood glucose and following the ABCDEs of diabetes care are the best treatments

What Is Acanthosis Nigricans?

Aconthosis Nigricans (Figures S-11 and S-12) causes the skin on the back of the neck, underarms, and groin to become thicker, darker, and velvety in appearance. This condition is extremely common in people with insulin resistance and can often be the first sign of underlying diabetes. Because of this, obesity is also significantly linked to acanthosis nigricans. Most adults who weigh more than 200% of their ideal body weight have some form of acanthosis nigricans.

Fortunately, this condition is mostly cosmetic and may completely disappear with weight control. Diet, exercise, and use of prescribed medications are critically important. Many people with acanthosis nigricans require high doses of insulin, while others may benefit from an oral medication, such as metformin. Otherwise, the only treatment is a topical agent such as retinoic acid, salicylic acid, lactic acid, and urea, if you want to improve the cosmetic appearance.

Acanthosis nigricans is uncommon in very thin patients. However, dramatic and unexplained weight loss that is combined with an abrupt onset of acanthosis nigricans needs medical evaluation. Rarely, acanthosis nigricans can also be a skin sign of internal cancer.

Do Medications for Diabetes Affect Your Skin?

Yes. The sulfonylurea class of oral medications can cause minor changes in your skin, and so can insulin.

Sulfonylureas

Sulfonylureas stimulate the beta cells in your pancreas to produce insulin. Skin rashes are the most common side effect in the first few months of therapy and are seen in 1–5% of cases. The rash often looks like measles. Also, be very careful in the sun. Hives and an allergic reaction can occur on sun-exposed skin, and extreme sunburns are a common side effect. The measles-like rash may disappear on its own even if you continue taking sulfonylureas, but other kinds of rashes may require you to stop taking this medication and seek help from a qualified health care professional.

Any alcohol that you drink may interact with a specific sulfonylurea—chlorpropamide—and cause flushing of your whole body and especially your face. Skin reactions and flushing are rare with the newer, second-generation sulfonylureas.

If you have a reaction to oral sulfonylurea drugs, you also run a greater risk of reacting to a number of related chemicals, including

- Permanent hair dye (paraphenylenediamine)
- A component of sunscreens called PABA (para-aminobenzoic acid)
- Local anesthetic creams (benzocaine)
- Some diuretic pills (hydrochlorothiazide)
- Sulfa drugs (sulfonamide antibiotics)

Insulin

Skin reactions to insulin are less common with newer, purer forms of insulin. Still, you may experience burning at the injection site, followed by a hive-like reaction that may fade over hours or days. Skin reactions may be immediate or delayed. Insulin can cause generalized hives and even respiratory or circulatory collapse due to insulin allergy, but this is extremely rare. These reactions are less common with human or synthetic insulin than the older beef or pork derivatives.

Occasionally, fat from the deeper layers under the dermis of insulin injections sites may decrease, causing little indentations on the surface (lipoatrophy), but this complication is much less common with newer purified insulin. If an insulin site is used repeatedly for years, the fat may actually increase in size, causing an elevated, thickened bump (hypertrophy). Darkening of the skin may also be seen at insulin injection sites.

Conclusion

As we have shown, there are a number of skin complications that can accompany diabetes and just as many ways to treat these complications. (See Table 22-1 for a summary of the skin conditions discussed here.) We've also discussed some general skin care steps you can take to prevent many of these conditions from appearing in the first place. Following are some "take-home" messages we hope you will consider after reading this chapter.

- Follow the ABCDEs. People with high glucose levels tend to have dry skin and less ability to fend off harmful bacteria. Both conditions increase the risk of infection.
- Keep skin clean and dry. Use antifungal or talcum powder in areas where skin touches skin, such as your armpits and groin.
- Avoid very hot baths and showers. *Do not soak your feet!*
- If your skin is dry, do not use bubble baths. Moisturizing soaps, such as Dove or Basis, may help. Immediately after bathing, pat the skin dry, and while still damp, apply a moisturizing cream (for example, creams with urea and lactic acid or moisturizers such as Lubriderm or Alpha-Keri).
- Use antifungal creams in your toe webs for active fungal infections and antifungal powders for prevention. *Do not use moisturizers in your toe webs!.*
- Avoid scratching your skin; you may cause open sores that will allow infection to set in.
- Moisturize your skin to prevent chapping, especially in cold or windy weather.
- *Treat cuts right away.* Wash minor cuts with soap and water. Do not use Mercurochrome antiseptic, alcohol, or iodine to clean skin because they are too harsh. Only use an antibiotic cream or ointment (double antibiotic cream or ointment-avoiding preparations with neomycin). Cover minor cuts with sterile gauze or Band-Aids containing mild antiseptics, such as the newer silver preparations. See a doctor right away if you get a major cut, burn, or infection with red areas extending beyond the margins of the cut.
- During cold, dry months, keep your home more humid. If possible, bathe less during times of lower relative humidity,

Table 22-1. Common Skin Problems Associated with Diabetes

Disease	Symptoms/Appearance	Treatment Comments
Dryness of skin	Cracking (fissure), scale	Hydration, proper soap, moisturizer
Itching of the skin	Generalized itching	Moisturizer cream, oral antihistamines
Dupuytren's contracture	Loss of skin flexibility, bending of the fingers	Blood sugar control or surgical correction
Yellow discoloration of the skin	Yellowish hue in the skin	No treatment
Diabetic dermopathy	Multiple dark skin spots mostly on the shins	Avoid trauma; apply moist interactive dressings for open areas
Necrobiosis Lipoidica Diabeticorum (NLD)	Red-yellow spots mostly on shins that may break down and scar	Avoid trauma; use topical or intralesional steroids, oral medications
Scleredema	Thickened skin on back, shoulders, and neck	No treatment; optimize diabetic control
Diabetic blisters	Blister on normal skin without cause	Avoid secondary infection with topical antimicrobials, avoid trauma
Xanthoma	Flat or elevated yellowish bumps	Diet, ABCDEs, local destructive treatments or surgery for the spots not associated with high fat–level group
Acanthosis Nigricans	Velvety dark areas on folded skin	Weight loss and blood sugar control
Bacterial infection	Redness, pain, edema	Topical or systemic antibiotics
Fungal infection	Redness and/or scaling on folded skin, maceration of toe webs, nail changes	Moisture control, topical or systemic antifungal drugs, keep folded skin dry and clean
Drug reaction	Rash, thinning of fat in the area of insulin injection	Antihistamines, consult with your physician to change the medication

and regularly apply moisturizers, especially if the skin is dry or chapped.

- Use mild shampoos. Do not use feminine hygiene sprays.
- *Take good care of your feet.* Check them every day for sores and cuts. Wear broad, flat shoes that fit well. Check your shoes for foreign objects before putting them on.
- See a dermatologist (skin doctor) about skin problems if you are not able to solve them yourself.

And finally, if there is one thing you take from this chapter, make it this: *Know your skin*. Check your skin monthly with a mirror. Know those hard-to-see spots. Be able to identify melanoma, the pigment cell skin cancer. Remember to check your feet after getting up in the morning, and prior to going to bed at night. *Know your feet, keep your feet*.

This chapter was written by Afsaneh Alavi, MD; Cathryn Sibbald, B. Pharm (C); R. Gary Sibbald, MD; Christopher M. Scott, MD; and William A. Burke, MD.

23

Bone Health

Are People with Diabetes More Likely to Have Fractures?

With age, the risk of having a broken bone or fracture increases for both men and women. In addition to age, there are other factors that increase the likelihood that a person will have a fracture, such as having had a previous fracture, having a family history of fracture, smoking, heavy alcohol use, and some medications. Having diabetes, both type 1 and type 2, also increases your chance of having a fracture. Maintaining healthy, strong bones is important. Since many fractures result from a fall, it is also important to maintain strength and balance to reduce your chance of falling.

How Do Bones Become Weaker and Susceptible to Fractures?

Although bones may appear to be solid and unchanging, they are actually dynamic tissues being torn down and rebuilt throughout adulthood. Cells in the bone called osteoclasts remove small sections of bone. These tiny pits in the bone are then refilled with new bone by other bone cells called osteoblasts. Over the course of about 10 years, all of the bone in an adult skeleton is replaced at least once. This replacement of bone, bit by bit, with new bone tissue is thought to allow repair of tiny cracks in the skeleton that occur with everyday wear and tear. The turnover of bone also helps your body maintain appropriate levels of minerals in your blood and other tissues. However, with older age, bone replacement by the osteoblasts starts to lag behind the removal of bone by the osteoclasts. Bone loss occurs and, if enough bone is lost, your bones become fragile, a condition called osteoporosis.

How Does Diabetes Affect Your Bones?

Lower bone density increases your risk of fracture. Studies have shown that those with type 1 diabetes tend to have lower bone mineral density than others the same age, a factor that probably contributes to their higher fracture risk. On the other hand, older adults with type 2 diabetes tend to have average, or even higher than average, bone density. This is probably because those with type 2 diabetes tend to be overweight, a factor that usually increases bone density. However, in spite of having average or higher bone density, those with type 2 diabetes still have a higher risk of fracture. This may be because people with type 2 fall more frequently. Also, even though older adults with type 2 diabetes on average have normal bone density, a significant proportion does have osteoporosis. Maintaining bone health is an important goal to prevent fractures for those with type 1 and type 2 diabetes.

Both the insulin sensitizing agents rosiglitazone and pioglitazone have been associated with increased risk of bone fractures. However, formal osteoporosis studies have not been completed. Nevertheless, if you have osteoporosis, you should discuss this matter with your doctor before starting either of these agents to treat your diabetes.

How Does Diabetes Affect Your Risk of Falling?

Falls are responsible for a large majority of bone fractures in older populations. Approximately 90% of hip fractures in the elderly result from a fall. About a third of older adults experience one or more falls each year, and about one in ten of those falls results in a fracture. Naturally, those who fall more often increase their chances of having a fracture. Unfortunately, older adults with diabetes are more likely to have a fall. Factors that can increase your risk of a fall include:

- Muscle weakness
- Poor balance
- Reduced vision
- Peripheral neuropathy

In addition, medications may increase your risk of a fall, especially those that may cause drowsiness or dizziness, such as sleeping medications, muscle relaxants, and some blood pressure pills.

When Should I Have a Test for Osteoporosis?

Until you suffer a fracture, osteoporosis does not typically cause symptoms. X-ray tests are needed to tell whether someone has low bone density. Bone mineral density (BMD) can be measured with dual X-ray absorptiometry (DXA). Based on the reading from a DXA scan, a physician can determine whether your bone density is

Factors That Increase Your Risk of Fracture

Older age

History of fracture with low or no trauma

Family history of fracture or osteoporosis

Heavy alcohol use

Smoking

Use of oral glucocorticoids ("steroids"), such as cortisone or prednisone

Low body weight

Frequent falls

Low bone density

normal, somewhat low (sometimes called osteopenia), or quite low (osteoporosis). Measurements of bone at the hip and spine are the most reliable for identifying low bone density.

There are a number of factors that increase your chances of having a fracture (see box, Factors that Increase Your Risk of Fracture). Low bone density is one important factor, but other factors, such as age, are also important. Most guidelines agree that women should get a DXA scan to screen for osteoporosis at age 60 if they have other risk factors for fracture, and age 65 if they do not. There are no consistent recommendations for men, although one organization recommends bone-density screening tests for men at age 70. A bone-density measurement is also recommended for any older adult who experiences a fracture caused by low or moderate trauma. If you have a variety of factors (see box) that increase your risk of fracture, you might consider bone density testing at a younger age.

What Can I Do to Help Keep My Bones Strong and Prevent Falls?

Eating healthy and exercising are two of the most important things you can do to maintain strong bones at all ages. Plus, there are additional steps you can take to keep your bones healthy and prevent falls.

Calcium and Vitamin D

Adequate supplies of calcium and vitamin D are essential to maintaining healthy bones. Good sources of calcium include:

- Dairy products
- Tofu (set with calcium)
- Black or navy beans
- Green, leafy vegetables
- Broccoli
- Almonds
- Dried figs
- Fortified foods such as calcium-fortified orange juice or cereal

Adults over 50 years old need a total of 1,200–1,500 mg of calcium a day, either through food, supplements, or a combination of both. There is no benefit in taking more than 1,500 mg per day and, at this level, urine calcium levels start to increase as the kidney eliminates the extra calcium. Taking excessive calcium on a regular basis may increase your risk of kidney stones.

Exposure to sunlight is an important source of vitamin D, because UV rays from the sun trigger vitamin D synthesis in skin. Season, geographic latitude, time of day, cloud cover, smog, and sunscreen affect UV ray exposure and vitamin D synthesis. In general, 10–15 minutes of daily sun exposure to the face, arms, hands, or back without sunscreen will provide enough vitamin D synthesis (and should be followed by application of a sunscreen with an SPF of at least 15 to protect your skin). If you have limited exposure to the sun, you need to include good sources of vitamin D in your diet, such as fortified milk, salmon, tuna, or sardines. Older men and women should get about 600–800 IU of vitamin D per day, which will probably require fortified foods or supplements. Most multivitamins will have 400 IU of vitamin D in them, and there are many calcium supplements that also provide vitamin D.

Physical activity

Adults should get 30 minutes of physical activity, such as walking, on most days of the week, preferably every day. Children need at least 60 minutes a day. Activities that are "weight-bearing" are especially beneficial, as they will help your body maintain bone density while also providing cardiovascular benefits. Examples of weight-bearing exercise are walking, jogging, dancing, and strength-training (resistance exercise). Regular exercise can reduce the chance of falling by improving and maintaining muscle strength and balance. Exercise may also reduce progression of peripheral neuropathy. Before starting any exercise regimen, however, consult with your health care team to make sure you develop an activity plan that is safe for you.

Vision

Protect your vision with regular eye exams and good glucose control. The better your vision, the less likely your chances of an accidental fall.

Medications that cause drowsiness or dizziness

Review your medications annually with your doctor. Changes in dose or timing may help decrease dizziness and reduce your risk of falls.

Smoking

Smoking increases your risk of bone loss and fracture. Keeping bones strong is one of many good reasons to stop smoking. There are medications and programs that can help you quit. Your doctor can tell you more about what is available in your area.

Maintain glucose control

Keeping your blood glucose levels under control will reduce complications—with vision, peripheral nerve function, and renal function—that can increase your risk of falls and fractures. Good control may also help to preserve bone density.

What About Medications to Treat Osteoporosis?

If your health care provider determines that you have a significant risk of fracture, several prescription drugs are available for treatment.

Bisphosphonates

Bisphosphonates work by slowing bone breakdown. There are three bisphosphonates that are approved by the FDA for osteoporosis:

- Alendronate (Fosamax)—taken orally daily or weekly
- Risedronate (Actonel)—taken orally daily or weekly
- Ibandronate (Boniva)—taken orally monthly or intravenously every 3 months

The bisphosphonate medications reduce spine fracture by 40–50%, though they vary in how effectively they treat other types of fracture. The oral preparations are difficult to absorb. The pills must be taken first thing in the morning on an empty stomach and washed down with two glasses of water. Then you must remain upright and wait 30–60 minutes before eating or drinking anything else. The main side effect to the oral drugs is a risk of irritation in the esophagus, the tube that connects the mouth to the stomach. When taken intravenously, about 15% of people will get flu-like symptoms, usually only after the first dose.

Selective estrogen receptor modulator

Raloxifene (Evista) is a selective estrogen receptor modulator (SERM). It acts like estrogen in some tissues, such as bone, and blocks estrogen action in other tissues, such as the breast. It has been shown to reduce spinal fractures by about 40%, but has not been shown to affect other types of fractures. It may also reduce your risk for breast cancer. The main side effect of raloxifene is an increased risk of blood clots, and it may lead to hot flashes, particularly in women who have recently gone through menopause.

Estrogen/progesterone

Estrogen/progesterone, or hormone replacement therapy (HRT), significantly reduced the risk of both hip and vertebral fractures by about 35% in the Women's Health Initiative (WHI) study. Because the WHI also showed increased risk of vascular side effects and breast cancer, estrogen has become a smaller part of osteoporosis prevention and therapy. It is currently used mostly during and immediately after menopause for women with symptoms such as hot flashes.

Calcitonin

Calcitonin (Miacalcin) also works by slowing bone breakdown. It reduces spinal fractures by about 30%, but has not been shown to affect other types of fractures. It is a once-per-day nasal spray that is well tolerated; the only side effect is possible nasal irritation. There is some evidence that calcitonin may help lessen bone pain from fractures.

Parathyroid hormone

Parathyroid hormone (PTH) (Forteo) is a daily injection that can increase new bone formation. It is usually reserved for those with severe osteoporosis or those who have not responded well to other medications. It has been shown to reduce spinal fractures by 65% and other fractures by 53%. There is a risk of high blood or urine calcium on PTH, and it can only be used for 2 years, as prolonged exposure to PTH in rats was associated with bone cancers. After PTH therapy, a different osteoporosis medication must be started, or the bone-density increases from PTH will be lost after a year or two.

Where Can You Learn More?

Further information about bone health can be obtained from the National Institutes of Health Bone Resource Center at www.osteo.org or the National Osteoporosis Foundation at www.nof.org.

This chapter was written by Ann V. Schwartz, PhD, and Deborah E. Sellmeyer, MD.

24

Oral and Dental Health

Case Study

PJ is a 19-year-old woman with type 1 diabetes. She has an abscessed (infected) wisdom tooth, and her dentist has recommended the removal of all four wisdom teeth. The oral surgeon, conferring with PJ's physician, may recommend a temporary reduction in insulin dosage after the extractions, because she won't be able to eat after the surgery. She will be closely monitored to prevent the development of DKA (chapter 4) or hypoglycemia (chapter 5).

Introduction

People with diabetes may develop a variety of oral problems, including gum disease and infections. Seemingly routine dental problems such as gum infections and abscesses from bad teeth can have a significant impact on blood glucose levels.

Toothaches, gum disease, or any oral condition that can interfere with your ability to eat take on added significance. Because healthy eating is such a key element to your control of the disease, it is even more important to maintain a healthy mouth. The key to good oral health is to focus on preventive care through regular checkups and cleanings and an oral hygiene program at home.

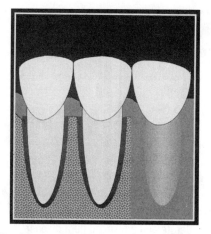

Figure 24-1. Anatomy of healthy teeth/gums/bone. Note the height of the bone and the tightness of the gums against the teeth.
Illustration by Julio Galvez, DDS

How Does Diabetes Affect Your Mouth and Teeth?

Diabetes affects the mouth in three ways:

1. High blood glucose has an effect on the small blood vessels of the body. In the mouth, it contributes to gum disease and slower healing.
2. People with diabetes have difficulty fighting off infections in the mouth. Their white blood cells show diminished capacity to fight off invading bacteria.
3. Diabetes can lead to an oral condition known as xerostomia, or dry mouth. This decrease in saliva production may be caused by autonomic neuropathy and can have several effects, including more cavities and oral fungal and bacterial infections.

What Is Periodontal Disease?

Periodontal disease may be referred to as gum disease, gingivitis, or periodontitis. These are all terms referring to the breakdown of the structures that support the teeth—the gums and bone.

In a healthy mouth, the roots of the teeth are solidly encased in bone. The soft tissue (the gums) covers the bone and wraps around each tooth up to the base of the crown (Figure 24-1). As a conse-

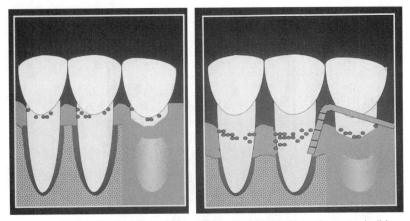

Figures 24-2 and 24-3. Moderate and advanced gum disease. Note the tartar buildup and the destruction of bone. We would expect the teeth in Figure 24-3 to be loose.
Illustration by Julio Galvez, DDS

quence, a space exists around the tooth between it and the gums, called the periodontal pocket.

Two types of material build up on the teeth above the gumline and below in the pocket: plaque and calculus (also called tartar). Plaque is a soft film that can be removed with normal brushing and flossing. Calculus is the harder material that is removed by dentists and dental hygienists during regular cleaning sessions. Both are rich in bacteria and cause irritation to the gums. If plaque and calculus are allowed to remain in contact with the teeth and gums, periodontal disease can develop and progress through several stages.

What Are the Symptoms of Gum Disease?

In gingivitis, the earliest stage of gum disease, the gums are red and swollen and bleed easily. After a thorough cleaning, the gums will return to normal. If the teeth are not cleaned, the gumline will begin to recede, exposing some of the root surface (Figure 24-2). As the gumline continues to move, the level of the bone starts to recede as well. Eventually, the teeth will loosen and need to be extracted or may come out on their own (Figure 24-3). At any point in this progression, a thorough cleaning and the implementation of good oral home care will stop the gum recession and bone loss. However, the lost gum and underlying bone cannot be replaced.

What Is the Connection Between Periodontal Disease and Diabetes?

According to data from the National Health and Nutrition Examination Survey, Americans with diabetes are more than twice as likely as the general population to experience some form of gum disease. Gum infections can, in turn, significantly raise your blood glucose levels.

How Is Gum Disease Diagnosed?

A thorough dental examination includes a visual exam, X-rays, and periodontal charting—a series of measurements including the depth of the pocket that surrounds each tooth (Figure 24-3).

What Is the Treatment for Gum Disease?

Treatment for gum disease can be as simple as routine cleanings performed every 3–6 months. If the amounts of plaque and calculus are more significant and/or the periodontal pockets are deeper, your dentist may recommend a scaling and root planing. This deep cleaning usually involves several visits and requires a local anesthetic. When completed, you may need to return more frequently than every 6 months for checkups.

In more severe cases, the loss of bony support for the teeth is more extensive, and the depth of the periodontal pockets makes it difficult or impossible to perform a thorough cleaning. You may be referred to a dental specialist concerned with gum problems—the periodontist. The periodontist uses many techniques, some of which involve surgical procedures. The major goals of periodontal surgery are to reshape the bone and reposition the gums for easier cleaning.

How Can You Prevent Gum Disease?

People with diabetes may develop periodontal disease and bone loss even without a buildup of plaque and tartar on their teeth. So, when plaque and tartar do accumulate, periodontal disease will progress much more rapidly than in those who do not have diabetes. The best defense against periodontal disease is the elimination of plaque and tartar from the teeth and gums. For most people, this is just a matter of brushing after meals and flossing daily. Electric toothbrushes may be helpful for people who have trouble with regular brushing and flossing. There are prescription products such as medicated rinses and toothpastes designed to kill bacteria and control bleeding and inflammation; these are available with a prescription from your dentist, who may also recommend more frequent cleaning appointments.

How Does Dry Mouth Affect Your Oral Health?

Xerostomia, or dry mouth, is thought to be due to autonomic neuropathy. While a lack of saliva is an annoyance in itself, it can also make you more likely to get cavities in your teeth.

How Is Dry Mouth Treated?

Your dentist may prescribe fluoride gels or rinses to strengthen the teeth and fill in small cavities. These products have more fluoride than over-the-counter toothpastes and should only be used with the advice of a dentist. Another prescription product is artificial saliva that can be sipped and swished to aid you in eating and speaking.

Nonprescription techniques include sugarless gum and candy, and drinking plenty of water. Chewing sugarless gum after meals decreases cavities and increases the flow of saliva. Sipping water throughout the day also helps.

Will Diabetes Interfere with Dental Treatment?

People with well-controlled diabetes can undergo dental treatment the same as anyone else, although some general precautions should always be taken. Local anesthetic with epinephrine should be avoided on many with diabetes, especially those who have had diabetes for a long time, because it causes a rapid heartbeat (tachycardia). Ask your dentist about this. It may be helpful to provide recent test results like blood glucose and A1C, which is a measure of your blood glucose over the past 2–3 months.

People who take insulin or oral medications are best scheduled for midmorning appointments, after taking their medication and eating a normal breakfast. Always ask how long the numbness will last—your dentist can use shorter-acting anesthetics so you don't have to skip a meal. For longer dental appointments, it may be necessary to monitor blood glucose during the appointment, and glucose tablets (or juice or cola) should be easily accessible in case symptoms of hypoglycemia arise.

People with uncontrolled blood glucose pose a challenge because of frequent fluctuations in blood glucose levels. Your dentist and physician should consult one another even for routine dental treatment. If you have heart valve disease, you may need protective doses of antibiotics. Always report any heart problems to your dentist.

What Happens After Your Dental Treatment?

Find out how long you can expect to be numb and whether there will be any discomfort as the numbness wears off. These two factors affect your ability to eat and affect blood glucose. You may need to switch to a soft or liquid diet temporarily, or in extreme cases, the dosage of your medication may need to be reduced. Consult with your physician before you do this. For some patients with diabetes, healing time may be longer. Your dentist may ask to see you for a follow-up visit or may prescribe an antibiotic.

* * * *

Good dental health will be a great benefit to your overall health. Regular check-ups, thorough home care, and good communication between you and your dentist and physician are the formula for a healthy mouth.

This chapter was written by Jeffrey A. Levin, DMD.

25

Anemia

What Is Anemia?

Anemia is a medical condition that occurs when a person does not have enough red blood cells in their bloodstream. Red blood cells play an important role in the body. They take the oxygen from the air we breathe into our lungs and stick it to a protein called hemoglobin. Red blood cells then carry their oxygen-rich hemoglobin, via circulation, to all parts of the body and release it for the cells to use. This oxygen provides the energy for all of the body's normal activities, from thinking to exercising.

Anemia means that less oxygen (energy) can be delivered to your body's muscles and organs. Therefore, if you are anemic, you have less energy and feel tired mentally and physically. Power supplied by the red blood cells to your body fades, and you feel as if your batteries are running low and need replacement.

Are You at Increased Risk for Anemia?

Anemia is a common finding if you have diabetes. Those with diabetes are nearly twice as likely to have anemia than those without diabetes. However, not everyone with diabetes will develop anemia. Anemia is largely seen in those who have diabetic kidney disease as a complication (see chapter 17). Chronic kidney disease (CKD) can be detected by testing the urine for increased levels of albumin, a protein normally found in the bloodstream, but found leaking into the urine in diabetic kidney disease. CKD can also be detected by a blood test that measures how well the kidney is filtering toxins from the body, called the glomerular filtration rate (GFR). People with protein in their urine or with a low GFR are five to ten times more likely to have anemia than those with healthy kidney function. Over 80% of all people with diabetes who also have anemia will have albumin in their urine or a low GFR.

Anemia is also more common in people with diabetes and heart disease, as well as the elderly, for whom any reduction in energy supply can make a big impact on activity levels and independence. Anemia may also be seen in those with type 1 diabetes and celiac disease. Anemia can also be caused by blood loss in the intestinal tract, for example, from an ulcer or cancer.

What Are the Symptoms of Anemia?

The symptoms of anemia can be difficult to detect at first because they are often mild and happen very gradually. Symptoms are also easily confused with the effects of diabetes or side effects of your medication.

Although fatigue does not affect everyone in the same way, people with anemia may feel weak or tired. They become easily exhausted, often when performing simple tasks like household chores. Often they seem to lose their breath, or become dizzy or faint after any exertion, such as climbing stairs or walking short distances. Sometimes this is associated with the sensation that the heart is racing (palpitations) or chest pains. Together these symptoms make it more difficult to find the energy to do normal activities. As a result, people with anemia become less active, something that is a major problem if you also have diabetes, because it affects your glucose control and blood pressure.

The lack of oxygen in patients with anemia also has a major impact on the ability to work and learn. Anemia can reduce your attention span and make it difficult to concentrate at work, home, or in the classroom. Sometimes it can lead to irritability, forgetfulness, or confusion, which can be dangerous under certain circumstances, such as when you're driving or operating machinery.

As the symptoms of anemia worsen, they can significantly affect many aspects of a person's quality of life. Although individuals with anemia may feel sleepy much of the time, often they actually experience difficulty sleeping. Low energy levels lead to a general reluctance to engage with others, so that anemic individuals may appear sad or depressed. Those with anemia may also lose interest in sex or become impotent. Other symptoms of anemia include headaches, leg cramps, and reduced appetite. People with anemia may also appear pale, particularly around the lining of the eyelids, lips, and nailbeds, which look less pink than usual.

It is not clear whether anemia makes the other complications of diabetes, such as eye, kidney and heart disease, any worse. However, people with anemia are much more likely to have these complications. For example, vision-threatening eye disease is over five times more common if you have anemia. Patients with diabetes and anemia also have an increased risk of developing end-stage renal disease or general mortality.

Why Does Anemia Make You Feel Unwell?

Oxygen provides the energy that the body needs for all of its normal activities. Anemia means less oxygen and, thus, less energy. Many of the problems caused by anemia are simply due to a reduction in energy supply.

When the number of red blood cells decreases in anemia, the body must work harder to try to compensate for the lack of oxygen. The lungs must work harder, so you feel short of breath and have an increased breathing rate, even at rest. The heart must also work harder, pumping extra blood to tissues to make up for the lack of oxygen. This makes the heart enlarge (hypertrophy) and beat faster (tachycardia). This can cause problems in persons with diabetes who have narrowing of the arteries to their heart, as the extra work can provoke chest pains (angina).

Why Does Anemia Occur?

There can be several reasons why the number of red cells in your bloodstream may be reduced. They can be lost as a result of bleeding or damage (hemolysis). Anemia can occur if the production of red cells in your bone marrow is reduced due to disease, or if the building blocks that are used to make red blood cells (including iron and certain vitamins) are deficient. Some drugs that are used to treat diabetes may also reduce the hemoglobin concentration in your blood.

CKD can also lead to anemia. This is because the kidney plays an important role in keeping the number of red blood cells in the circulation at a constant level, ensuring that the oxygen (energy) supply to the body also remains constant (Figure 25-1).

For example, if you were to donate a pint of blood, your kidneys would immediately sense the difference and produce a hormone called erythropoietin (EPO), which stimulates your body to make more red cells. And soon enough, your red blood cell levels would

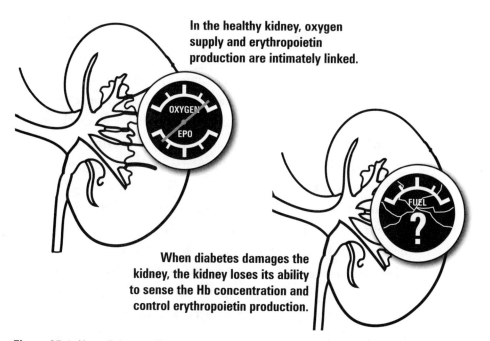

In the healthy kidney, oxygen supply and erythropoietin production are intimately linked.

When diabetes damages the kidney, the kidney loses its ability to sense the Hb concentration and control erythropoietin production.

Figure 25-1. How diabetes affects EPO production in the kidney.

be returned to normal. However, if you have CKD, your kidneys lose their ability to sense the number of red blood cells in the circulation. It is like the fuel gauge is stuck, and the kidney has no idea how much is left in the tank. The kidney can still blindly make a constant amount of EPO, but if energy levels fall, a damaged kidney cannot increase its production of EPO to compensate and, as a result, anemia develops.

This form of anemia, where EPO levels are stuck at normal when they should be high, is the most common cause of anemia in people with diabetes. However, other causes of anemia, including blood loss or iron and vitamin deficiency, should always be ruled out before attributing anemia to CKD.

How Do You Detect Anemia?

As the symptoms of anemia are similar to those you might observe in diabetes and its many complications, the diagnosis depends on blood tests performed as part of a routine check-up. You may notice that your doctor will perform a complete blood count (CBC) to look for abnormalities in your blood. This test provides a count of all the cells in your bloodstream, including the number of red blood cells that carry oxygen (red blood cell count), the percentage of the blood that consists of red blood cells (hematocrit), and the concentration of hemoglobin in your blood. A value below the normal range for your age and gender indicates anemia. A CBC is usually very quick, and typically results are ready within a few hours of receiving the sample.

This check is different from the one your doctor commonly uses to measure your glucose control, which is called the A1C. This test measures how much glucose is stuck to the hemoglobin in your red blood cells, but not the hemoglobin levels themselves. It is dependent on glucose control over the past few months. However, if you have anemia, your A1C can sometimes be falsely low because you have less hemoglobin for glucose to stick to. This can lead to misleading results for you and your doctor and affect the management of your diabetes.

If you are found to have anemia on a routine blood check, other diagnostics will often be requested. These include checks of your iron stores, such as ferritin levels and transferrin saturation (TSAT), in your body, which can help to determine whether your anemia is due to iron deficiency. Levels of vitamin B12 and folate are also often tested. Sometimes your doctor will wish to exclude internal bleeding as a cause of anemia, particularly if iron stores are low or the red blood cell count has dropped suddenly. All patients with type 1 diabetes and anemia should be tested for celiac disease, a common but often undiagnosed partner of type 1 diabetes.

How Should Anemia Be Treated?

If you are found to have anemia, it means there is an increased risk of having or developing complications of your diabetes. These complications include eye disease, kidney disease, and heart failure. A finding of anemia therefore means it is even more important to keep your blood pressure, lipids, and glucose levels under control. It also means your health care team should check you for these complications if this has not already been done.

There are many treatments available for restoring the red blood cell count back into the normal range. These interventions can diminish fatigue and improve the quality of life in those with anemia. These same medications are often described as "performance-enhancing drugs" when taken by those who do not have anemia. By increasing energy levels in the body, performance is significantly improved. Although in an athlete, this might give an unfair advantage, in someone whose performance is already impaired as a result of their anemia, correcting the level of red blood cells can help restore a normal level of function and help retain independence. This is especially the case in those with diabetes and heart failure, where treating anemia has been shown to improve shortness of breath and keep those with diabetes out of the hospital.

The most widely used class of drugs for treating anemia are the EPO analogues. These drugs are hormones that have been engineered to be similar to the natural EPO produced by kidneys. These injections essentially supplement what the undamaged kidney would normally be manufacturing, much in the same way that taking insulin substitutes for the product of a healthy pancreas. Increased EPO levels then stimulate red blood cell production in the bone marrow and increase your energy level.

EPO is always given with iron therapy (injections or tablets). This is because iron is an important building block of hemoglobin. Even with high levels of EPO, it is impossible to make more red blood cells if iron is not available.

What Are the Risks of Treating Anemia?

Although there is plenty of evidence that treating anemia can make you feel better, it can also cause problems. Every time the red blood cell count is increased, the blood becomes slightly thicker and, consequently, blood pressure often rises. This is a problem particularly for those with diabetes and CKD, who struggle to keep their blood pressure under control every day. There may be an increased risk of blood clots, and in some studies, a small rise in hemoglobin has been associated with an increased risk of heart disease. The balance of risk and benefits in treating anemia in diabetes is currently being tested in a large, international trial. Hopefully, the answer to this important question will be available soon.

This chapter was written by Merlin Thomas, MD.

Associations with Diabetes

26

The Metabolic Syndrome

Case Study

A 43-year-old woman with high blood pressure, Ms. G, is seen by her physician. After checking her blood pressure, which is now controlled with one medication, her doctor reviews her laboratory report and makes the comment, "It looks like you have the metabolic syndrome."

Ms. G: What is that?

Dr. M: Well, it means that you have high triglycerides (fats in your blood), and your high density lipoprotein (HDL) is low. HDL is sometimes called the "good cholesterol" and the higher the better. It is believed that by lowering your triglycerides and increasing your HDL, you will get more protection from heart attacks, strokes, and other vascular problems.

Ms. G: How is that a syndrome?

Dr. M: You're considered to have the metabolic syndrome when you are overweight and carry your weight in your abdomen. Add hypertension, high triglycerides, and low HDL for a woman, and you have most of the elements of the metabolic syndrome.

Ms. G: If I don't have all of the elements, how can I have this syndrome?

Dr. M: Metabolic Syndrome is defined as having any three of the five problems listed in Table 26-1.

Table 26-1. Criteria for the Metabolic Syndrome

To be diagnosed with the metabolic syndrome, you must have three of the following.

Issue	Measurement	Ms. G's Measurement
Central obesity	Waist circumference bigger than 35 inches (88 cm) in women, 40 inches (102 cm) in men	Waist: 38 inches
High triglycerides	Greater than 150 mg/dL or on drug treatment for elevated triglycerides	Fasting triglycerides: 221 mg/dL
Low HDL	Less than 40 mg/dL in men, 50 mg/dL in women	Fasting HDL: 37 mg/dL
High blood pressure	Higher than 130/85 mmHg, or taking a medication	BP: 128/78 mmHg and on medication
High fasting glucose	Greater than 100 mg/dL or previously diagnosed with type 2 diabetes	Fasting glucose: 88 mg/dL

Ms. G: I know that my lipid levels aren't perfect, and I've had high blood pressure for 3 years. What difference does it make to be told that I have this metabolic syndrome?

Dr. M: The metabolic syndrome is a cluster of abnormalities that occur together in some individuals. These abnormalities are risk factors for heart disease and stroke. Finding them together makes me concerned that your risk of a vascular event is increased.

Ms. G: How do you know someone's risk of a "vascular event"? And I assume that you mean a heart attack or stroke, by the way.

Dr. M: You are correct. Heart attack and stroke are among the most devastating vascular events. It is also possible to get blockages in the blood vessels to your legs. As for your risk of a vascular event, we don't know exactly what your risk is, but we can estimate it by using a scoring system called the Framingham Risk Score. It will tell you your 10-year risk of having a heart attack. You can do a web search for this to find an online calculator.

Ms. G: But I feel fine. Do I really need to worry about this?

Dr. M: The problem with risk factors for heart disease and stroke is that they do not cause any symptoms. High cholesterol, high blood pressure, and even early diabetes can be completely silent (meaning they have no symptoms). It is important to have these risk factors checked out now and then and to treat the problems if necessary.

Ms. G: Do I need treatment for this metabolic syndrome?

Dr. M: Well, you don't treat the metabolic syndrome itself; you treat the underlying conditions that make up the syndrome. But experts agree that when you have these conditions clustered together as the metabolic syndrome, you should begin treating them right away.

Ms. G: What's the treatment? Medication?

Dr. M: Treatment consists of making changes in your diet and increasing your physical activity by exercising.

Ms. G: Exactly what am I supposed to do about my diet?

Dr. M: You are overweight and have been for a number of years. Start by reducing your calories by 300–500 kcal per day. Other changes are recommended for treating high triglycerides.

Ms. G: This is too vague. What type of diet is the best for me?

Dr. M: Several diets work well for the metabolic syndrome. Following a Mediterranean dietary pattern—more fruits, vegetables, grains, nuts, legumes, dairy, and olive oil, with small portions of poultry, fish, and red meat along with red wine—has worked for the metabolic syndrome. Another diet that was tested for hypertension, called the D.A.S.H. diet, has also improved some of the metabolic syndrome conditions.

Ms. G: What about low-carb, high-protein diets?

Dr. M: Well, there has been some indication that a low-carb diet can be helpful, but you need to keep an eye on saturated fats as well. And many low-carb diets don't do that. Why don't I have you see a dietitian to go over things carefully? This may take more than one visit, so be ready with your questions. Exercise is also important. Are you getting any exercise?

Ms. G: I chase around after the kids and sometimes walk at work.

Dr. M: Aim for 30–60 minutes of dedicated exercise 3–5 times per week. This exercise should cause you to sweat and should get your heart rate up. Exercise has a beneficial effect on your blood pressure and your ability to use insulin, and may lower your cholesterol and triglycerides. However, we will need to talk about whether you should get a stress test done before you start your exercise program.

Ms. G: I'm not sure that I can handle all of these things at once.

Dr. M: It can be overwhelming, but you'll have lots of support. A good dietitian will help you make small changes that add up to big improvements in your diet and lifestyle. You can start exercising 10 minutes per day and work your way up. You'll find that exercise feels good to do, and most people increase their time if they stick to it. Walking is fine, but some strengthening exercises are helpful as well.

Ms. G: Is there anything else that I need to do or to take?

Dr. M: Currently, there are no specific medications for the metabolic syndrome. Some are being considered, but none are available right now. Like I said earlier, we approach the metabolic syndrome by treating each of the risk factors that make up the syndrome. For example, your blood pressure is well controlled. I recommend continuing your blood pressure medication as you are doing now. Your LDL (low density lipoprotein) cholesterol is acceptable at 117 mg/dL, but I will watch it carefully. You are at higher risk than normal for developing diabetes, so we will watch your blood glucose more carefully. I want you to return for further testing in 6 months after making every effort to start dietary changes and lose a few pounds. The real culprit causing the metabolic syndrome is excess weight. Even modest weight loss will help reduce your risk factors significantly.

Ms. G: You haven't mentioned anything about my low HDL. What can I do to bring it up?

Dr. M: Raising your HDL can be a challenge. I am concerned about your low HDL, especially with the other abnormalities in your lipid profile. Lifestyle changes can increase your HDL level by a modest amount. Some drugs can increase HDL levels, and may be worth trying in your case. I will prescribe a long-acting niacin, which has a side effect of facial flushing. If you take an aspirin before taking the niacin, it often helps to reduce the flushing sensation.

Managing lipid levels (cholesterol, LDL, triglycerides, and HDL) is important for reducing risk, so I have provided a chart of the most commonly used drug classes to lower cholesterol (Table 26-2). We may need to consider using another of these agents in the future.

Because I know your medical history and that it would be safe for you, I would like you to begin taking a baby aspirin every day, if you are not already doing so. Baby aspirin is 81 mg in the United States and should be taken daily to reduce blood clotting tendencies. By keeping platelets—clotting particles in the blood—less sticky, it prevents them from attaching to the blood vessel walls and causing clots to form.

Ms. G: This is really quite enough news for one day and enough things to do. Is there anything else that you are concerned about with the metabolic syndrome?

Dr. M: People with the metabolic syndrome run a higher risk for some forms of liver disease caused by a buildup of fat in the liver. There are types of kidney disease that are also associated with obesity. I certainly recommend that you consider making the lifestyle changes that can prevent further weight gain and potentially help you lose some extra pounds.

Table 26-2. Drug Classes Commonly Used to Treat Cholesterol

Drug Class	Total cholesterol	LDL	Triglycerides	HDL
Statins[1]	↓↓	↓↓	↓	↑
Fibrates[2]	↓	↓	↓↓	↑
Ezetimibe[3]	↓	↓	↓	~
Niacin[4]	↓	↓	↓↓	↑↑↑
Fish oil[5]	↓	↓	↓↓	↑

1: Statins are mainly used to lower your cholesterol levels by decreasing how much cholesterol your liver makes.

2: Fibrates are mainly used to lower your triglyceride levels.

3: Ezetimibe is mainly used to lower your cholesterol levels by decreasing the amount of fats you absorb from your meal.

4: Niacin is a B-vitamin that helps control your blood lipid (fats) levels, especially HDL cholesterol (the good cholesterol).

5: The American Heart Association recommends that patients with heart disease take at least 1 gram of fish oil containing elements of EPA and DHA (special types of fatty acids). Patients who need to lower their triglycerides should take 2–4 grams a day, but should do so only under the advice of a physician.

Ms. G: I'm not sure that I like having the metabolic syndrome, but I appreciate the way that you explained it. I am happy that it is something that I can work toward, as I am overdue for restarting an exercise program and improving my diet. Thank you for the advice and encouragement.

This chapter was written by Janet McGill, MD.

27

Polycystic Ovary Syndrome

What Exactly Is Polycystic Ovary Syndrome?

Polycystic ovary syndrome (PCOS) is a clinical syndrome, not a disease, and the key to understanding PCOS lies in understanding the concept of a clinical syndrome. Doctors can often diagnose a specific disease when they have a good understanding of the cause and the expected effects resulting from it. But sometimes things aren't so clear. That's when we have a syndrome, a group of findings that tend to occur together. But we don't know precisely which one is the cause and which ones are the effects. That's what happens in PCOS. The following things tend to occur together in PCOS:

1. Irregular menstrual periods or even lack of menses altogether
2. Increased levels of male hormones in the blood and ovaries
3. Ovaries with many cysts

Not every woman has all of these features. But more than 5% of women have PCOS.

Is It Normal for Women to Have Male Hormones?

Actually, all women have some male hormones (called androgens) and, conversely, all men have some female hormones (called estrogens). But in PCOS there are more androgens than usual. This can cause excessive hair growth on the face and trunk, acne, and even some male-pattern balding. Fortunately, androgens can be lowered by treatment.

How Is PCOS Diagnosed?

As you might expect, there is no single test for PCOS. Instead, making the diagnosis involves putting together several clinical clues by taking a thorough history, performing a physical exam, and getting a few simple blood tests. A personal history usually reveals irregular or missing menstrual periods, and elevated androgens can be either inferred from unwanted hair growth or measured directly in the blood. Interestingly, locating ovarian cysts by an ultrasound test is not always helpful. Some women with PCOS do not actually have ovarian cysts, while those women without PCOS sometimes do. So the observation of ovarian cysts may not be as important to the diagnosis as other data. There are also other rare disorders that may be confused with PCOS that physicians will take into consideration. These include excessive production of adrenal hormones, increases in the hormone prolactin, thyroid disease, or even tumors of the ovary or adrenal glands. These can usually be ruled out by history and blood testing.

How Does PCOS Affect Those with Diabetes?

Although most people think of PCOS as a gynecological disorder, it is strongly related to diabetes. Most women with PCOS are also resistant to insulin, which means that their pancreas can make insulin, but the insulin it is not very effective. This leads to high blood insulin levels, just like in many people with type 2 diabetes. High insulin levels cause the ovary to make too much androgen and cause the androgens in the blood to be more active in body tissues. In susceptible women, excessive internal insulin can trigger PCOS.

Are Those with PCOS at Increased Risk for Developing Diabetes?

Yes. Type 2 diabetes tends to develop in stages. The first stage is insulin resistance with normal blood glucose, followed by small increases in blood glucose levels (sometimes referred to as pre-diabetes), and finally full-blown type 2 diabetes. For those with PCOS, the risk of developing high blood glucose levels or type 2 diabetes may be as high as 40% by age 40. There is also an increased risk of gestational diabetes. For many women, PCOS is a warning that diabetes may be developing.

Can PCOS Be Treated?

Fortunately, there are effective treatments for PCOS. Weight loss and exercise form the basis of all therapies for treating PCOS. Rapid weight loss may affect your menstrual periods and is not recommended, but gradual weight loss spread over months reduces insulin and androgen levels. Exercise for 60–90 minutes on most days has similar effects. These lifestyle changes are also the most effective ways to prevent diabetes and are more effective than drugs.

If additional treatment is required, it needs to be tailored to your life goals and planned carefully with the medical team. Drugs that improve insulin sensitivity, such as metformin, rosiglitazone and pioglitazone, also reduce blood androgens and insulin and can lead to normal menstruation. Oral contraceptive pills can regularize periods and reduce blood androgens. However, excessive hair growth tends to respond poorly to these treatments and often needs separate treatment with drugs or procedures to remove the hair.

If you plan to become pregnant, discuss your situation with your doctor before you start any treatments. Since lifestyle interventions or insulin-sensitizing drugs can improve fertility, there may be a need for contraception after treatment.

Should I Be Screened for Diabetes If I Have PCOS?

The American Diabetes Association recommends that any woman with PCOS who is over her ideal body weight be screened for diabetes every 3 years. It is also recommended that pregnancy be planned with the help of your health care team.

This chapter was written by Richard E. Ostlund, Jr. MD.

28

Cancer

Introduction

There will be nearly one and a half million new cases of cancer diagnosed in the U.S. this year. The probability of being diagnosed with any cancer over your entire lifetime is one in two if you are a man, and one in three if you are a woman. Cancer is a common disease, and diabetes prevalence is steadily increasing, which leads to the conclusion that more and more patients will be coping with the management of both diabetes and cancer. Numerous studies are actively looking at a possible link between diabetes and cancer, yet there has been no consensus as to whether diabetes actually puts you at a higher risk of being diagnosed with cancer. There is, however, some evidence to suggest that type 2 diabetes may be related to certain types of cancer, such as cancers of the pancreas, endometrium (or uterus), prostate, liver, colon, and rectum.

What Is Cancer?

Cancer refers to a group of diseases characterized by abnormal cells that grow and divide uncontrollably, often leading to the formation of a tumor. Cancer cells have two key features: the ability to invade locally into neighboring tissue as well the ability to spread to distant parts of the body. This latter process, spreading to different parts of the body, is called "metastasis."

Another way to think about cancer is at the cellular level. Each cell in your body is regulated by a set of genes, which are encoded in your DNA. When cancer begins to develop, DNA has often become damaged and cannot repair itself. Cells containing the abnormal or mutated DNA may continue to grow uncontrollably, replacing normal cells and forming cancerous tumors.

Many different classes of genes play a role in whether cancer develops or not. Some genes help to repair DNA once it is damaged in the cells, while others work to process and clear the body of toxins and other hazardous materials to which cells may be exposed. However, there are two special classes of genes that function in the earliest stages of cancer—proto-oncogenes and tumor suppressors.

Proto-oncogenes

Proto-oncogenes function normally to help cells grow and divide. When these genes are damaged, they can become oncogenes, and the outcome is the rapid growth typical of cancer cells. If you were to think of cellular growth and cancer as a car, oncogenes would be the gas pedal.

Tumor suppressors

In keeping with the car analogy, the second class of genes would be considered the brakes of the car. Tumor suppressor genes act to control the rate at which cells divide. They also function in programming the death of cells when they become damaged and cannot repair themselves. When tumor suppressor genes are inactivated (the brakes fail) and proto-oncogenes are turned on (foot on the gas pedal), the result is an uncontrolled, accelerated division of cancer cells.

What Causes Cancer?

We have just described how cancer begins in the body, but what actually causes these mutations to happen in the first place? Some cancers are caused by inherited genetic mutations. But many cancers occur when normal cells will mutate for no apparent reason at all, which is often referred to as a "sporadic" mutation. Though the source of these sporadic mutations is not always clear, we are exposed to many things in our environment, either intentionally or unintentionally, that increase our risk of cancer.

Tobacco

Cigarette smoking is currently the leading preventable cause of cancer death among men and women in the United States. For example, it is estimated that nearly 90% of lung cancer deaths are attributed to tobacco use, which includes those inhaling "environmental tobacco smoke" either directly from the cigarettes or from the exhaled smoke of nearby smokers. Tobacco is linked to a number of other cancer sites, including bladder, kidney, pancreas, stomach, liver, esophagus, larynx, pharynx, and oral cancers. There has been a steady decline in smoking rates in the United States since the middle of the 1960s. However, these rates have stopped dropping, which indicates a continued need for education programs in youth and tobacco-cessation programs for all smokers.

Obesity

The prevalence of obesity in this country is at an epidemic proportion. Obesity and physical inactivity are important factors and have been linked to cancers of the colon and rectum, prostate, endometrium, stomach, breast (specifically the type of breast cancer occurring after menopause), ovary, and esophagus. In the United States, nearly 20% of all cancer deaths are estimated to be specifically due to excess body weight.

Other lifestyle risk factors

Other major lifestyle factors that have been shown to be related to cancer include diet (particularly diets high in saturated fat intake and low in consumption of fresh fruits and vegetables), alcohol use, post-menopausal hormones, and oral contraceptives, as well as excessive exposure to the sun's ultraviolet (UV) rays. Importantly, lifestyle factors can often be modified and thus have significant public health implications.

Environmental factors

There are a number of environmental factors that people are inadvertently and often unknowingly exposed to in their home or workplace. Radon—a colorless, odorless gas present in the ground, water, and air—is a result of the natural breakdown of uranium in soil and rocks. It is also a known cause of lung cancer. Low levels of radon are present in most homes in the United States, but some homes may accumulate hazardous levels of radon. High levels of arsenic are another cause of cancer and even low to moderate levels, such as those commonly found in household drinking water samples, have been linked to bladder and skin cancers. Additionally, a number of occupations have been connected to cancer. Workers exposed to certain pesticides, asbestos, benzene, solvents, medical X-rays, and even hair dyes while on the job have been shown to be at an increased risk for certain types of cancer.

Infections

Viral and bacterial infections are also known to cause certain cancers. Infectious agents that increase the risk of cancer include, but are not limited to:

- Human papillomavirus (HPV) and cervical cancer
- *Helicobacter pylori* bacteria and stomach cancer
- Epstein Barr virus (infectious mononucleosis) and lymphomas
- Hepatitis B and C and liver cancer

Diabetes and Cancer

If diabetes does in fact increase your risk for cancer, how this happens is still unknown. However, it may be a consequence of high levels of insulin in the bloodstream (hyperinsulinemia). Insulin may influence cancer risk in several ways and is likely to operate differently depending on the type of cancer. Normal cells grow and divide more quickly in the presence of high levels of insulin. Insulin is also thought to act to promote the reproduction of cells once they mutate to form cancer; in a way, feeding the cancer so that it may continue to grow and spread. And, since type 2 diabetes is tightly linked to being overweight, the additional hormonal abnormalities that are associated with obesity—altered levels of estrogen, testosterone, and more—may compound the effects of insulin for certain cancers.

With all of this in mind, it is still difficult to state with certainty that diabetes causes cancer. There are alternative explanations for the link between diabetes and cancer that should be considered. Cancer is generally a disease with a long period of latency, meaning there can be a lot of time from formation of the first cancer cell to the onset of signs or symptoms. This makes it difficult to determine whether diabetes occurred before the earliest phases of cancer or the cancer preceded the development of diabetes. For example, prostate cancer is a disease of older men and is often relatively slow growing. After the introduction in the late 1980s of widespread screening for early detection of prostate cancer, many cases of prostate cancer have been caught before they showed any symptoms or became a serious problem. It is possible, then, that any link between diabetes and cancer may be a matter of improved early screening. Furthermore, many researchers believe that the metabolic alterations in diabetes may cause an early cancer to develop more quickly into an aggressive cancer.

Still, there is evidence to suggest a link between some types of cancer and diabetes. Below we'll discuss additional risk factors and the proposed connection with diabetes by cancer site.

Pancreatic cancer

Cancer of the pancreas is a particularly lethal form of cancer. It so lethal, in fact, that it is difficult to study the risk factors associated with the development of the disease as patients often die within months of diagnosis. Fortunately, pancreatic cancer is relatively rare, accounting for just 2% of all new cancer cases diagnosed in the United States. Since the pancreas is the organ that produces insulin, the relationship between diabetes and pancreatic cancer is a problematic one. There are studies that suggest that people with diabetes have an elevated risk, but other studies suggest that type 2 diabetes may actually be a consequence of pancreatic cancer.

Endometrial cancer

Endometrial (uterine) cancer is the fourth most common cancer in women and mostly affects post-menopausal women. In the United States, approximately 40–50% of all cases are attributed to obesity. Endometrial cancer has also been linked to use of "estrogen-only" hormone replacement therapy (HRT), therapy that has waned since the early 1980s, when it was replaced by a combined estrogen-plus-progesterone therapy. Diabetes has been shown to have a modest effect on your risk for endometrial cancer. Recent studies suggest that the observed increase in endometrial cancer risk associated with diabetes is highest among women who are also morbidly obese or have high blood pressure.

Liver cancer

In this country, liver cancer is very rare, though it is a very common cancer internationally. Most cases are linked to a chronic infection of either hepatitis B (HBV) or C (HCV) and/or alcohol-related liver damage or cirrhosis. The disease is much more common in developing countries and eastern Asia, where HBV and HCV infection rates are high. Studies suggest that people with type 2 diabetes are at an increased risk of liver cancer, but there is some question as to whether the relationship has more to do with cirrhosis or is perhaps partly explained by obesity and dietary factors.

Prostate cancer

Prostate cancer is the most common cancer diagnosed among men in the United States, with one in six men diagnosed during their lifetime. Prostate cancer risk is highest among older men, those with a family history of prostate cancer, and African American men. Obesity has also been linked to a higher risk of aggressive cancer. Studies looking at the relationship between diabetes and prostate cancer have produced conflicting results, some indicating an elevated risk with others suggesting men with diabetes actually have a lower risk of prostate cancer. The studies that point to a lower risk suggest that the medications used to treat diabetes or its complications, such as metformin, may offer a protective benefit against this form of cancer.

Colorectal cancer

Cancers of the colon and cancers of the rectum are typically considered as one disease because the underlying causes are suspected to be very similar. Colorectal cancer is commonly diagnosed in the United States and is the second and third leading cause of cancer death in men and women, respectively. Diabetes and colorectal cancer share many of the same risk factors—obesity; a sedentary or inactive lifestyle; a diet high in animal fat, red meat, and refined sugar—and many researchers suggest that there is a causal link between the two diseases.

Managing Diabetes and Cancer

Many people will be diagnosed and treated simultaneously for cancer and diabetes simply because the conditions are so prevalent regardless of whether there is a direct causal relationship. In general, when there is a new and potentially serious cancer diagnosis, this takes precedence over close diabetes management. For example, treatment of some cancers may require a defined period of chemotherapy treatment. During this time, there may be periods of nausea and decreased appetite. Certain foods may no longer seem appetizing. The goal during this time period is to maintain weight, sometimes at the cost of tight glucose control. It should also be noted that some of the medications commonly used during cancer care may affect blood glucose levels. For example, glucocorticoids are often prescribed during cancer treatment to control nausea and pain. Unfortunately, if you have diabetes, these medications will increase blood glucose levels.

With this in mind, it is still important to work with your health care team to develop a treatment plan that treats both conditions in the long term.

This chapter was written by Jennifer L. Beebe-Dimmer, MPH, PhD, and Kathleen A. Cooney, MD.

29

Sleep Disturbance

Introduction

Sleep disturbances are not mentioned in today's guidelines for the treatment of diabetes. Yet, evidence from multiple sources shows that sleep deprivation aggravates insulin resistance and its various components, including high blood pressure, elevated blood glucose, and blood lipids. Sleep deprivation is also associated with obesity. We've all recognized the need for good diet and exercise to help with diabetes. The third component is sleep—being rested, being refreshed.

Lack of sleep is especially common in adults with type 2 diabetes. This is partly because there is more obesity in this group, and partly because of other factors, not fully understood, about diabetes. Accordingly, it is important that every person with diabetes have an understanding of sleep issues and whether they affect them. This chapter will review the various causes of sleep deprivation, show how it affects diabetes, and suggest how you can manage it.

What Are the Consequences of Sleep Disturbance?

Daytime drowsiness is the most obvious consequence of poor sleep. This is not only unpleasant, but it's been shown to raise your risk of accidents, produce errors in judgment and performance, and lead to poor eating habits. The majority of fatal car accidents—not related to alcohol—are believed to be caused by people either falling asleep at the wheel or being too tired to handle a situation. Medical interns and residents are no longer allowed to work as many hours per week as in the past because it was shown that they begin to make mistakes when fatigued, mistakes that can have grave consequences. Airline pilots have long recognized this.

Most interesting is research that shows we eat differently when we are sleep-deprived. In carefully conducted experiments, healthy volunteers were deprived of half their usual sleep time for a matter of days. They began to eat more and to eat more calorie-dense food (junk food) compared to those who were well rested. All of us know that it is difficult to exercise as hard or as long when we are tired, so if we're eating poorly as well, it's easy to see how lack of sleep can clearly sabotage lifestyle control of diabetes.

In addition to disrupting lifestyle modifications, sleep deprivation also creates a physical response in your body that raises your major risk factors for heart disease. These risk factors include:

- Elevated blood pressure
- Elevated triglycerides (fats)
- Lower HDL cholesterol (the good cholesterol)
- Elevated inflammation
- Elevated blood glucose

Successfully treating sleep problems improves all of these risk factors.

What Types of Sleep Disturbances Are There?

Perhaps the most common cause of sleep deprivation in the United States is self-inflicted. We simply don't give ourselves enough time to sleep, or we allow too many distractions during sleep, such as pets, children, TV and radio, etc. Many of us stay up late at night for work or entertainment, and then force ourselves awake with an alarm clock and coffee. As a population, we sleep, on average, almost 90 minutes a day less than our grandparents.

People who travel among time zones have long recognized the impact of jet lag. A similar phenomenon occurs in people who work alternate day and night shifts. The quality of sleep you get varies with stress and environmental factors. Caffeine and alcohol can disrupt sleep, as can eating a heavy meal or exercising right before bed.

Insomnia and fitful (fragmented) sleep is a common complaint. The overwhelming number of advertisements for sleep aids is evidence of how disturbing a problem this can be. Restless leg syndrome (RLG) is increasingly being recognized as a medical cause of sleep disturbance, and medication can be quite successful in relieving it. However, one of the most common and best characterized forms of sleep disturbance is sleep apnea.

What Is Sleep Apnea?

Sleep apnea refers to a condition where, numerous times during sleep, an individual stops breathing and is then awakened by the need for oxygen. Since the episode of awakening is very short, the individual usually doesn't know she has lost sleep, only that she wakes up tired and stays tired all day. Because it's difficult to recognize sleep apnea, you need to look for other symptoms that generally accompany it. Very loud snoring is one indication that sleep apnea is present.

The most common type of sleep apnea is obstructive sleep apnea (OSA), caused by physical obstruction of the airway during sleep. OSA is more common in obese individuals, in men, and in the elderly. One study of adults with type 2 diabetes found that while fewer than 20% of women below age 65 had OSA, over 60% of men above age 65 did.

There are excellent studies showing that treating OSA in individuals with diabetes can lower fasting glucose, post-meal glucose, and A1C as much as or even more than any oral medications available. Unfortunately, effectively treating OSA is the difficult part. The usual treatment for OSA, continuous positive airway pressure (CPAP), is sometimes less than successful, so there is more research to be done.

How Is a Sleep Disturbance Diagnosed?

When attempting to diagnose a sleep disturbance, the first question should be, "Do you wake up refreshed?" That, more than the absolute hours a person sleeps, indicates whether a sleep disturbance is significant. Insomnia or fitful sleep is usually obvious, but people may be reluctant to mention it because they either think nothing can be done or they fear medical sleep aids. Additionally, it's difficult to report some symptoms, since they occur during sleep. The spouse or bed partner is usually needed to report on abnormal breathing or movement during sleep.

If you have sleep apnea, your history probably reveals very loud snoring, the kind that is heard throughout the house. Your spouse or bed partner (if not forced away by the snoring) typically observes periods of not breathing followed by loud grunts and gasps for breath. This usually goes on all night. You probably also have severe daytime drowsiness, falling asleep whenever it's quiet. When a person falls asleep in the waiting room, that's usually a clue (a good specialist won't let you wait too long for an appointment).

Many sleep disturbances can be diagnosed with home tests or with a careful history. However, if the issue appears to be sleep apnea or restless leg syndrome, you may be referred to a sleep specialist. Physicians of many different backgrounds have begun to specialize in sleep disturbances, while more and more health care professionals recognize the need for consultation. The specialist may chose to do an overnight study in a sleep lab, which will resemble a hotel more than a laboratory. Depending on the suspected culprit, the study may include measurements of oxygen in the blood, brain waves, movement, and more. If the specialist suspects you have sleep apnea, you may begin a trial of treatment (see below) right away.

How Are Sleep Disturbances Treated?

Perhaps the toughest disturbance to treat is voluntary sleep deprivation. Just like diet and exercise, people just don't change their sleep habits easily. At the very least, people are encouraged to try increasing their sleep time by going to bed at least one hour earlier for a week. When this "prescription" is followed, the results are sometimes dramatic and avoid the hassle and expense of multiple tests.

Controversy continues over the use of pharmacologic sleep aids, but most clinicians are comfortable with them. The more recent aids, including zolpidem (Ambien), pyrazolopyrimidine (Sonata), eszopiclone (Lunesta), and ramelteon (Rozerem), do not appear to have a large risk of dependency or addiction, and two are even approved for continuous daily use (eszopiclone and ramelteon). However, sleep aids still carry a stigma, mainly because of older agents, such as Valium or barbituates, that clearly had addiction potential.

Fatigue from jet lag or changing work shift times is difficult to treat, and so there are numerous proposed remedies. Most would agree that avoiding caffeine and alcohol helps and, for jet lag, shifting to the new time zone on arrival is a good strategy. Prescription sleep aids can help, but so can simple aids such as neck pillows and eye shades for sleep during travel.

Restless leg syndrome can be successfully treated with medications, and safety issues are being resolved.

Obstructive sleep apnea is currently best treated by CPAP, which consists of a device, worn over the nose, that blows air with a high enough pressure to keep the airway open. It is not always easy to get the right level of comfort and effectiveness, and some people simply cannot tolerate it. But when CPAP is successful, it can dramatically improve a person's quality of life. For certain subgroups with OSA, surgery to widen the airway, or even devices that reposition the jaw, may be appropriate.

Conclusions

Sleep disturbances are very common in people with diabetes, and they are usually readily diagnosed and successfully treated. This is a matter of both quality of life and basic health issues so critical to cardiovascular health. Glucose control, blood pressure, lipids, and virtually all factors associated with diabetes are affected. Future guidelines for diabetes should take sleep disturbances into account.

This chapter was written by Daniel Einhorn, MD, FACP, FACE.

30

Infections

Introduction

Infectious diseases can be caused by a large variety of microorganisms, including viruses, bacteria, fungi, and parasites. People with diabetes can get the same infections as everyone else, but certain infections tend to occur more frequently or more severely in people with diabetes. This chapter explains how and why infections may present a special problem for you.

How Does Your Immune System Deal with Infections?

Our bodies are surrounded by, and covered with, vast numbers of microorganisms that would like to use us as a source of food and housing. Some of these are harmless, or even helpful, but some cause infections. To prevent infection, our bodies have developed a remarkably effective system of defenses. Infections develop only when these defenses are breached. The first lines of defense are anatomical (such as our skin) and physiological barriers (such as the acid in our stomach). In addition, we have a complex inner immune system that helps detect invading microorganisms and destroy them.

White blood cells are produced in your bone marrow and circulate in the bloodstream until they are needed to fight an invading microorganism. These cells are attracted to an infected area by chemicals that are released when tissue damage occurs. Our immune system also makes antibodies that recognize foreign invaders and help kill them.

What Are the Symptoms of Infection?

When an organism such as a bacterium or virus enters your body, it triggers a series of events designed to fight the invasion. This process may produce some of the findings of inflammation, such as pain, tenderness, redness, warmth, or swelling. Pain is caused by three things: chemicals produced in your body to attract white blood cells, the release of toxins (a type of poison) from the invading germs, and the destruction of the tissues under attack. These chemicals and toxins, and the battle between your defenses and the germs, help produce the heat associated with an infection. As more chemicals are released, the small blood vessel (capillary) beds near the infection expand to allow more white blood cells to enter the infected area. This increase in blood supply contributes to the warmth and redness that is associated with an infection.

As the infection progresses, a thick, cloudy fluid called pus may form. This is made up of white blood cells, germs, tissue debris, and fluid from the blood vessels. Unlike the clear, yellow drainage in many uninfected wounds, the presence of pus is usually evidence of an infection. As pus accumulates under the skin, it may cause a swelling called an abscess. This requires surgical drainage.

How Are Infections and Blood Glucose Control Connected?

Poor blood glucose control over several years probably increases your risk for developing certain infections. High blood glucose levels can impair your white blood cells' ability to digest and kill bacteria. In addition, glucose levels can rise dramatically when the body is under stress, such as when it is fighting an infection. Among other responses, stress increases the secretion of various hormones, including cortisol and glucagon. These, in turn, increase the release of glucose from the liver, so the blood glucose level goes even higher.

Does Insulin Help You Deal with Infections?

Not directly, but insulin does help lower blood glucose, which is usually higher during an infection. When people who use insulin are admitted to the hospital for treatment of a severe illness, they may require increased insulin doses to lower high blood glucose levels. Patients with type 2 diabetes who do not use insulin may temporarily need insulin to reduce their hyperglycemia. Once the infection or stress is under control, diabetes treatment can usually go back to normal.

Is the Immune System of People with Diabetes Different from Those of People Without Diabetes?

Diabetes can alter your immune system, making it more difficult for you to detect or fight infections. First, diabetes can impair the production and effect of many infection-fighting components of your immune system, such as white blood cells and antibodies. Second, there are complications of diabetes, such as blood vessel diseases, that hinder your body's ability to deliver these infection fighters. Lastly, diabetes complications, such as neuropathy, can inhibit your ability to sense the infection. By the time you notice the findings of inflammation, the infection can be quite severe.

Can Normal Microorganisms Cause Infections in People with Diabetes?

Bacteria and fungi that are routinely found on certain parts of your body are called normal flora. Areas where these organisms grow include the skin, mouth, and intestinal tract. These organisms actually help prevent infection, but in certain situations the normal flora can also cause infections. This may occur when there is an overgrowth of these organisms at a site where they are normally found (for example, oral thrush, which is caused by an overgrowth of a common, yeast-like fungus called *candida*) or when they invade a site where they are not normally found (for example, skin bacteria infecting bone at the base of an open foot ulcer). Infections, unlike normal microorganism growth, are characterized by the presence of pus or by the signs of inflammation. Diabetes can raise your risk for infections from organisms that rarely cause infections in people who do not have diabetes.

How Are Different Types of Infections Diagnosed?

Many different microorganisms can cause infection, but bacteria are the most important. Only about a dozen types are common causes of infections. We classify bacteria by several characteristics. Two of the most useful are 1) whether the bacteria need oxygen (aerobic) or do not need oxygen (anaerobic) to grow and 2) whether they appear purple (gram-positive) or pink (gram-negative) on slides containing specially stained smears of body specimens. These classifications help predict the course of the infection and the most appropriate antibiotics to use for treatment. The specific organism causing an infection is identified by culturing (growing in the lab) a specimen from the affected area—for example, from urine, pus, or mucus. The most frequent bacterial types that cause infections in patients with diabetes are aerobic gram-positive organisms, specifically a bacterium called *staphylococcus*. Aerobic gram-negative organisms are most common in urinary tract infections. Anaerobic organisms (both gram-positive and gram-negative) are usually found with other bacteria in deep soft-tissue infections, and they are often associated with a foul odor. Each antibiotic acts against a specific group of organisms. Organisms that grow on the cultures can be tested against various antibiotics to determine how susceptible they are to each one.

What Types of Infections Are Common in People with Diabetes?

People with diabetes are more likely to develop several specific types of infections. In addition, some infections may be more severe or cause complications more often in people with diabetes. There are also some very rare, but serious, infections that occur almost exclusively in people with diabetes. See Tables 30-1, 30-2, and 30-3 for more on these types of infections.

Table 30-1. Common Infections in People with Diabetes

Infection	Description	Common organism(s)	Typical signs and symptoms	Treatment
Urinary tract infection	Infection of the bladder (cystitis) or kidney(s) (pyelonephritis)	Bacteria or fungi	Painful, frequent, urgent urination; blood or pus in urine	Antibiotics or antifungal drugs (oral or intravenous)
Foot infection	Skin infection often related to a diabetic foot ulcer (see chapter 15)	Bacteria	Red, painful, warm, swollen foot; pus drainage	Antibiotics (oral or intravenous)
Onychomycosis	Fungal infection of fingernails or toenails	Fungi	Thickened, yellow nails that sometimes separate from the skin	Antifungal drugs (oral or topical)
Tinea pedis	Fungal infection of skin between the toes	Fungi	Cracks in toe web skin, itching	Antifungal drugs (usually topical)

Table 30-2. Infections That Are Often More Severe in People with Diabetes

Infection	Description	Common organism(s)	Typical signs and symptoms	Complications with diabetes	Treatment
Influenza	"The Flu"; Upper respiratory infection occurring in late winter/ early spring	Influenza A or B virus	Fever, headache, muscle aches, fatigue, cough, sore throat	Pneumonia from influenza or bacteria	Antiviral drugs (zanamivir, oseltamivir) can reduce the severity and duration of symptoms

Infection	Description	Common organism(s)	Typical signs and symptoms	Complications with diabetes	Treatment
Pneumonia	Infection of the lung	Bacteria (occasionally viruses or fungi)	Fever, cough with sputum, malaise	Can spread to bloodstream, increased risk of severe infection	Antibiotics (oral or intravenous)
Cellulitis (skin) & soft tissue infections	Infections of the skin and underlying tissues	Bacteria, especially *streptococci* or *staphylococci*	Fever and/or painful, red skin, sometimes with blisters	Necrotizing fasciitis, a rapidly spreading soft tissue infection	Antibiotics and surgical removal of infected and dead tissue

Table 30-3. Rare Infections Nearly Exclusive to People with Diabetes

The following infections usually require hospitalization

Infection	Description	Common organism	Symptoms	Treatment
Malignant otitis externa	Severe external ear canal infection that can spread to bone	Bacteria (especially *pseudomonas*) or fungi	Severe earache, pus or foul smelling drainage from the ear, fever, hearing loss	Antibiotics, sometimes surgery
Rhinocerebral mucormycosis	Infection of the sinuses or palate of the mouth associated with diabetic ketoacidosis	Rhizopus (fungus)	Pain in eyes or sinuses, yellowish-white nasal discharge, swelling around the eyes	Antifungal drugs usually with removal of dead or infected tissue
Emphysematous cholecystitis	Severe infection of the gallbladder with gas in the wall of the gallbladder	Gas-forming bacteria	Pain in the right upper abdomen, nausea, vomiting, fever	Surgical removal of the gallbladder (cholecystectomy), intravenous antibiotics
Emphysematous pyelonephritis	Severe infection of the kidney(s) with gas in the kidney(s)	Gas-forming bacteria	Fever, pain in the flank/back, nausea, vomiting	Intravenous antibiotics, sometimes surgical drainage

What Type of Urinary Tract Infections Might You Be More Likely to Develop?

Cystitis (bladder infection)

This is an infection of the lining of the urinary bladder. Symptoms of acute (sudden-onset) cystitis include pain or burning on urination, increased frequency of urination, pain over the bladder (above the pubic area), and sometimes fever. Your urine may be cloudy, have a foul odor, or even contain some blood. Most bladder infections are caused by bacteria and respond to oral antibiotics within a few days. Antibiotics are usually given for 3–7 days. Patients with diabetes are also more likely to have urinary tract infections caused by fungi, which require antifungal agents. Fungi can occasionally form a large mass called a fungus ball. These can occur anywhere in the urinary tract and may require surgical removal. Rarely, patients develop a severe form of bladder infection that is characterized by air in the bladder wall, called emphysematous cystitis (see Table 30-3). This usually requires hospitalization and possibly surgery.

Pyelonephritis (kidney infection)

Infected urine from the bladder can go up the ureters (the tubes connecting the bladder to the kidneys) to cause an infection of the kidneys called pyelonephritis. Acute pyelonephritis typically causes fever, chills, nausea, vomiting, and severe side (flank) or upper-back pain. These symptoms may occur simultaneously with, or soon after, symptoms of cystitis.

Patients with pyelonephritis may be treated at home if they are not experiencing severe symptoms, such as high fever, severe high blood glucose levels, or vomiting. Otherwise, hospitalization with intravenous therapy is needed for a few days. The total duration of antibiotic therapy is usually 2 weeks.

If your health care provider suspects that you have pyelonephritis, especially if your symptoms have persisted for several days, he or she may suggest an X-ray or ultrasound test to look for emphysematous pyelonephritis. This unusual, but serious, complication is diagnosed by the presence of gas in the kidneys. Most cases of emphysematous pyelonephritis occur in people with diabetes, perhaps because high blood glucose levels in the tissue allow bacteria or fungi to produce the gas. As with emphysematous cystitis, this infection requires immediate hospitalization, and sometimes surgical drainage.

Other complications of kidney infections include infection of the tissues surrounding the kidney (perinephric abscess) and death of tissue in the kidneys (renal infarction). After an episode of pyelonephritis has been treated, some may be evaluated for abnormalities of the urinary tract that may make them more likely to get infections in the future. This evaluation may include an ultrasound examination of the kidneys, measurement of urinary flow, an excretory urogram (an X-ray with an injection of dye), or cystoscopy (looking into the bladder with a special instrument).

Why Are Foot Infections So Common in People with Diabetes?

People with diabetes are prone to foot infections, most often related to a foot ulcer. This is related to several factors.

1. Diabetes can damage your sensory nerves, particularly in your feet. This decreases sensation so much that you might not feel when you cut your foot or when sores develop from improperly fitted shoes. Once there is a break in the skin, you are at risk of bacteria invading your skin and causing an infection in the unattended sore.

2. Diabetes can cause peripheral arterial disease (see chapter 10), or clogging of your arteries, resulting in decreased blood flow to your feet. This will make it more difficult for wounds to heal and can reduce the delivery of antibiotics and white blood cells to infected sites.

3. Diabetes can suppress your immune system, making it more difficult for you to fight infections.

Depending on the severity of the foot infection, treatment usually consists of antibiotics (either pills or intravenous) and removal of any dead or infected tissue. It is crucial to keep pressure off the infected wound. This may require bed rest, a wheelchair, crutches, casting the foot and leg, or special foot wear. Sometimes, narrowed arteries may need to be bypassed or widened to help wounds heal. Without proper treatment, foot infections can quickly progress and lead to amputation of the foot or leg, or even death. Unfortunately, diabetes greatly increases the risk of foot amputation. Fortunately, most amputations can be prevented by good foot care.

What Is Onychomycosis?

Onychomycosis is a fungal infection of the nails, most commonly of the bigger toes. It can affect other nails of the feet and sometimes the hands. The fungus causes the nails to become rough, thickened, and yellow. Eventually, the entire nail may become soft and crumbly and may fall off. Many people are simply disturbed by the appearance of the nail, but the infection can lead to ulcers and infection of the toe itself.

Nail fungus can be treated by oral antifungal drugs, such as terbinafine (Lamisil) or itraconazole (Sporanox). These prescription drugs have potential side effects that you should discuss with your provider. The medications are relatively expensive and must be taken for 12 weeks. While the success rate for treatment is up to 80% of nails treated, infection frequently returns. Also, it takes a new toenail 18 to 24 months to grow out normally after the fungus has been treated.

What Is Malignant External Otitis?

Malignant, or invasive, external otitis is a serious type of external ear infection that occurs almost exclusively in people with diabetes. The name refers to the severity of infection; it is not a cancer. This infection begins in the external ear canal, then involves the soft tissue next to the ear, and may eventually spread to the bone located near the ear canal. Most people with diabetes who develop this infection are older than 65 years of age, are men, and have long-standing diabetes.

Signs of malignant external otitis include severe, persistent earache, festering and sometimes foul-smelling ear discharge, and possibly hearing loss. As the infection progresses, it may involve the base of the skull or even the facial nerve, which may cause drooping of facial muscles. Patients may also have systemic signs of infection, such as fever, and elevated glucose levels and white blood cell count. Making a diagnosis may require special X-rays or scans.

Once diagnosed, therapy usually requires more than 6 weeks of antibiotics, and surgical removal of infected tissue or bone may also be necessary. Despite appropriate therapy, the infection may come back.

What Is Rhinocerebral Mucormycosis?

This is an uncommon fungal infection that occurs in people with diabetes, especially those who have had episodes of ketoacidosis (chapter 4). It involves your nasal sinuses or the palate (roof) of your mouth. The fungi that cause this infection can grow rapidly in the presence of high glucose and in an acid environment—such as in ketoacidosis. This infection advances rapidly and, if not quickly diagnosed and properly treated, it can be life-threatening.

The first symptoms are usually pain in your eyes or face, followed by yellowish-white or blood-tinged nasal discharge, swelling around the eyes, increased tearing, visual blurring, and sinus or nasal tenderness. Physical examination by your doctor may disclose a darkening or ulceration in the nasal passages or palate; imaging tests (X-rays, scans) may be needed to confirm the diagnosis.

Therapy must be started early and be aggressive, to prevent spread of the infection to the brain. The dead and infected tissue must be surgically removed, and antifungal and antibiotic medicines must be given.

What Is Emphysematous Cholecystitis?

Emphysematous cholecystitis is a severe infection of the gallbladder caused by gas-forming bacteria. It tends to occur in men and has high rates of complications, such as gangrene or perforation of the gallbladder. Up to 15% of people with this infection will die from it. Although having gallstones is the usual underlying factor for developing acute cholecystitis, emphysematous cholecystitis is associated with gallstones only about half of the time. Usually, the infection is caused by a several different bacteria. Prompt surgical removal of the gallbladder and antibiotic therapy are necessary to treat the infection.

How Can People with Diabetes Lower Their Risk of Having an Infection?

The infections discussed in this chapter can be severe and frightening. The good news is that they are usually preventable. Good hygiene is recommended for everyone to reduce the spread of infection. Washing hands frequently and covering the mouth/nose when sneezing or coughing can help reduce the spread of many respiratory infections, both to and from you and others. You can reduce the risk of infections by keeping your blood glucose levels as normal as possible, by eating a healthy diet (rich in fruits and vegetables and low in refined carbohydrates) and properly using medications that lower blood glucose levels. Since you may lack normal sensation in your feet, you need to be particularly careful about keeping your feet clean and dry. You should inspect your feet regularly for any sores or cuts. It is also important to wear properly fitting shoes, avoid walking barefoot outside, and test the bath (or hot tub) water temperature with your hands. Also, check your shoes for any objects that may have fallen in.

Vaccines can reduce your risk of developing certain infections and can also reduce their severity if you are infected. People with diabetes (who are not allergic to eggs) should receive the influenza vaccine every year. Those who are 50 years or older can also be given the pneumococcal vaccine, which may reduce their risk of developing severe symptoms or complications from pneumococcal pneumonia (pneumonia due to the bacterium, *streptococcus pneumoniae*). Since protection lessens over time, a booster of the vaccine is recommended every 5 years.

If you travel to other countries, you can contact your local travel agent, public health department, or the Centers for Disease Control and Prevention to learn which vaccinations are recommended for your protection in the countries you'll be visiting. The hepatitis A vaccine is often recommended, as is a tetanus shot if you haven't had one in the past 10 years. Some people, especially those at risk of exposure to blood, may need hepatitis B vaccinations. New vaccines that help prevent shingles (a reactivation of the chicken pox virus) and whooping cough (pertussis) may also be appropriate.

Are You More Susceptible to Infections from Antibiotic Resistant Organisms?

Since people with diabetes often have regular contact with hospitals or clinics, and they are at a higher risk of developing some infections, they are also more prone to infections caused by organisms that are resistant to the antibiotics usually used to treat those infections. This antibiotic resistance may lead to inadequate treatment, resulting in more complications and worse outcomes. Methicillin-resistant *staphylococcus aureus* (MRSA) has emerged as an important cause of skin and soft tissue infections in the United States in recent years, and people with diabetes are at an increased risk of infection with this bacterium. There are new antibiotics that can effectively treat MRSA, as well as most other resistant bacteria. One important way to decrease your risk of antibiotic-resistant infections is to avoid taking antibiotics when you do not need them, such as for colds or uninfected skin ulcers.

This chapter was written by Traci A. Takahashi, MD, MPH, and Benjamin A. Lipsky, MD.

31

Dementia and Alzheimer's Disease

Case Study

LK is 71 years old and was diagnosed with type 2 diabetes 4 years ago. She has maintained good blood glucose control. Recently she has been forgetting her appointments and losing her car keys. She is worried that she may have dementia or Alzheimer's disease, as she has heard that people with diabetes have a higher risk of memory problems. She wants to be referred to a neurologist. The neurologist obtained blood tests and a magnetic resonance imaging (MRI) scan of her brain. The MRI and blood tests ruled out other possible causes of dementia, and a series of cognitive tests confirmed the diagnoses of dementia and Alzheimer's disease.

What Is Dementia?

Dementia is not a disease itself but a syndrome that refers to a cluster of symptoms that cause memory and cognitive problems, such as difficulty with orientation, attention, language, and problem solving. These difficulties should also exhibit a progressive cognitive decline above and beyond normal age-related changes. In addition to the more apparent cognitive problems, dementia is also associated with an increase in mortality, morbidity, and health care utilization, not to mention the enormous burden on caregivers and family members.

More than 33% of women and 20% of men aged 65 and older will develop dementia during their lifetime, and many more will develop a milder form of impairment. As a large proportion of the population in the United States begins to age, and life expectancy continues to increase, the cases of dementia are projected to rise. Estimates suggest that there will be a 50% increase in the total number of people with cognitive impairment in the next 25 years.

Dementia is due to a variety of causes, but the two most common are Alzheimer's disease and vascular dementia. Less common causes include Parkinson's disease, HIV-associated dementia, Down syndrome, Huntington's disease, thyroid disorders, vitamin deficiency, depression-induced pseudodementia, head trauma, and syphilis. Because people with diabetes are more likely to have the most common causes of dementia, Alzheimer's disease and vascular dementia, only these types of dementia will be covered in this chapter.

What Is Alzheimer's Disease ?

Alzheimer's disease, also referred to simply as Alzheimer's, is the most common type of dementia. Over half of all dementia is due to Alzheimer's disease, a condition characterized by memory loss, cognitive decline, and, ultimately, severe behavioral changes and complete loss of the ability to care for oneself. The first symptom noticed is usually short-term memory loss, which progresses from simple forgetfulness to a consistent loss of short-term memory. Eventually the condition will progress to the most devastating part of the disease, the loss of familiar and well-known skills and the ability to recognize people.

The prevalence of Alzheimer's increases with age. Among people 65 years and older, one in ten has the disease, while 50% of those aged 85 years and older have symptoms of Alzheimer's. The risk of having Alzheimer's doubles every five years after the age of 65.

Alzheimer's is a neurodegenerative disease, which means that there are changes in the brain happening as part of the progression of the disease. People with Alzheimer's lose neurons (nerve cells) and develop brain atrophy, a sign of neuordegeneration. People with Alzheimer's also develop other physical abnormalities in their brains (such as amyloid plaques and neurofibrillary tangles), though how these affect the condition is not clearly understood.

The usual course of the disease is 5–10 years, although there have been reports of people living longer with the disease. The sooner Alzheimer's is diagnosed, the more effective treatment can be. Therefore, as with most diseases, early detection is crucial.

What Is the Cause of Alzheimer's Disease?

The ultimate cause of this disease is unknown, though there are several risk factors that are discussed later in this chapter. While genetic factors play a large role in the very rare early-onset familial Alzheimer's disease (Alzheimer's before age 60, which accounts for only 5% of Alzheimer's cases), genes seem to play a smaller role in the more common late-onset Alzheimer's, which genearally appears after age 60. However, one confirmed susceptibility gene, ApoE, has been associated with a greater chance of developing Alzheimer's.

Women and African Americans are more likely to get Alzheimer's disease, though the exact reason is unknown. Since the chances of Alzheimer's increase with age, and women tend to live longer, this may explain their greater risk. Along the same lines, African Americans are more likely to have hypertension and diabetes, both of which increase the risk of dementia.

Large population-based studies also suggest that people with diabetes are more likely to get Alzheimer's disease than people without diabetes.

What Are the Symptoms of Alzheimer's Disease?

It is perfectly normal to occasionally forget a meeting, an appointment, or what day of the week it is. What is abnormal is for these events to occur more frequently and to progressively worsen, as this could potentially be a sign of impending dementia. (See the box Ten Warning Signs of Alzheimer's Disease for more.) As Alzheimer's progresses, the symptoms associated with the disease generally become more severe. The following are characteristic for different stages of the disease.

Ten Warning Signs of Alzheimer's Disease

- **Recent memory loss that impairs one's ability to complete routine assignments at work and/or function effectively at home.** May frequently forget names, phone numbers, and work tasks and have trouble remembering them even when reminded.

- **Problems with language.** May progressively forget simple words, substitute inappropriate words, and/or make statements that don't make sense.

- **Disorientation in time and space and getting confused or lost in a familiar place.** May leave home and then forget an intended destination, or become lost on a nearby street and not know how to get home.

- **Difficulty completing familiar tasks.** May, for example, prepare a meal but forget to serve it—or even forget that it was made.

- **Distorted judgment.** May dress inappropriately, completely forget what was set out to do mid-task, or forget key routine tasks, such as keeping set appointments or caring for a pet.

- **Problems with abstract thinking.** May have trouble with simple mathematical calculations, such as balancing a checkbook or remembering a familiar, often-used phone number.

- **Misplacing things.** May put things in inappropriate places, such as putting keys in the microwave, a toothbrush in the kitchen cabinet, or a briefcase in the refrigerator.

- **Repeated and sudden changes in mood and behavior.** May begin exhibiting out-of-character rapid mood swings for no apparent reason.

- **Changes in personality.** May start to act in ways that are counter to one's usual personality style, for example, acting suspicious, fearful, or confused.

- **Loss of initiative to do things.** May become passive, unresponsive, express little interest in previously enjoyed activities and require real encouragement to get involved.

Mild

At the early stage of the disease, people have a tendency to become less energetic or spontaneous, though changes in behavior often go unnoticed even by a person's immediate family. This stage of the disease is sometimes referred to as Mild Cognitive Impairment.

Moderate

As the disease progresses to the middle stage, a person might still be able to perform tasks independently, but needs help with more complicated activities

Severe

As the disease progresses from the middle to late stage, the person will undoubtedly not be able to perform even the simplest of tasks on his or her own and will need constant supervision. He or she may even lose the ability to walk or eat without help from a caregiver.

What Is Vascular Dementia?

Vascular dementia is the second most common type of dementia in elderly people. It refers to a number of syndromes that lead to vascular lesions in the brain, most often a series of small strokes. Early detection and accurate diagnosis are highly crucial, since vascular dementia is somewhat preventable.

Multi-infarct dementia is the most common form of vascular dementia and accounts for 10–20% of all cases of progressive dementia. It usually affects people between the ages of 60 and 75 and, unlike Alzheimer's, is more likely to occur in men than women.

Multi-infarct dementia is caused by a series of strokes that disrupt blood flow and damage or destroy brain tissue. (See chapter XX for more on strokes). A stroke occurs when blood cannot get to part of the brain, for instance, when a blood clot or fatty deposit (called plaque) blocks the vessels that supply blood to the brain. A stroke also can happen when a blood vessel in the brain bursts. A number of conditions can lead to a stroke, such as high blood pressure (hypertension), diabetes, high cholesterol, or heart disease. However, of these conditions, hypertension is the most important risk factor for multi-infarct dementia.

What Is the Cause and What Are the Symptoms of Vascular Dementia?

Multi-infarct dementia is often the result of a series of small strokes. Some of these small strokes produce no obvious symptoms and are noticed only on brain imaging studies, so they are sometimes called "silent strokes." A person may have several small strokes before noticing serious changes in memory or other signs of multi-infarct dementia. Sudden onset of any of the following symptoms may be a sign of Vascular Dementia:

- Confusion and problems with recent memory
- Wandering or getting lost in familiar places
- Moving with rapid, shuffling steps
- Loss of bladder or bowel control
- Laughing or crying inappropriately
- Difficulty following instructions
- Problems handling money

Since strokes happen suddenly, cognitive changes also occur quite quickly. People with multi-infarct dementia may even have some improvement before declining again after subsequent strokes.

Are People with Diabetes at a Greater Risk of Alzheimer's Disease, Vascular Dementia, or Cognitive Impairment?

Several large studies have shown that people with diabetes are at a higher risk of developing vascular dementia, Alzheimer's disease, and cognitive impairment. The exact reasons for this are unknown, although research suggests that vascular risk factors such as high cholesterol and hypertension increase the risk of not only vascular dementia but Alzheimer's disease as well. Indeed, Alzheimer's disease and vascular dementia often coexist in people, so controlling vascular risk factors is a good approach to reducing your risk of *both* types of dementia.

Blood glucose control is also critical, as poorly controlled blood glucose can interfere with cognitive functioning, which may also contribute to the development of dementia. Episodes of severe low blood glucose (hypoglycemia) can also damage the blood brain barrier, which may also play a role in dementia.

Ways You Can Lower Your Risk of Dementia

- Maintain a healthy A1C level (<7% for most individuals)

- Control your hypertension

- Follow a healthy diet

- Maintain a healthy weight

- Do your best to avoid episodes of hypoglycemia and hyperglycemia

Can Dementia or Cognitive Impairment Be Prevented?

There is no cure for dementia, however there are several things one can do that will reduce your chances of developing it (see box).

What are the Risk Factors for Dementia that You Cannot Change?

- **Age**. This is the biggest risk factor.
- **Gender.** Women are more likely than men to get Alzheimer's disease, though men are more likely to get vascular dementia.
- **Genetics.** One major susceptibility gene, apoE, has been identified for Alzheimer's disease.
- **Education Level.** Those with fewer years of formal education have a higher risk of dementia.

What Are the Risk Factors for Dementia That You Can Change?

- **Mental Agility.** Engaging in mentally challenging activities may lower your risk. Studies have shown that cross word puzzles, reading, playing a musical instrument, and other cognitively stimulating activities can reduce your risk.
- **Physical Health.** Studies have shown that obesity and overweight increase the risk of dementia. Physical activity, however, lowers your risk. Physical activity has beneficial effects on vascular risk factors and there is also evidence that it directly supports brain function.
- **Cardiovascular Risk Factors.** Try to maintain healthy cholesterol levels, blood pressure, and blood glucose levels.

Conclusion

Dementia and Alzheimer's disease affect those with diabetes at a much higher rate. However, by knowing your risk factors and the early symptoms of these conditions, you can actively work to lower your risk and/or begin treatment of the disease early, thus minimizing the negative effects associated with these diseases. If you or a family member is having what you think are symptoms of dementia or Alzheimer's disease, make an appointment with a neurologist. The earlier you begin treatment, the better your long-term outcomes will be.

This chapter was written by Rachel A. Whitmer, PhD.

32

Psychosocial Complications

Introduction

There is a wealth of scientific knowledge about diabetes and its physical complications (for example, eye problems, nerve problems, heart problems, kidney problems, etc.). Much of this knowledge has helped people with diabetes take better care of themselves and prevent the physical complications of diabetes. There is also scientific knowledge about another category of diabetes complications—psychosocial complications. However, since the general public is not as aware of psychosocial complications as they are about physical problems related to diabetes, not as much is being done to prevent and/or deal with psychosocial complications. In this chapter we will review psychosocial complications in order to better inform you about this area and to present a problem-solving model for preventing and dealing with these complications.

What Are Psychosocial Complications?

Psychosocial complications can be either a consequence of physical complications or a direct result of having diabetes. Think of psychosocial complications as psychological barriers to good self-care. These barriers can be emotional, social, or behavioral.

Emotional barriers

Emotions that we experience can at times be positive and can have a protective effect on us. For example, in some situations, fear may prevent us from entering an unsafe situation. However, fear may also present a psychological barrier to doing everything that is necessary to take good care of yourself. For example, fear of hearing bad news may prevent some people from going to the doctor for regular check-ups. Fear of low blood glucose may prevent you from following recommendations from your doctor for medication or insulin management. Other emotions can just as easily act as a barrier to good self-care. For example, anger about having diabetes may make it difficult to accept the need for lifestyle changes. Sadness or depression about your diabetes can result in giving up or thinking that making changes is hopeless.

However, just as emotions can present a barrier to good diabetes care, they can also help you take better care of yourself. For example, optimism about your lifestyle changes can result in success and better health. Feeling proud that you achieved one or more of your lifestyle goals can result in maintenance of those goals. We will help you identify when an emotion may be presenting a barrier to good care, show you how to deal with that emotion, and then convert it into an emotion that will lead to better care and prevention of complications.

Social barriers

Psychological barriers can also be social in nature. How much we reach out to others or are supported by others varies from person to person, but in general we are social beings. As such, we are vulnerable to social barriers. For example, we can be over-concerned about social acceptance. If someone with diabetes is concerned about what people think of them, they may be less likely to complete aspects of diabetes care that make them stand out. This is a problem that often affects adolescents with diabetes, as they are particularly concerned about what their friends think of them. Lack of social support can also be a social barrier. Making lifestyle changes can be particularly difficult, and a lack of close family members and/or friends to cheer you on or join you in making changes can result in giving up or not making positive changes.

However, there are also social factors that can result in better self-care. Social support from friends and family can have an extremely positive effect. Many studies have shown that support from friends and family results in fewer psychosocial complications (for example, less depression) and can also result in better physical health. Although friends and family are the most likely individuals who support you, there are many other potential sources of support, including your physician and health care team, your religious leader, and other people in your community.

There are many types of social support that you may receive from friends, loved ones, and health care professionals. The four main categories of support are:

1. **Emotional**— Emotional support involves helping you deal with your emotions. Listening to you or encouraging you are two ways of offering emotional support.
2. **Informational**—Informational support occurs when you are given written resources such as pamphlets or books about how to best take care of diabetes.
3. **Tangible**—Tangible support refers to someone doing something specific to help you take care of your diabetes. This type of support includes buying supplies, giving insulin injections, or helping with blood glucose testing.
4. **Companionship**—Companionship support refers to someone joining with you to help make diabetes care easier. Examples include exercising with you or following your meal plan with you.

Behavioral barriers

Psychological barriers to better health can also be behavioral in nature. Many of us behave in ways that do not improve our health and may in fact put as at risk for physical harm. For example, most of us drive faster than we should, eat more fast food than we should, and exercise less often than we should. We may engage in some of these behaviors because of a tendency to act that way, or we may have learned those behaviors from others around us. However, no matter how these behaviors have started, they have typically become habits by adulthood. Habits are behaviors that we have done so often that they have become automatic. It may be difficult, and at times a long process, but habits can be changed! You can choose behaviors that will bring about better health and will prevent physical and psychological complications.

How Do You Deal with the Psychosocial Complications of Diabetes?

Throughout the rest of this chapter we will help you to identify ways to deal with the psychological complications of diabetes. In general we will focus on helping you use the following problem-solving process:

1. Recognize when an emotional, social, or behavioral barrier is present.
2. Deal with that barrier.
3. Turn the barrier into a situation that leads to better diabetes care.

This process will be discussed across several diabetes-related concepts, including receiving the initial diagnosis of diabetes, making lifestyle changes, following the diabetes treatment regimen, and managing good health over a lifetime. Lastly, we'll discuss special considerations related to diabetes in adolescence.

Dealing with the diagnosis of diabetes

A diagnosis of diabetes can create a complex set of emotions. Many people describe first feeling concern and anxiety. Others, particularly those who have relatives with diabetes, may not be as distressed. Most studies have shown that mild depression may follow a diagnosis of diabetes, but that most people rebound, or return, to their typical mood state as they adjust to the diagnosis and the day-to-day changes it involves. So, what is the best way to deal with being diagnosed with diabetes?

As a first step, monitor yourself and try to identify the three types of psychological barriers to good health that you may be encountering. In other words, identify the emotional, social, and behavioral barriers that you are experiencing. The primary barriers in this area tend to be emotional. Many people report feeling overwhelmed and, consequently, they will shut down. Another common emotional barrier may be anxiety, anger, or a similarly intense emotion that may interfere with how you process information about diabetes or how you act on this information. In order to prevent these emotions from affecting your physical and psychological health, you must deal with these emotions. Dealing with these emotions may involve talking with a psychologist or a social worker about your feelings. Talking about your reactions with your endocrinologist or family physician may offer some relief as well. Family and friends are also important sources of support; they may act as a sounding board for your feelings and may be able to provide comfort in this regard.

Although emotional barriers to good health are the most common responses to a diagnosis of diabetes, also think about social and behavioral barriers that you may be experiencing. Many people encounter the social barrier of withdrawal. Feeling overwhelmed and depressed may cause some to withdraw from others just at the time they most need support. Think carefully about the ways in which you could use help, and then ask specifically for that kind of support. It may also help to have others advocate on your behalf and help to arrange for social support. If you continue to experience withdrawal, however, it may be time to seek professional help from a trained mental health provider.

Making lifestyle changes

For most, a diagnosis of diabetes means a need to make lifestyle changes, such as diet and physical activity. Making changes to your lifestyle has proven to be one of the most difficult challenges of good diabetes management. First and foremost, there are many behavioral barriers to making lifestyle changes, and many of these behaviors have become habitual. Our eating and exercise habits are established very early in life and are continually reinforced throughout our lives by those around us. When we are young, we watch our parents and other family members and tend to adopt their habits with regard to eating and exercise. If you have a parent who often eats potato chips and drinks regular soda, it is likely that you will adopt those same habits in childhood and will continue with those habits throughout your adult years. Likewise, having parents who are inactive and prefer watching TV may result in children who grow up also preferring leisure time to exercising. There are even more behavioral barriers to exercise today than when we were growing up. Most of the things that make our lives easier—cell phones, televisions, computers, and cars—encourage a more sedentary lifestyle.

What is the best way, then, to change from an unhealthy to a healthy lifestyle? First, identify the emotional, social, and behavioral barriers in your life that are making it difficult for you to make lifestyle changes. Write down each of these barriers so that you can deal with each one. For example, you may identify that you eat for comfort or for stress-relief, which is an emotional barrier. You may also identify the social barrier of having no one to help motivate you to exercise. Lastly, you may identify the behavioral barrier of snacking on high-calorie foods whenever you are watching TV.

As you try to identify barriers to lifestyle change, you'll find that most will be behavioral. Writing down a plan for change with specific goals outlined is the most effective way to make behavioral changes in your diet and physical activity. For example, if you have been eating a diet high in fat and sugar, you may want to outline healthier choices that are *reasonable to make* (unreasonable goals are often abandoned quickly) given your current lifestyle and the day-to-day demands of your life. Keeping these dietary goals on paper with you when you go out to eat or go shopping will help remind you to make healthy choices and can guide you in deciding what a healthy choice might be. As stated previously, habits tend to be automatic. In other words, you tend not to think about what you are doing with habits such as eating and exercise—you just do it. Your dietary goal sheet will help you to stop and think before you act. In this way, behavioral barriers will slowly become healthy behaviors that help bring about positive change.

Although there are many behavioral barriers to exercise, there are also social barriers, such as not having an exercise partner or someone to encourage you. You can change behavioral and social barriers within this area. Just as with eating, goals for exercise should be written down. Exercise goals should be modest, you should build up slowly, and your doctor should approve your exercise plan. You can lift social barriers by involving someone else in your exercise program. This type of involvement from others helps on many levels. First, it provides support for your healthy changes. Second, it turns the often-unpleasant experience of sweating and working your muscles into a social event. Finally, having others involved in your physical activity plan holds you accountable. For example, if you are not feeling up for a brisk walk around the neighborhood, you will be more likely to go if your walking partner shows up expecting you to join him or her.

Turning barriers into healthful lifestyle behaviors requires a plan. This plan should be reasonable given your current lifestyle and day-to-day responsibilities. Regular monitoring of your plan will help keep you on track and will prompt you to remember to make the changes in your diet and exercise that you are working on. Finally, involving others in your changes provides support and holds you accountable for the changes you are making.

Handling the demands of the diabetes treatment regimen

In addition to making lifestyle changes, diabetes means you will need to follow a recommended diabetes treatment regimen. Such a regimen may include taking medication or insulin, blood glucose testing, or adjustments in insulin, among other demands. Studies have shown that following your doctor's recommendations leads to better health and fewer physical complications. What are the psychological barriers to following a prescribed regimen?

As with diagnosis and lifestyle change, many barriers are a combination of emotional, social, and behavioral barriers. For example, one common barrier is confusion as a result of the overwhelming amount of information that has to be considered when deciding what and when to eat, how much and what kind of medication to take, and how to best handle changes in daily routines. In addition, competing demands at home, work, or school make it easy to be distracted and overlook diabetes self-management needs. We know that monitoring blood glucose levels closely through frequent checking, along with appropriate adjustments in insulin or medication, can help keep blood glucose in the normal range. However, it is difficult to have the time or resources to check frequently, and without knowing blood glucose patterns, it is difficult to adjust medication appropriately.

Having so much information to sift through and having to deal with general, day-to-day demands can make it difficult to follow the treatments as your doctor has prescribed them. However, you can deal with the regimen barriers you have identified and instead turn them into positive ways to improve your health and prevent complications. The first and most important step is to be honest with yourself and your health care provider about what you are actually doing. If you aren't honest with your health care provider about your diabetes self-management, then your doctor will be making recommendations that may not be in your best interest because they are not based on what you are actually doing. This, in turn, may make your diabetes worse.

When you are honest with your health care provider, the two of you can form a plan that will help you reduce your barriers to good care. Once again, this plan should be written down. Making behavioral changes will be much easier if there is a plan to follow. The plan should be posted in places where it will remind you at the times (or in the places) that you need reminders about your diabetes regimen. Dealing with the emotional and social barriers will also be easier if you recruit social support and this social support is active. In other words, the person who is supporting you may do things for you that make it easier to take care of your diabetes. For example, those who are supporting you may draw up your insulin for you, buy supplies or groceries, or prepare blood glucose testing materials when it is time to be tested. They may even help with other tasks so that you have more time to deal with your diabetes regimen. Lastly, it will help you to feel less overwhelmed if you are also receiving emotional support to help you deal with the demands of diabetes.

As before, a written plan and social and emotional support are the keys to overcoming the barriers that keep you from following your diabetes care plan. Remember to *keep your goals realistic* and to move toward your final goal in small steps. Any small changes in your diabetes self-management should be experienced as a success in order to motivate you to move forward. Try to appreciate the fact that there will be times when you can do it all, and other times when you will just be getting by.

Dealing with having diabetes for life

At this point, there is no known cure for type 1 diabetes. Although type 2 diabetes can be improved with the right diet, exercise, weight loss, and medication, these lifestyle changes must last a lifetime. Consequently, diabetes is a chronic health condition that will need to be dealt with for a person's entire life. The long-term demands that diabetes and diabetes care places on an individual can result in the psychosocial diabetes complication of "burnout." Burnout is loosely defined as psychological exhaustion and decreased performance caused by being overworked or being exposed to stress over a long period of time. Much has been written about burnout in regard to taking care of diabetes. In fact, the topic is so important that the American Diabetes Association published an entire book, *Diabetes Burnout*, by Dr. William Polonsky, about this psychosocial complication of diabetes. Dr. Polonsky explains that burnout involves dealing with the emotions and behaviors that come with realizing that diabetes will forever be a part of your life and that, even with optimum care, your diabetes may not always be in control.

There are many approaches to managing and minimizing burnout with diabetes. First and foremost is the need to take on an effective, problem-solving approach to dealing with the ups and downs of diabetes. The problem-solving model we have presented for other barriers in this chapter may help you to deal with many of the difficulties you will encounter in taking care of diabetes. However, there are times that you will not be able to solve a particular problem. At these times, it will eliminate a great deal of frustration if you become focused on diabetes-related problems that you can solve versus focusing on those situations that may be out of your control. This requires some acceptance on your part. Accepting that you will have diabetes the rest of your life may be a huge burden lifted off of your shoulders and will allow you to focus on what it is about diabetes that you can control.

Finally, at times it may be helpful to employ a cost/benefit approach when dealing with the long-term requirements and complications of diabetes. Sometimes good diabetes self-care affects your quality of life in a significant way. For example, you may have noticed that avoiding sugary foods at all costs diminishes your quality of life so much so that you are not a happy person. But, because of the way candy, cookies, and cake make your blood glucose levels harder to control, you have tried to avoid eating these foods. Using the cost/benefit approach, you may choose to eat sugary foods on holidays, birthdays, and other special occasions, accepting the trade-off that it may make diabetes self-care more difficult on these occasions.

What Psychosocial Considerations Are There for Adolescents?

There are special considerations related to having diabetes in adolescence, and we will focus on three of those here: responsibility for self-care, family conflict, and peer pressure.

Having diabetes while being an adolescent is not easy. Adolescents are typically wanting and needing greater independence from their parents and, in most healthy families, this process takes place gradually over the course of the teen years. Responsibility for diabetes care can also be gradually transferred from parents to adolescents, but research has shown us that this transfer of care needs to be matched closely with adolescents' level of maturity. Giving adolescents higher levels of responsibility and independence than they are ready for can result in poor diabetes care and more frequent hospitalizations. Thus, a barrier to good care is premature transfer of responsibility from parents to adolescents. When parents maintain their involvement throughout adolescence and slowly turn over tasks as adolescents mature, this barrier changes into a situation that helps support diabetes care.

This can be a difficult balancing act. Diabetes care issues can often lead to greater family conflict, and family conflict can affect diabetes outcomes. Conflict may relate directly to diabetes, such as disagreement over who is responsible for what. Conflict may also be about other topics, such as curfews or chores, but may indirectly affect an adolescent's diabetes self-care. Thus, family conflict can present a barrier to good self-care. Conversely, positive family factors, such as parental support, family communication, and family problem-solving skills, can lead to better diabetes care. Thus, for adolescents and their families, the focus should be on addressing the barrier of family conflict by working on better communication and problem-solving skills. Families with intense conflict may benefit from guidance from a psychologist.

Although family relationships remain important, social relationships outside of the family—friends, girlfriends, boyfriends—assume increasing importance throughout adolescence. Greater interest in peer relations and increased desire for independence may negatively affect diabetes self-care. Specifically, fitting in with peers may be more important than meeting the demands of a diabetes regimen. Adolescents may not want to stand out by testing their blood glucose, administering insulin, or eating or drinking something different. Thus, this concern about what peers think, as well as direct peer pressure from friends, can be serious barriers to good diabetes care. Coping with these barriers involves helping adolescents take better care of themselves even when around friends. Research has shown that talking directly with at least one good friend and teaching that friend about diabetes helps adolescents with diabetes stick more closely to their diabetes care regimen. Friends can be a good source of social support. They may offer emotional support or other types of support, such as companionship support. For example, they may join their friend in making exercise and dietary changes. Teaching at least one good friend about diabetes and encouraging adolescents to access social support from friends can help overcome social barriers.

Conclusion

We hope this chapter leads to a greater understanding of psychosocial complications. However, simply knowing about the barriers to good diabetes care is useless without a corresponding desire and intent to act on this knowledge. Identifying psychosocial complications is only the first step in the problem-solving model. The second step involves dealing with that barrier, and the third and final step involves turning the barrier into a situation that supports better diabetes care. By following this problem-solving model, adults and adolescents with diabetes alike have the power to bring about a happier and healthier approach to diabetes care over their lifetime.

This chapter was written by Michael A. Harris, PhD, and Peggy Greco, PhD.

Confounders of Diabetes and its Complications

33

Obesity

Case Study

DL was a 57-year-old obese male who weighed 215 pounds with a Body Mass Index (BMI) of 32 and a waist circumference of 45 inches. He had a previous history of hypertension and high cholesterol, and had 2 coronary stents for atherosclerotic heart disease. Although he had not been previously diagnosed with diabetes, a lab report revealed an elevated fasting glucose of 158 mg/dL and an elevated A1C of 6.7%. He reported taking Norvasc, Benicar, Vytorin, Foltex, and Niaspan. The obesity specialist, working with his primary care physician, prescribed a starting dose of metformin twice daily, along with a low glycemic load diet and exercise, to stabilize and decrease his glucose levels. At a later appointment, DL reported a greater sense of fullness and ability to stick with his diet than he had experienced in past attempts at weight loss. Within 3 months of beginning his treatment, he weighed 198 pounds, and his fasting glucose went from 158 mg/dL to 100mg/dL while his A1C decreased from 6.7% to 5.7%. After 9 months, his glucose is in an excellent, manageable state, and he has maintained a total weight loss of 22 pounds, 10% of his total body weight, while reducing his waist circumference to 43 inches. While he continues to take metformin at a full dose, he is no longer taking Norvasc or Niaspan, and the dose of his other medications, Benicar and Vytorin, were decreased. He continues to receive regular follow-up care to monitor his labs. He feels well and is physically more active than before.

Introduction

The dramatic increase in cases of diabetes in the last 20 years is undoubtedly due to the dramatic increase in obesity over that period of time. Obesity, an excess of body fat, is now one of the major risk factors for developing diabetes. In fact, studies show that 90% of the people who are diagnosed with type 2 diabetes for the first time are also overweight. Men and women who are 35–60 years of age and who have gained 10–20 pounds since age 18–20 have three times the risk of developing diabetes than those who have kept their weight within a few pounds. Further, the odds of developing diabetes increases with weight gain, especially abdominal weight gain. If you are overweight or obese, losing 5–10% of your body weight and preventing weight regain in the future can help you control your blood glucose levels and may even help you avoid diabetes-related complications.

What Complications Can Develop from Obesity?

Being overweight or obese is associated with more than 50 illnesses. The most serious include the many complications associated with type 2 diabetes, such as peripheral arterial disease (chapter 10) and stroke (chapter 11). Other related health problems include sleep apnea (chapter 29) and cancer (chapter 28). The combination of diabetes and obesity can put you at even greater risk because you are more likely to have high blood pressure and high blood lipids. Having high blood pressure, diabetes, and obesity at the same time significantly raises the potential for added pressure on blood vessel walls and increased heart rate. This makes high blood pressure even more serious for someone with diabetes who is overweight.

What Is BMI and Why Is It Important?

Body Mass Index (BMI) is a way of measuring your weight compared to your height (see Figure 33-1). A BMI of 25–29.9 is considered overweight, while a BMI of 30 or higher is considered obese. Generally, if your BMI is higher than 25, you are at a greater risk for developing diabetes and other complications.

Because BMI simply calculates your weight compared to your height, it doesn't take into account how that weight is distributed. Athletes and those with a lot of muscle mass may have an "overweight" BMI, even though they are in good physical shape. Those who are very tall or very short can also have misleading BMI numbers. Still, this calculation works well for the vast majority of people, and your health care provider can help clarify any potential issues.

What About Your Waist?

Many diabetes and obesity specialists believe your waist circumference is a vital sign, like your temperature, pulse, or blood pressure. While there is a relationship between BMI and diabetes risk, the presence of extra fat inside your abdomen, as measured by your waist circumference, is just as significant. In fact, your waist size is an even more important measure of diabetes risk than your weight, because fat inside the abdomen (adipose; see box) is riskier than fat under the skin (subcutaneous). For women, a waist bigger than 35 inches puts you at greater risk for diabetes; for a man, risk increases at more than 40 inches. Some populations, like Asians, are at risk at an even smaller waist circumference, so speak with your health care provider for measurements specific to you.

Adipose Tissue

Fat is stored in cells that are known collectively as adipose tissue. While the main purpose of adipose tissue is to store energy in the form of fat for times of need, adipose tissue also produces hormones

BMI

Height				Good Weights					▶ 27					Increasing Risk								
	\multicolumn{22}{c}{Weight (in pounds)}																				
	19	**20**	**21**	**22**	**23**	**24**	**25**	**26**	**27**	**28**	**29**	**30**	**31**	**32**	**33**	**34**	**35**	**36**	**37**	**38**	**39**	**40**
4'10"	91	96	100	105	110	115	119	124	129	134	138	143	148	153	158	162	167	172	177	181	186	191
4'11"	94	99	104	109	114	119	124	128	133	138	143	148	153	158	163	168	173	178	183	188	193	198
5'	97	102	107	112	118	123	128	133	138	143	148	153	158	163	168	174	179	184	189	194	199	204
5'1"	100	106	111	116	122	127	132	137	143	148	153	158	164	169	174	180	185	190	195	201	206	211
5'2"	104	109	115	120	126	131	136	142	147	153	158	164	169	175	180	186	191	196	202	207	213	218
5'3"	107	113	118	124	130	135	141	146	152	158	163	169	175	180	186	191	197	203	208	214	220	225
5'4"	110	116	122	128	134	140	145	151	157	163	169	174	180	186	192	197	204	209	215	221	227	232
5'5"	114	120	126	132	138	144	150	156	162	168	174	180	186	192	198	204	210	216	222	228	234	240
5'6"	118	124	130	136	142	148	155	161	167	173	179	186	192	198	204	210	216	223	229	235	241	247
5'7"	121	127	134	140	146	153	159	166	172	178	185	191	198	204	211	217	223	230	236	242	249	255
5'8"	125	131	138	144	151	158	164	171	177	184	190	197	203	210	216	223	230	236	243	249	256	262
5'9"	128	135	142	149	155	162	169	176	182	189	196	203	209	216	223	230	236	243	250	257	263	270
5'10"	132	139	146	153	160	167	174	181	188	195	202	209	216	222	229	236	243	250	257	264	271	278
5'11"	136	143	150	157	165	172	179	186	193	200	208	215	222	229	236	243	250	257	265	272	279	286
6'	140	147	154	162	169	177	184	191	199	206	213	221	228	235	242	250	258	265	272	279	287	294
6'1"	144	151	159	166	174	182	189	197	204	212	219	227	235	242	250	257	265	272	280	288	295	302
6'2"	148	155	163	171	179	186	194	202	210	218	225	233	241	249	256	264	272	280	287	295	303	311
6'3"	152	160	168	176	184	192	200	208	216	224	232	240	248	256	264	272	279	287	295	303	311	319
6'4"	156	164	172	180	189	197	205	213	221	230	238	246	254	263	271	279	287	295	304	312	320	328

BMI ≥27 are highlighted because health risk escalates rapidly above this level.

Figure 33-1. Determine your BMI by finding your height and weight, and then matching those to the corresponding BMI number.

that regulate blood pressure, insulin sensitivity, clotting, and inflammation. If you gain too much weight for your body to handle, the "overflow" of adipose tissue accumulates in your abdomen. Not only do your pants not fit, but you also produce excessive amounts of the regulatory hormones mentioned above, which leads to many of the diseases we associate with obesity.

Although some adipose tissue is essential, having *too much* inside the abdomen is associated with insulin resistance. Insulin is a hormone responsible for helping the body turn glucose into usable energy. Insulin resistance is a condition in which muscle, fat, and liver cells are unable to use insulin properly. Since diabetes is a complication of insulin resistance, and insulin resistance stems from abdominal fat, the link between diabetes and excess abdominal adipose tissue is strongly lined to type 2 diabetes risk. By measuring your waist circumference, your physician can help you determine your degree of abdominal obesity.

What Are the Benefits of Weight Loss?

It is widely known that losing just a small amount of weight can improve blood glucose levels for those with diabetes. Experts have recently discovered that when you lose weight, the first fat to go is adipose tissue inside your abdomen. Researchers have shown that the adipose tissue in your abdomen can be reduced by one-quarter to one-half with just a 10% loss of body weight! Remember, the fat inside your abdomen increases insulin resistance and worsens your blood glucose, blood pressure, and other problems. Dropping approximately 10% of your body weight will reduce your abdominal adipose tissue, which can improve your body's sensitivity to insulin, making it easier for your body to convert glucose to usable energy.

If you are overweight or obese, weight loss is an important step toward improving your overall health. In addition to improving the chronic illnesses we've already mentioned, studies have also shown that moderate amounts of weight loss can improve physical health, increase mobility, improve emotional well-being, and even extend your life expectancy.

How Can You Improve Your Diet?

With the many diet plans being promoted today, you may find it difficult to determine which plan is the best choice for you. The diet that will be most effective for you is the diet that you like the best and feel is the easiest to follow given your personal lifestyle. Remember, a meal plan is something that needs to work for a lifetime. Many diets claim quick weight loss, but can't be followed in the long term and usually lead to lost weight eventually being gained back. Working with a health professional, such as a registered dietitian (RD), may help your weight loss by providing expert guidance and positive reinforcement.

Three basic concepts seem to be most helpful for people with diabetes—the glycemic load, choosing foods with low energy density (see Table 33-1), and thinking long-term.

The glycemic load

The glycemic load, derived from the glycemic index, describes how much certain foods, particularly carbohydrate-containing foods, will raise your blood glucose. Low glycemic–load diets contain lower levels of easily digestible carbohydrates and build in foods that help maintain stable blood glucose levels. In particular, foods that contain fiber and protein tend to raise blood glucose at a lower rate, thus less insulin is produced. High levels of insulin can make you feel hungry, making it harder to lose weight. By reducing hunger and even promoting feelings of "fullness," low glycemic foods may be the key to helping you lose weight and keeping it off. However, the glycemic index is not perfect. When you mix foods with different glycemic values, it can make your actual glycemic load hard to determine. Still, when used as a piece of your total meal plan, it can offer benefits.

Low energy density

Foods with a low energy density contain fewer calories per gram. We tend to eat roughly the same weight of food each day, so eating foods that contain fewer calories per gram may help you lose weight. These foods can fill you up without adding extra calories. In general, foods with a lot of water and fiber have less calories per gram. Fruits, vegetables, and whole grains contain a lot of water and/or fiber and will help you feel full while consuming fewer calories. On the other hand, foods that have a high fat content are packed with calories in a small volume. Desserts, candies, and processed foods have a higher energy density and will offer more calories per gram.

Table 33-1. Sample Food Recommendations:
Low Glycemic Load and Low Energy Density

Low Glycemic Load (serving size)	Low Energy Density (calories per gram)
Whole-Grain Bread (1 slice)	Lettuce (0.1)
Brown Rice (1/3 cup steamed)	Carrots (0.4)
Raisin Bran Cereal (1/3 cup)	Chicken Soup (0.5)
Spinach (3/4 cup raw)	Orange (0.5)
Lettuce (1 cup)	Oatmeal, Prepared with Water (0.6)
Black Beans (1/2 cup)	Apples (0.6)
Spit Pea Soup (1 cup)	Grapes (0.7)
Apple (1 medium)	Green Peas (0.8)
Blueberries (1 cup)	Cheerios Cereal with 1% Milk (1.1)
Grapefruit (1 cup)	Turkey Breast, Roasted, No Skin (1.4)

Thinking long-term

Trying to lose weight quickly is tempting, but it may also be less healthy and less permanent. Remember, it is often more difficult to stick to extreme diets as they may drastically limit portion size and even exclude certain foods entirely, leaving you hungry and unsatisfied. You will be more likely to lose weight and keep it off by making manageable changes instead. Try things like:

- Portion control—use a smaller plate than normal (10 inches or smaller)
- When arranging food on your plate, make 1/2 the plate vegetables, 1/4 protein, 1/4 carbohydrate
- Eat your vegetables first
- Increase your fiber intake—select whole-grain foods over refined products
- Use less fat and use healthy fats like olive or canola oil
- Choose low-sodium foods—sodium contributes to high blood pressure
- Drink fewer calorie-rich beverages, such as soda and juices—they can add hundreds of calories to your diet
- Eat whole fruit—it's a source of natural fiber and has fewer calories than fruit juices
- Read the Nutrition Facts label—this will help you determine the fat, cholesterol, sodium, fiber, and sugar content of your foods

What Are the Benefits of Physical Activity?

Building exercise into your daily routine is an equally important step toward improving your health, your blood glucose, and your weight. Not only does exercise burn calories and increase your endurance, it can also increase your body's ability to use glucose effectively. Even further, exercise improves your body's sensitivity to insulin by reducing the amount of adipose tissue in your abdomen. Finally, increased physical activity raises your levels of good (HDL) cholesterol, which in turn, can help lower your risk of heart disease and stroke.

Be creative in your exercise regimen, and find activities you enjoy—this will certainly help you succeed in your quest to lose weight and better manage your diabetes. And remember, exercising doesn't mean you have to join a gym. Walking is a great activity! Below are some examples of how you can fit walking into your daily routine:

- Start with 30 minutes a day—you can break this up into two 15-minute walks
- Motivate yourself and others—join or start a walking group with co-workers, friends, or family
- Track your progress—use a pedometer to work your way up to 10,000 steps a day
- Set new goals—gradually increase and vary your pace

Precautions to take with physical activity

Since each person's body will respond differently, it is best to consult with your doctor before starting an exercise regimen. With medical supervision, you and your doctor can learn the effect of exercise on your individual blood glucose levels. During physical activity, your body, especially the muscles, needs extra energy and uses glucose for fuel. However, this uptake of glucose by the muscles can lower your blood glucose to unsafe levels (hypoglycemia) if you are taking certain diabetes medications. In addition, your body may interpret prolonged exercise as stress and release hormones into the blood that increase the glucose available to your muscles, thus raising your blood glucose levels. Adding exercise into your daily routine should be a gradual process—overstepping your bounds may discourage you from continuing with your regimen or, worse, cause injury.

Can Medication Affect Your Weight?

The side effects of certain prescription medications, including some diabetes medications, may make it difficult to lose weight or may even cause weight gain. Insulin, sulfonylureas (such as Glipizide), and thiazolidinediones (such as Actos and Avandia) have all been associated with weight gain, even though they may have proven health benefits. Talk to your doctor about your diabetes medications. By modifying your diabetes therapy, you may find it easier to lose weight. Note that if your blood glucose is very high and you have been losing weight as a result, the use of any medicine may cause weight gain, but it's alright—you are gaining back tissue you have lost to the metabolic problems of diabetes.

Some prescription medications are considered "weight neutral," meaning they will not have an impact on your weight, or will result in only minimal weight change. Metformin is an oral medication often prescribed for people with diabetes who are overweight or obese. Metformin will not lead to hypoglycemia because it does not cause your body to produce additional insulin (as opposed to sulfonylureas). By improving insulin sensitivity without storing more calories as fat, metformin canusually leads to a modest weight loss. Alpha-glucosidase inhibitors, such as Acarbose, are also weight neutral. They work by slowing the absorption of carbohydrate calories from the intestine and may have additional health benefits. There are some new choices as well. Sitagliptin (Januvia) is a medication that prolongs the effect of an intestinal hormone that helps control blood glucose and does not cause weight gain. Exenatide (Byetta) is an injectable diabetes medication that functions by allowing the insulin in your body to work more effectively and by suppressing glucagon secretion. This medication is thought to slow the progression of food from the stomach into the small intestine, which may help you feel full more quickly and maintain your fullness level for longer periods, possibly leading to weight loss.

Are There Medications that Can Help You with Weight Loss?

Orlistat (Xenical) is a prescription medication that helps reduce fat absorption in the gastrointestinal tract. In addition to promoting weight loss by removing some of the ingested fat in your bowel, orlistat can reduce glucose levels, especially when used in combination with metformin. Orlistat also lowers LDL ("bad") cholesterol, which can reduce your risk of developing heart disease. However, it is associated with frequent loose bowel movements and occasional soiling of pants.

Sibutramine (Meridia) is an appetite suppressant that helps reduce cravings and can help you feel full throughout the day. This prescription medication has also been shown to reduce blood glucose and A1C levels for people with diabetes. While sibutramine can help you lose weight on its own, research has shown that combining it with lifestyle modification (such as diet and exercise) leads to the greatest percentage of weight loss. A proportion of people on sibutramine will have increased blood pressure and heart rate.

Phentermine is another agent approved by the FDA for weight loss for short-term use. Increases in blood pressure are seen in some people with this medication as well.

Can Over-the-Counter Products Help You Lose Weight?

The only FDA-approved weight-loss medication approved for over-the-counter use is orlistat (Alli). It is half the dose of Xenical, but may provide up to 85% of the weight loss of the higher dose used in the full prescription strength. Alli comes with a lifestyle program designed by professionals and is meant for people who are committed to reducing fat in their diet and adhering to the program. Eating too much fat while taking Alli will produce gastrointestinal side effects.

On the other hand, despite what the public has been led to believe, no other over-the-counter weight-loss products, including dietary supplements, have been approved by the FDA. In fact, no weight-loss supplements have been shown to be safe and effective based on the type of credible medical research studies currently used. While these supplements claim to reduce your weight quickly and without much effort, there is actually no evidence that they work as promised. This includes products like hoodia, "cortisol-reducers," and more. Furthermore, some supplements and pills can be dangerous, since the ingredients often include unnamed stimulants, such as synephrine (often listed as "bitter orange"), which has been shown to raise blood pressure dramatically. With safe options available for weight loss, using non-FDA approved weight-loss schemes is both unnecessary and ill advised.

What Is Bariatric Surgery?

If you find that exercise, diet, and/or medications do not have an impact on your weight, bariatric surgery is an option that can decrease your weight and may improve your diabetes. Bariatric surgery is another name for weight loss surgeries, with gastric bypass and gastric banding as the most popular selections.

Gastric bypass

In gastric bypass (Figure 33-2), a small pouch is created from the stomach and this new pocket serves as the permanent, new stomach. The small intestine is then connected to the pouch, bypassing the remainder of the old stomach. With a drastically smaller stomach, you cannot consume as much food, but will still feel full after small meals. Of note for people with diabetes, bypassing the upper part of the intestine, the duodenum, seems to improve blood glucose remarkably. Studies have shown that after surgery, 84% of those with type 2 diabetes will be off all diabetes related medication and have normal fasting blood glucose and A1C levels.

Gastric banding

Although a gastric banding (Figure 33-3) procedure will limit the amount of food you can eat, it will not change your normal digestive functions since the entry point of food into the small intestine is not repositioned. In this case, surgeons create a small pouch by placing a band around the upper part of the stomach. The small pouch slows the movement of food into the rest of the stomach, causing the patient to feel full more quickly. In those with type 2 diabetes who have undergone gastric banding, research has demonstrated that 48% will be free of their diabetes and diabetes related medication with this procedure.

Who Qualifies for Bariatric Surgery?

In order to qualify for bariatric surgery, you must have a BMI of 40 or above. However, those with a BMI of 35–40 who have severe

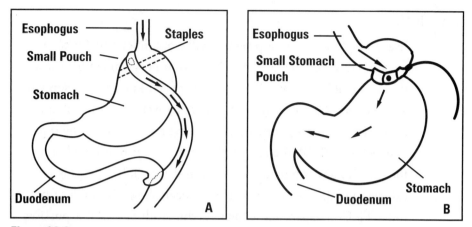

Figure 33-2.
A. Gastric bypass creates a small pouch in the stomach and connects the small intestine to this new pouch, bypassing the old stomach. **B.** Gastric banding creates a small pouch at the top of the stomach, limiting how much a person can eat.
Figures adapted from National Institutes of Health. 2004. *Gastrointestinal Surgery for Severe Obesity*

complications of obesity, including diabetes and sleep apnea, also qualify for surgery. In many cases, you must follow a medically supervised weight-loss program for approximately 6 months before becoming eligible for surgery.

What Are the Risks Associated with Bariatric Surgery?

While the statistics on weight loss and diabetes improvements are rather remarkable with bariatric surgery, there are still considerable risks that must be weighed. As with any other surgical procedure, there are risks with anesthesia and the possibility of infection of the surgical site, or the need for another operation. Patients who have this surgery must take vitamin and mineral supplements for life. Other common complications may include vomiting and nutritional deficiencies due to incomplete absorption of iron, calcium, and other nutrients. Your physician can provide more information on the specific complications and/or side effects of each procedure, and together you can weigh the risks and the benefits.

Conclusion

Every weight loss diet or program will work differently for each person. However, the Diabetes Prevention Program (DPP) showed that a weight loss of just 7% after 1 year (or 14 pounds for someone who weighs 200 pounds), with 4% of that weight loss maintained after 4 years (just 8 pounds), reduced the risk of developing type 2 diabetes by 58%! The results illustrated that people could reduce their risk of developing diabetes and lose weight by engaging in exercise and diet. Similar results have been shown in studies from India, Finland, Japan, and China. As this study shows, it is possible for people to lose weight and maintain it through exercise and diet, and thereby reduce their risk of developing diabetes.

Remember, before starting any new weight-loss plan, whether diet or exercise, be sure to talk to your primary doctor or endocrinologist! He or she can answer questions or can refer you to another health professional who can provide more information. If you have diabetes and are overweight or obese, just losing 5–10% of your body weight may produce many beneficial results, but it is important to talk with your doctor to determine the best course of action, whether it be diet, exercise, medication, surgery, or a combination of any of the above.

This chapter was written by Louis J. Aronne, MD, FACP ; Guadalupe D. Minero, MPH; and Quinn T. Leslie.

34

Smoking

Introduction

Cigarette smoking is the most significant cause of preventable illness and death worldwide. In the United States alone, we have 48 million smokers, and we spend more than $100 billion each year to treat health problems caused by smoking. Currently about 20% of adult men and women in the United States are smokers. Tobacco use kills nearly half a million Americans every year and brings disability and suffering to countless others.

Type 2 diabetes is one of the most common chronic diseases around the world and affects more than 15 million Americans. The numerous complications associated with diabetes are discussed throughout this book. Unfortunately, diabetes control can be compromised in smokers, and the consequences of tobacco use are much more serious for people with diabetes. In spite of this, the proportion of people with diabetes who smoke is similar to the proportion in the general population.

Most people are aware that smoking cigarettes significantly raises their chances of developing chronic respiratory diseases, lung cancer, other types of cancer, and cardiovascular diseases, including heart attacks and strokes. What most people don't know are the metabolic effects of smoking. Many people do not realize that tobacco use interferes with blood glucose control and also contributes to some of the other hazards associated with diabetes.

How Does Smoking Affect Metabolism?

Smoking can promote metabolic changes in people without diabetes that are similar to those seen in type 2 diabetes, including problems with high blood sugar and blood lipid levels. Studies find that following the same intake of oral glucose, both blood sugar and insulin levels are higher after smoking, even in people without diabetes. Even though insulin levels are elevated, smokers experience insulin resistance, and they are less sensitive to the actions of insulin. Diminished blood flow to skeletal muscles and changes in the blood vessels caused by smoking are thought to add to this insulin resistance.

Smoking is associated with increased abdominal fat deposits and increased waist-to-hip measurements, which also predispose smokers to develop abnormalities in glucose and lipid metabolism. Compared with nonsmokers, people who smoke have higher levels of the low density lipids (LDL, or "bad" cholesterol) and plasma triglycerides. They also have lower levels of the high density lipids (HDL, or "good" cholesterol). These changes in the blood lipids mean that smokers are more likely to develop atherosclerotic changes in their hearts and blood vessels. These lipid abnormalities are most common in those who smoke more than one pack per day.

If You Have Diabetes, Does Smoking Affect You Differently?

People with diabetes who smoke are more likely to experience metabolic problems, including high blood glucose, insulin resistance, and elevated lipid levels. Tobacco use is seen more often among people with higher A1C levels. The number of cigarettes smoked each day can be linked to the severity of the insulin resistance and the lipid abnormalities.

Those with diabetes are already at increased risk of developing cardiovascular problems such as heart attacks, strokes, and peripheral arterial disease. About 65% of deaths among those with diabetes are due to cardiovascular diseases. Poorer metabolic control means that if you have diabetes and you smoke, you are more likely to experience these complications.

Tobacco use also increases the odds of suffering from the microvascular complications of diabetes, including damage to the eyes, nerves, and kidneys. Retinal damage is more common if you smoke and advances at a faster pace. Damage to the kidney's filtering system and the associated protein loss in the urine progress faster in smokers, even if they have well-controlled blood pressure. Peripheral nerve damage occurs about twice as often in smokers with diabetes as compared to nonsmokers.

Is Smoking the Actual Cause of These Complications?

Chemicals found in tobacco, such as nicotine and carbon monoxide, damage the pancreas and impair beta cell function and insulin receptor sensitivity. Smoking creates a higher proportion of LDL cholesterol, lower levels of HDL cholesterol, and greater elevations in blood triglycerides after eating. These toxic effects directly impair your body's regulation of blood glucose and insulin levels. They also lead to additional lipid abnormalities, including those associated with insulin resistance, such as high circulating levels of free fatty acids and triglycerides. Smoking also raises circulating levels of certain blood proteins that increase your risk of forming blood clots inside arteries, veins, and coronary vessels.

When compared to people with diabetes who do not smoke, those who do smoke have an increased chance of developing diabetes complications, even when their blood glucose and blood pressure readings are similar. In the absence of hypertension, hypercholesterolemia, and obesity, smoking has been identified as an independent risk factor for premature death. All mortality rates are increased if you use tobacco.

Can Smoking Cause Diabetes?

Smoking does not appear to influence the development of type 1 diabetes, which is caused by an autoimmune response that destroys pancreatic beta cells and eliminates all insulin production in the body. On the other hand, evidence from several studies indicates that smoking does increase your risk of developing type 2 diabetes. This is not surprising, since so many of the metabolic consequences of smoking actually mimic the symptoms of type 2 diabetes (impaired insulin secretion, insulin resistance, etc.). Most of these studies demonstrate a direct relationship between the number of cigarettes smoked each day and the likelihood of developing diabetes, particularly in those who smoke more than one pack per day. Compared with those who have never smoked, men who smoke more than one pack per day are about twice as likely to develop diabetes. The total number of packs ever smoked ("pack-year" history) also influences the incidence of diabetes. The risk in men was shown to be affected by the amount of nicotine and tar consumed on a daily basis, not just the cigarette count.

Does Quitting Smoking Help?

Yes. Quitting smoking greatly reduces your risk of developing type 2 diabetes. Women who quit smoking for more than 5 years, and men who quit for more than 10 years, will have about the same odds of developing diabetes as if they had never smoked.

If you already have diabetes, giving up cigarettes immediately improves metabolic control and reduces your cardiovascular risk factors. Furthermore, the risk of experiencing other problems from smoking diminishes over time. Weight gain after quitting can be a concern, but in most cases, the health benefits of quitting smoking will more than compensate for the disadvantages of gaining weight. Insulin requirements may also decrease after you quit smoking.

What Is the Best Way to Quit Smoking?

Quitting smoking is never easy, but a number of helpful strategies are available. Attempting to quit without assistance ("cold turkey") is difficult and has the poorest long-term results. Professional counseling sessions, even brief ones, have been shown to improve quit rates. Also, the American Cancer Society (1-800-ACS-2345 or cancer.org) and many state agencies sponsor Tobacco Quit Lines, which provide helpful tips and suggestions to callers, making it easier to stop smoking. Useful information can also be accessed at no charge by visiting www.smokefree.gov, which is a website developed by a branch of the National Cancer Institute.

There is also a growing list of medications that make quitting easier, usually more than doubling success rates. Fortunately, these products are safe for those with diabetes. Although some treatments are available without a prescription, it is a good idea to discuss your plan to quit smoking with your doctor. He or she can help you select the most appropriate method and offer advice that will improve your odds of success.

Currently approved treatments for smoking cessation include nicotine replacement therapies (NRT) such as the nicotine patch, gum, lozenges, inhaler, and nasal spray. Two prescription medications, bupropion (Zyban) and varenicline (Chantix), are also safe and effective. Bupropion and some forms of NRT may be useful for those with diabetes, as they have been found to minimize weight gain after quitting. However, varenicline has been found to be more effective in helping people quit than bupropion. Two other drugs, nortriptyline (a tricyclic antidepressant) and clonidine (a blood pressure medicine) may help some people quit smoking, but they do not appear to be as effective as other methods and are not considered "first-line" therapy for smoking cessation. New medications are being studied to determine whether they offer any advantages over treatments that are currently available.

Conclusion

Smoking is a serious, but modifiable, health risk. Quitting smoking is especially beneficial if you have diabetes. In fact, if you have diabetes and you smoke, you'll reap greater health benefits from quitting smoking than you would from simply improving control of your blood glucose, cholesterol, or blood pressure levels. Many effective treatments have been designed to assist smokers who are motivated to stop. If you have diabetes and you smoke, now is a great time for you to stop smoking and start enjoying the rewards of a healthier lifestyle!

This chapter was written by Anne Autry, MD, and Robert M. Anthenelli, MD.

35

Transplants:
Kidney, Pancreas, and Islet Cells

When Should You Consider a Kidney Transplant?

The kidneys are small organs that sit on either side of your spine. Their main functions, though they perform many, are to filter your blood and excrete waste products. For those with diabetes, kidney function often becomes compromised over time, and kidney disease is quite common (see chapter 17). Once you've been diagnosed with kidney disease, you and your health care team should begin to explore the option of a kidney transplant. The main objective is to get you a new kidney before you need dialysis, a process where your blood is purified through a machine. Dialysis becomes necessary once your kidney disease progresses to end-stage renal disease (ESRD), and at that point, it or a kidney transplant will be your only two treatment options. A kidney transplant is nearly always preferable to dialysis, as the death rate over time is lower with a transplant, and the quality of life is much better.

Before you reach ESRD, you will see other warning signs of kidney insufficiency, such as chronic fatigue, high blood pressure, anemia, and swelling. A chemical in your blood called creatinine will also begin to rise. Your doctor should perform a creatinine check regularly, and especially if you begin to show other signs of kidney disease. Once you begin to show symptoms and experience a rise in creatinine, your physician should refer you to a kidney specialist, or nephrologist. The nephrologist will do an evaluation to see if you are a candidate for a transplant.

If you have a living donor for a kidney, such as a relative or friend, you can do the kidney transplant before you need to go on dialysis or with only a short period on dialysis. If you do not have a living donor, you will likely need to wait 2–5 years for kidneys from someone who has died under circumstances where his or her organs can be obtained for transplantation. Donors such as this are referred to as "deceased donors" and have either given permission in advance for their organs to be taken for transplantation at the time of death or have relatives who gave permission immediately after death. Either way, the wait for a deceased-donor kidney illustrates why it's a mistake to wait until you've begun dialysis to consider a transplant.

What Happens During an Assessment for a Kidney Transplant?

A kidney transplant assessment usually requires several visits or days to complete. Blood will be drawn, X-rays will be taken, and you will consult with physicians from several specialties, including a cardiologist to check your heart and a surgeon to review the risks and complications of a transplant. You may also see a social worker.

Your blood type (A, B, AB, or O) will be confirmed to match you with potential donors. You can receive a transplant from anyone with your blood type or with an O blood type (O is the universal donor type), but if you are O, your donor can only be O. You will also be tissue typed for what are called human leukocyte antigens (HLA), used to determine the degree to which you genetically match potential donors.

Most people with diabetes referred for kidney transplantation are found to be suitable candidates, though sometimes conditions are uncovered that need to be treated before a transplant can be performed. The most common of these conditions is heart disease, which if present might require what is called an angioplasty or a bypass procedure (see chapter 6). People with diabetes and kidney disease often have a higher rate of heart disease than those without diabetes. By treating this heart condition, the risk of a heart attack at the time of or after the transplant can be greatly reduced.

Once your physicians are satisfied with your test results, you can be placed on the waiting list for a deceased-donor kidney transplant or proceed to a living-donor kidney transplant if you have a suitable volunteer.

What Is Involved in Kidney Transplant Surgery?

A kidney transplant is major surgery and requires you to be in the hospital for at least a week. During the procedure, the donor kidney artery and vein are attached to the blood vessels above your groin and your ureter, the tube that carries the urine to your bladder (see Figure 35-1). Your own kidneys are usually not removed. After the transplant, you will take drugs that suppress your immune system so that your body will not reject the new kidney. However,

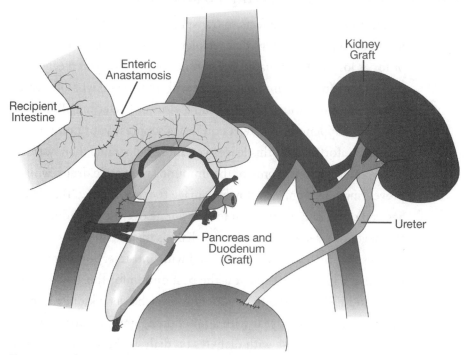

Figure 35-1. Graft sites for kidney and pancreas transplants.

these immunosuppressant drugs can have side effects, which are discussed below.

How Does a Kidney Transplant Help?

A kidney transplant, whether from a living or deceased donor, nearly always immediately relieves the symptoms of kidney insufficiency or failure and eliminates the need for dialysis. We now know that those with diabetes and kidney failure who receive a kidney transplant are more likely to stay alive than those who are on the waiting list but stay on dialysis. In fact, the dramatic improvement shown by the most successful transplant recipients is an impressive demonstration of the best in modern medicine. For example, women who have undergone a successful kidney transplant can go on to have a successful pregnancy, a feat that's nearly impossible while on dialysis.

Are There Drawbacks to Having a Kidney Transplant?

The most serious side effects to transplant surgery come from the immunosuppressive drugs that recipients must take for a lifetime, or for as long as the donated organ functions. When you receive a donated organ, your immune system will try to expel what it sees as a foreign invader, much like it would a virus or bacterium. To keep this from happening, anti-rejection drugs suppress your immune system. Unfortunately, this leaves you more vulnerable than normal to certain infections. Some of the immunosuppressive drugs, while preventing rejection, also slowly damage the new kidney. This damage can cause kidney function to deteriorate over time, leading to the need for a second transplant or dialysis treatment.

Despite the drawbacks associated with anti-rejection drugs, it's clear that a kidney transplant is the best option for those with diabetes and ESRD. More than 90% of those who get a kidney transplant survive the first year with a functioning graft, compared to only an 80% for those with diabetes on dialysis. At four years, more than 80% of transplanted kidneys are functioning, and at 10 years, more than 50% are functioning. Some kidney transplants have been known to function more than 40 years. (The function rates are somewhat higher for transplants from living donors as opposed to those from deceased donors.) Age is becoming less of a factor as well. Though transplants are rarely done in people over age 70, older and older patients are undergoing successful transplants every year.

What Happens After a Kidney Transplant?

You will work with your primary physician and the doctors and nurse coordinators at the transplant center to maintain your kidney graft function. Directly after your operation, you will have frequent clinic appointments. You will be informed of the drugs and doses you must take to prevent rejection of the new organ and reminded of the importance of not skipping doses. You will be instructed to do blood and urine tests that help detect rejection, the most important of which is the blood creatinine check. When a kidney is rejected, creatinine levels rise. This may need to be confirmed by a needle biopsy of the kidney transplant. If your body does begin to reject the new organ, you will receive a temporary increase in the doses of your current drugs or the temporary addition of another drug to reverse the process. You will also be monitored for complications from the immunosuppressive drugs, including infections, certain cancers (most often of the skin), bone disease, high cholesterol, and others.

These days, most kidney transplant recipients enjoy long-term function of their new organ. However, if the kidney fails, a retransplant is usually possible and can be planned for long before dialysis is necessary.

What Is a Pancreas Transplant and How Can It Affect Diabetes?

The pancreas is an organ the size and shape of a banana that resides inside your abdomen, under your stomach. It is connected to your intestine by a tube called a duct and is connected to your bloodstream by capillaries. The pancreas has two major duties. One is to help digest food by secreting enzymes into your intestine via the duct. The other is to secrete insulin into your blood stream to maintain normal blood glucose levels.

For glucose to enter muscle, liver, and other cells and supply your body with energy, you need insulin. Without insulin, blood glucose becomes dangerously high. Insulin is produced by cells in the pancreas called beta cells that reside in clusters called the islets of Langerhans. The islets are scattered throughout the pancreas, but make up only 2% of the organ. When a person has diabetes, his or her beta cells are destroyed (type 1) or don't meet the body's insulin needs on their own (type 2). In a fully functioning pancreas, the beta cells always secrete just the right amount of insulin, something that is very difficult to duplicate by insulin injections or with medication, even with the most careful monitoring. Thus, successfully transplanting either the pancreas or islets isolated from the pancreas can restore blood glucose to constantly normal levels in someone with diabetes.

Who Should Consider a Pancreas Transplant?

Pancreas transplants aren't for everyone with diabetes. If you have type 2 diabetes that you can control through diet, exercise, and oral medication, or if you have well-controlled type 1 diabetes using insulin, it doesn't make sense to undergo a pancreas transplant. However, for those who need a kidney transplant, and will have to take anti-rejection drugs anyway, a pancreas transplant may make sense. It is also a viable option for those who have "brittle" diabetes, with frequent highs and lows in their blood glucose levels in spite of their best attempts at control. Finally, pancreas transplants are especially suited for those with severe hypoglycemic unawareness, to the point that they often need help from those around them.

Unlike kidneys, most pancreases come from deceased donors. While it's possible to function with half a pancreas, thus making a living donor possible, the risk of diabetes developing in the donor makes this difficult. Pancreases for transplantation are usually obtained from donors who have given permission in advance and die under circumstances where their organs are suitable for removal. There is not a severe shortage of pancreases like there is with kidneys, so a whole pancreas from a deceased donor is often available for a transplant.

How Is a Pancreas Transplanted?

A transplanted pancreas is placed in the abdomen through an incision, and its blood vessels are usually connected to the blood vessels in the pelvic area, similar to what is done in a kidney transplant (see Figure 35-1). A small portion of donor intestine (duodenum) that is connected to the pancreatic duct is usually included with the graft, and it is connected to either the recipient's intestine (as illustrated) or bladder. The blood vessel connections allow the new pancreas to secrete insulin into the recipient's bloodstream on demand, normalizing blood glucose levels and eliminating the need for insulin injections.

Does a Pancreas Transplant Really "Cure" Diabetes?

In the sense that it eliminates the need for insulin injections and normalizes blood glucose levels, a pancreas transplant does "cure" diabetes. But the word "cure" is perhaps overly optimistic, since the complications of diabetes that affect other organs (kidneys, nerves, eyes) that are already present at the time of the transplant will persist or improve only very slowly over a long period of time. Also, there is the possibility that your body will reject the pancreas and your need for insulin injections would return. And even if the new organ isn't rejected, immunosuppressive (anti-rejection) drugs replace insulin as a daily medication regimen.

What About an Artificial Pancreas?

Many people are excited about the possibility of an "artificial pancreas," an implantable insulin pump that would deliver precisely the right amount of insulin to your bloodstream by using a continuous glucose monitor (CGM) to sense glucose levels automatically (though the name is a little bit of a misnomer, because this artificial pancreas would only handle insulin secretion and not the remaining functions of your pancreas). The big advantage of an artificial pancreas over an islet cell or pancreas transplant? No need for immunosuppressive drugs, since there's no organ to be rejected.

Right now the pump technology exists, but the CGM technology has not advanced to the point where a durable and reliable glucose meter that can be implanted and coupled to a pump exists. Progress is being made in this area, but much of the information is owned by the companies working on the devices, so it's difficult to say when this could actually be tested in humans. However, this technology seems very achievable, and it's hoped that within a few years we may have a functioning device available.

Where Are Pancreas Transplants Available?

For ESRD patients with type 1 diabetes, combining a pancreas transplant with a kidney transplant from the same deceased donor is now done routinely at most transplant centers in the United States. Occasionally, both organs (one kidney, half a pancreas) are transplanted simultaneously from a living donor. Or, if the ERSD patient has a living donor for only the kidney, this kidney can be transplanted first, with the option of receiving a deceased-donor pancreas transplant later. In some cases, a deceased-donor pancreas may be available at the time of a living-donor kidney transplant, so if you are scheduled for a kidney transplant, you can check with your transplant center about getting a pancreas as well. If a pancreas transplant is not offered at your hospital, you may want to locate a center that does offer this, or do the kidney first and than go to another center for the pancreas. Pancreas-kidney recipients are not only dialysis free but they're insulin free as well, so the change in quality of life when both are successful can be quite dramatic.

What Are the Long-Term Results of Pancreas Transplants?

Generally, kidney transplants function better over time than pancreas transplants, primarily because there are more surgical complications associated with a pancreas transplant, leading to a higher rate of removal early on for reasons other than rejection. A recent analysis was done of more than 6,000 simultaneous pancreas and kidney transplants from deceased-donor organs in the United States from 2000 to 2007. The results showed that 95% of the recipients were alive at 1 year and 88% at 4 years, with the pancreas functioning at 85% after 1 year and 74% after 4 years. Research in a few centers seems to show that some complications of diabetes can improve over time after a successful pancreas transplant, particularly neuropathy-related complications. Those who receive just a pancreas transplant may see an improvement in kidney disease, but this can be offset by the side effects of the anti-rejection drugs, some of which can damage kidneys. Some observations also suggest that normal blood glucose levels from a pancreas transplant can stop the progression of blood vessel complications from diabetes, but more research needs to be done to know for sure.

Pancreas transplants for those without kidney disease

Currently, only about 10% of pancreas transplants are performed in those who have diabetes but do not have kidney disease, and nearly all of these are in people who have brittle diabetes with hypoglycemia unawareness. In the past, for unexplained reasons, the rejection rate was higher for pancreas transplants alone than for pancreas-kidney transplants, but new anti-rejection drugs have reduced this discrepancy. Since pancreas-kidney transplants give two benefits—becoming insulin independent as well as dialysis free—for the price of anti-rejection drug therapy, it makes sense to recommend pancreas transplants to those who are already getting a kidney transplant. However, new drugs are now so effective in preventing rejection that we may see more single pancreas transplants in the years to come.

What Are the Risks of a Pancreas Transplant?

Anytime an organ is transplanted from one person to another, anti-rejection drugs are needed. These drugs can make it more difficult to fight off certain infections, and the rate of certain types of cancer, particularly of the skin, is increased over time. These risks are common to all organ transplants. Surgical complications are also a risk in any transplant procedure; however, they are much higher for pancreas transplants than they are for kidney procedures. Surgical complications serious enough to require removal of the organ graft occur about 10% of the time for a pancreas transplant, whereas it is around 1% for kidney transplants. Other reversible complications (such as bleeding or infection) may also require another operation. Any candidate for a pancreas transplant must be aware of these possibilities. There is also a risk that the pancreas transplant will simply stop working; usually because it is rejected by the body. However, a second pancreas transplant can be done when the first fails.

What Are the Benefits of a Pancreas Transplant?

If a pancreas transplant is successful, you will no longer be required to take insulin. The quality of life improvement here is obvious, especially if you have difficult-to-control glucose levels and hypoglycemia unawareness. If you receive a simultaneous kidney transplant, your new pancreas can lower your risk for developing kidney disease in your new kidney (a situation that happens to about 30% of those with diabetes who get just a kidney transplant). In fact, with the blood glucose control that comes with a functioning pancreas, you can prevent most diabetes complications, as long as they have not begun to develop before the operation. Again, these benefits have to be weighed against the side effects of the anti-rejection drugs and the very real possibility that the pancreas will not function as well over time.

What Are Islets and What Is an Islet Transplant?

The Islets of Langherhans (commonly just called "islets" and pronounced "eye-lets") are clusters of cells that are scattered throughout the pancreas. There are about a million islets in the pancreas, but they are tiny and together make up only 2% of the organ. Islets are composed of beta cells that make insulin, alpha cells that make glucagon (which also helps blood glucose regulation), and delta cells that make somatostatin (another important hormone). Islets work to control blood glucose levels in your body by secreting insulin to lower glucose levels and glucagon to raise glucose levels. In type 1 diabetes, beta cells are either totally destroyed or reduced to such a small number that not enough insulin is produced to drive glucose into the cells of the body for energy. As a result, people with type 1 diabetes require insulin injections. To do an islet transplant, the islets need to be extracted from the pancreas of a donor so that they can be injected into the recipient (see Figure 35-2), a much less invasive proce-

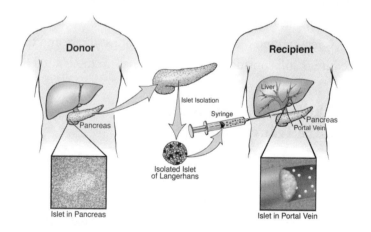

Figure 35-2. Islet cell extraction and transplant process.

dure than a whole pancreas transplant (compare to Figure 35-1). If successful, an islet transplant eliminates the need for insulin injections just like a pancreas transplant does.

How Are Islet Cells Transplanted and How Is This Different Than a Pancreas Transplant?

A pancreas transplant means a whole or part of a pancreas is transplanted by major surgery. An islet transplant means that only the islets, which contain the beta cells that make insulin, are transplanted. And, instead of the incisions and grafting required in an organ transplant, islets are transplanted by a simple injection (see Figure 35-2).

An islet transplant is done under local anesthesia, where a small area of skin on your abdomen is numbed for the procedure. A radiologist injects the islets through a small tube into your liver via your portal vein (see Figure 35-2). The islets stick in your liver and are nourished by your liver's blood supply. The islets may work right away and start making insulin, but it often takes a few days or weeks for them to start functioning optimally. Thus, you can't stop insulin injections right away, but as islet function improves, you can gradually reduce your insulin dose. If the transplant is a success, you can eventually stop injections altogether. Most patients are in the hospital only 1–3 days with an islet transplant, unless they are asked to stay longer for research studies.

Keep in mind that islet transplants are still rare and that the procedure is still considered "investigational" in the United States.

Where Do the Islets Come From?
How Many Are Transplanted?

Islets are usually obtained from a deceased-donor pancreas. Great care is used to select a healthy pancreas for an islet transplant. Special solutions and procedures are used to free the islet cells, which can be seen only under a microscope, from the donor pancreas. The processing of islets takes 6–8 hours.

About 10,000 islets per kilogram of body weight need to be transplanted for someone with diabetes to become free of insulin injections. For a person weighing 154 pounds, that would be approximately 700,000 islets. Even though this is only 70% of the usual number of islets in a pancreas, it may take two to four pancreases to get that many islets because so many are lost during isolation. Thus, you might need more than one islet transplant procedure to become insulin-injection free. However, even if you can't give up insulin injections entirely, the islets from even one donor can improve your diabetes control, reduce the amount of insulin you need, and take care of brittle diabetes swings. Occasionally, some recipients are able to give up insulin injections entirely after islet transplants from one donor.

Can a Living Family Member or Friend Donate Islets?

Living donors have been used as a source of islets for transplantation. Only half of the donor pancreas is removed for islet isolation and, since the organ is entirely fresh, the islet yield may be high. However, as of 2006, this has only been done three times and only once was the procedure successful enough to eliminate insulin injections. Thus, living-donor islet transplantation is definitely in its infancy, in contrast to half-pancreas transplants from living donors, which are usually successful. However, even living-donor half-pancreas transplants are infrequent, since there is a risk of diabetes to the donor and deceased-donor pancreases are relatively plentiful.

How Successful Are Islet Transplants?

Islet transplants have become increasingly successful in recent years, but in the United States, it is still a rare and investigational procedure, done at only a few specialized centers, and conducted in what are called clinical trials. The less insulin one needs before the islet transplant, the more likely the transplant is to eliminate the need for injections, so most centers only accept patients who need less than 40 units per day.

The islet transplants done so far do not appear to be as durable as pancreas transplants. Even though 70% of islet recipients don't need insulin injections at 1 year, at 4 years this percentage is only 20%. In contrast, at 4 years more than 70% of pancreas transplant recipients are still off of insulin. However, most of the islet recipients who had to go back on insulin continued to have some islet function, and the diabetes was easier to control than before the transplant.

What Are the Benefits of an Islet Transplant?

If completely successful, an islet transplant will work just as well as a successful pancreas transplant and eliminate your need for insulin injections. A partially successful islet transplant will reduce the amount of insulin you need and improve your blood glucose control. Studies have also shown that, in general, the quality of life improves after an islet transplant for the few patients who have undergone a successful transplant.

What Are the Risks of an Islet Transplant?

Since the procedure is much less invasive, the surgical risk of an islet transplant is much lower than it is for a pancreas or kidney transplant. Still, the risk is not zero, and complications, such as bleeding, can occur at the site of islet injection. Since the islets are injected into the liver, the possibility of liver damage exists, though the problems appear minor so far. Blood clots, infections, and, rarely, death are also possibilities, but the observed rate of these complications has been very minimal.

The main risk for islet cell transplants is the need for immunosuppressive drugs to prevent rejection of the islets, the same as for whole-organ transplants. The anti-rejection drugs can impair the immune system and increase the rate of certain infections. Over time, the rate of certain cancers, such as of the skin, is also increased.

What Happens After an
Islet Transplant?

You will need frequent clinic visits and blood tests to check how well the islets are working and to see if there are any side effects from the transplant or the medications. You will still have to check blood glucose levels frequently to make sure the islets are still functioning or to adjust your insulin dose if injections are still necessary. The doses of the anti-rejection drugs you are taking also have to be adjusted, so the levels of these medications in your blood will need to be checked weekly in the beginning and then monthly later on.

Most of the centers currently doing islet transplants have research money to pay for the cost of the anti-rejection medications for about a year, but patients (or their health insurance companies, if the policy allows) will need to cover the high costs of medications afterward. People interested in getting an islet transplant should talk with doctors conducting islet transplant studies and with their health insurance company about whether any financial help is available. The hope is that islet transplants will become more common. If this procedure becomes routine care, insurance companies will likely pay from the beginning.

Will an Islet Transplant Cure Diabetes?

A successful islet transplant is as much of a "cure" as a successful pancreas transplant. It may eliminate the need for insulin injections, but the regimen of anti-rejection drugs you'll need to take makes it only a partial cure at this time. Additionally, many people eventually return to insulin injections. However, a successful islet transplant, even one that does not completely eliminate insulin injections, can improve your diabetes control significantly. One does not need to be "cured" to experience a benefit.

Could a Stem-Cell Transplant Cure Diabetes?

Stem cells are immature cells that have the potential to develop into any kind of cell in the body. Research is underway to determine if stem cells can develop into pancreatic beta cells that can then be transplanted to cure diabetes. If this method were to prove successful, the need for islet cell donors would disappear. Unfortunately, little progress has been made in humans so far. A few researchers have successfully reversed diabetes in mice with stem cells, so there is hope. However, it is thought that it will be several years or decades before stem-cell transplants will be viable in humans.

What Is Happening in Islet-Transplant Research?

Since islet transplants are still at the forefront of transplant procedures, a lot of research is still ongoing. Some research is focused on improving methods to prevent rejection and finding anti-rejection drugs that do not harm islet function. One of the problems with islet transplants is that some of the anti-rejection drugs are what are called "diabetogenic"; that is, they either impair islet function or increase your need for insulin. Naturally, this is a problem when the point of the transplant is to *decrease* your need for insulin. Different combinations of drugs to prevent rejection are being explored, but none are totally satisfactory yet. Nevertheless, better drug combinations seem to be leading to more successful islet transplants from fewer donors.

Would You Like to Participate?

The National Institutes of Health has sponsored an islet transplantation trial involving several centers called the Clinical Islet Transplantation Consortium. As of the printing of this book, candidates for islet transplantation are being recruited. If you are interested, you can find more information at the consortium's web site at www.citisletstudy.org. If you participate in a study, you will be informed of the risk and benefits of an islet transplant by the health care professionals conducting the investigation, and you will sign a consent form allowing you to be in the study or to withdraw at any time. The results of these studies will help determine whether islet transplants can become a treatment of choice for type 1 diabetes in the future.

Other researchers are working on coating islets in a way that prevents the white blood cells and other antibodies from rejecting the foreign islet cells. If it works, this strategy could eliminate the need for anti-rejection drugs. Stem cells are also being investigated for their capacity to evolve into beta cells (see box on pg 403). Another possible unlimited source of islets could come from animals, and several groups are working on using pig islets. Your body will reject animal tissues at a much higher rate than human tissue, so it will take several years before all the problems involved with animal islets are solved and transplants in humans can begin.

This chapter was written by David E. R. Sutherland, MD, PhD, and Annelisa Carlson, MD.

Appendix

Medications and Blood Glucose:

A review of diabetes medications and their effects on blood glucose

Introduction

While diabetes can be an overwhelming diagnosis, it is by no means a disease you should fear. There are several aspects of diabetes that may be confusing. Without guidance, attempting to understand the disease can grow increasingly more complex. It is helpful to be reminded that you are not alone. With friends, family, a supportive network of health care professionals, and your own accumulated knowledge, you can become your own best advocate. By reading this book, you are taking steps to ensure a quality life with diabetes.

Your health care team members are an important component for understanding the disease. However, it is easy to forget that you are the most important player on the team. Without active involvement from your physician, nurse, pharmacist, or dietician, your diabetes care will not be as effective. Therefore, it is important that you understand all your medications, both old and new, including how they function in your body.

Research results show that medications will work if a patient takes them as prescribed. The purpose of this appendix is to help you understand the treatment plan so that you have the knowledge base required for better health. The tables below discuss medications prescribed for both type 1 and type 2 diabetes. A brief discussion of the various tables explains how a person with diabetes ought to use them. Ultimately, the purpose of this appendix is to encourage you to have a conversation with your health care provider to understand where the different pieces of the puzzle fit together.

The following tables are not all-inclusive. It is safe to say that the treatment of diabetes is dynamic and requires an ever-changing approach. At the time of publication, only a select list of the more common types of diabetes agents was included. For more specific information on medications, including those not listed in the chart, contact your physician or pharmacist.

How Do You Use the Tables?

Table A-1

Table A-1 presents the different kinds of insulin that are currently used to treat type 1 and type 2 diabetes. Insulin is the first treatment option for type 1, but can be an important cornerstone for the treatment of type 2 diabetes as well. This table includes certain characteristics, such as how quickly a medication begins to work (onset), how long the medication takes to have the greatest effect (peak), and how long the medication lasts in the body (duration). These characteristics help determine which insulins could be included in your treatment plan.

The insulin products, Humulin R and Novolin R, are examples of regular insulin (Table A-1). Typically, they begin to work within 30 minutes to an hour after they are injected into the body. Their peak effect occurs 2–3 hours after injection. This takes place usually when your body is absorbing the digested food, and its effect may last for an additional 3–6 hours to allow coverage as your body continues to digest the food.

Table A-2

Table A-2 lists oral and injectable medications that are primarily used to treat type 2 diabetes with a single drug. The injectable medications may be also used to treat type 1 diabetes. These medications work both to help the body produce more insulin and to make better use of injected insulin. The upper section of the table presents more "traditional" treatments that require taking medications orally. Although these medications are quite successful in helping control blood glucose levels, some of the agents are often used in combination with other medications to help make the most of the different mechanisms of action.

A select few medications are offered as combination products to help reduce the number of tablets taken at one time. Similar to Table A-1, a discussion on the duration of the medication is offered to help you understand how long a particular medication works. The bottom half of the table lists medications that have made headway into the market most recently. They are listed as miscellaneous agents, because when added to a therapy plan, they proved beneficial in helping control a higher blood glucose. At the very bottom of Table A-2 is a list of medications that are about to be approved by the FDA and could be on the market shortly.

Tables A-3 and A-4

It is now common knowledge that when a patient takes a medication, there is always the possibility that it may interact with other medications that the patient is currently taking. These drug-drug interactions occur by a number of processes. For example, drug A may interfere with the body's ability to remove drug B. The final outcome is that there is an accumulation of drug B in the body until drug A has either been removed by the body or has been discontinued. The data presented in Table A-3 are an example of such an interaction. In this table, drugs in the top row are medications used to treat diabetes. Drugs listed in the row to the left indicate drugs that inhibit, or prevent, the removal of diabetic agents. Thus, these drugs can cause increased hypoglycemia to varying degrees.

The data in Table 4 list the medications that should be avoided while taking oral diabetes tablets. It is important to note that only drug interactions with a very high degree of severity are listed.

When taking any combination of the drugs in these tables it is important to more closely monitor your blood glucose until you know how it will be affected.

Obviously, there are numerous medications that should be avoided but are not listed in this table. Many of these drug-drug interactions are well documented and understood. To ensure the best medical care possible, you need to let your physician and pharmacist know what other medications you are taking before starting new drug therapy. These medications include items that are termed over-the-counter (OTC) products (for example, aspirin and acetaminophen) or herbal supplements (such as ginkgo biloba and ginseng). *However, do not abruptly discontinue medications, regardless of drug interactions, without first consulting your physician.*

Tables A-5.1, A-5.2, A-6.1, and A-6.2

These tables list medications that *may* increase or decrease blood glucose levels to varying degrees. However, just because a medication is listed in these tables does not necessarily mean that it will alter your blood glucose. In fact, you may experience no effect whatsoever. A few points to note regarding the tables:

- Table A-5.1 lists drugs that may increase blood glucose levels and are organized by their active ingredients.
- Table A-5.2 is identical to Table A-5.1 except that it lists the drugs by the more common brand names.
- Table A-6.1 lists drugs that may decrease blood glucose levels and are organized by their active ingredients.
- Table A-6.2 is identical to Table A-6.1, except that it lists the drugs by their more common brand names.

It is important to reemphasize that this list of medications does not include all medications that should be avoided. To be more precise, this is a list of medications that gives you a general idea about how to monitor your blood glucose levels more closely. It is recommended that you test your blood glucose before taking the new medication, followed by further tests every couple of hours. Continue monitoring for several days, and keep track of your blood glucose test results.

Note: The same drug may be listed as a causative agent for both an increase and a decrease in blood sugar levels, since reactions may differ from individual to individual.

Furthermore, it is important to note that the use of some medications, especially OTC products, may require a visit to your physician to discuss a possible change in drug therapy or of your diabetes therapy plan. It may also be beneficial for you to test your blood glucose level more than once throughout the day before taking a new medication to see if there is any impact on your blood glucose level. Doing this may help you identify another medication not listed in these tables.

One Final Note

Optimal health care results from the collaboration among you and your health care providers to formulate the best treatment plan tailored to your needs. The following tables are not specific guidelines to be closely followed in every situation. Instead, they serve as tools to help you understand the use of specific medications for a more effective outcome. Remember that you are an active participant in your treatment plan. It is expected that the information presented here will prove useful in helping to better inform you about diabetes and how to approach the use of your medications.

This appendix was written by Majid-Theodore R. Tanas, MS, PharmD Candidate; Jason M. Lund, BS, PharmD Candidate; Danial E. Baker, PharmD, FASHP, FASCP; and R. Keith Campbell, BPharm, FASHP, FAPhA, CDE.

Table A-1. Different Types of Non-Oral (Injectable) Medications Used to Treat Diabetes

TYPES OF INSULIN

Type of Insulin	Name	Onset[1] (hours)	Peak[2] (hours)	Duration of Effect[3] (hours)	Appearance
Rapid-Acting Insulin	Novolog (insulin aspart)	0.5	1–2	3.5	Clear
	Humalog (insulin lispro)	<0.25	0.5–1.5	3–4	Clear
	Apidra (insulin glulisine)	0.2–0.5	0.5–1.5	3–4	Clear
Short-Acting Insulin	Humulin R (regular insulin)	0.5–1.0	2–3	3–6	Clear
	Novolin R (regular insulin)	0.5–1.0	2–3	3–6	Clear
Intermediate-Acting Insulin	Humulin N (isophane insulin)	2–4 2–4	6–10 6–10	10–16 10–16	Cloudy Cloudy
	Novolin N (isophane insulin)	3–4	6–8	6–23	Clear
Long-Acting Insulin	Humulin U (ultralente)	6–10	10–16	18–20	Cloudy
	Lantus (insulin glargine)	4		24	Clear
	Levemir (Detemir)				

COMBINATION PRODUCTS

Type of Insulin	Name	
Lispro-Lispro Protamine	Humalog Mix 75/25 Humalog Mix50/50 Novolog Mix 70/30	The purpose of the combination products is to combine different types of insulin in order to reduce the number of injections. Usual combinations include a rapid- or short-acting insulin combined with an intermediate-acting insulin to provide initial coverage that continues until the next injection.
Aspart-Protamine		
NPH-Regular Combinations	Humulin 70/30 Novolin 70/30 Humulin 50/50	

1 Onset is a measurement of how quickly the insulin will begin to work.
2 Peak is a measurement of when the maximum affect of the medication will occur.
3 Duration of Effect is a measurement of how long the insulin will work.

Table A-2. Agents Used to Treat Type-2 Diabetes

TYPES OF ORAL AGENTS

Generic (Trade)	Duration (hours)	Mechanism of Action
Sulfonylureas (1st Generation)		Sulfonylureas work to increase the amount of insulin the pancreas releases into the bloodstream.
Acetohexamide (Dymelor)	12–18	
Chlorpropamide (Diabinese)	24–72	
Tolazamide (Tolinase)	12–24	
Tolbutamide (Orinase)	6–12	
Sulfonylureas (2nd Generation)		See above.
Glimepiride (Amaryl)	18–28	
Glipizide (Gluctrol, Glucotrol XL)	10–24	
Glyburide (DiaBeta, Micronase)	18–24	
Glyburide, Micronized (Glynase)	18–24	
Short-Acting Insulin Secretogogues		Short-acting insulin secretogogues work in a similar way to sulfonylureas by stimulating pancreatic insulin secretion.
Nateglinide (Starlix)	4	
Repaglinide (Prandin)	4	
Biguanides		Biguanides reduce the liver glucose production and increase the ability of your body to use glucose. Metformin beneficially affects lipids and cholesterol.
Metformin (Glucophage)	8–12	
Metformin Extended Release (Glucophage XR)	~24	
Alpha-Glucosidase Inhibitors		Alpha-Glucosidase Inhibitors prevent the breakdown of complex carbohydrates and sucrose in your digestive tract and ultimately decrease the amount of post-meal sugar that is absorbed.
Acarbose (Precose)	4–6	
Miglitol (Glyset)	4–6	
Thiazolidinediones ('Glitazones')		'Glitazones' increase insulin sensitivity throughout your body.
Pioglitazone (Actos)	16–24	
Rosiglitazone (Avandia)	12–24	
Sitagliptin (Januvia)	18–24	Inhibits the breakdown of the incretin hormones GLP-1 and GIP, which regulate gastric emptying and glucagon secretion.

COMBINATION ORAL AGENTS

Generic (Trade)	Duration (hours)	Mechanism of Action
Metformin; Glipizide (Metaglip) Metformin; Glyburide (Glucovance) Metformin; Pioglitazone (Actoplus Met) Metformin; Rosiglitazone (Avandamet) Glimepiride; Rosiglitazone (Avandaryl) Glimepiride; Pioglitazone (Duetact) Sitagliptin; Metformin (Janumet)	See individual agents.	See individual agents.

MISCELLANEOUS AGENTS

Generic (Trade)	Duration (hours)	Mechanism of Action
Exenatide (Byetta)	Up to 10 hours	Exenatide enhances glucose-dependent insulin secretion and other antihyperglycemic actions of incretins.
Pramlintide (Symlin)	3 hours	Mimics normal pancreatic secretions, which slows down stomach emptying time, reduces after-meal glucagon secretion, and reduces caloric intake through centrally-mediated appetite suppression.

Table A-3. Drugs to Avoid While on Oral Diabetes Drugs [1]

Diabetes Medication	Drugs to avoid
Acarbose	Amylase; Cellulase; Lipase; Protease Charcoal Digoxin Ethanol Pancreatin Pancrelipase Sacrosidase
Acetohexamide	Methotrexate
Chlorpropamide	Methotrexate
Glimepiride	Methotrexate
Glipizide	Methotrexate
Glyburide	Bosentan Methotrexate
Metformin	Dofetilide Radiopaque Contrast Agents
Miglitol	Amylase; Cellulase; Lipase; Protease Charcoal Digoxin Pancreatin Pancrelipase Sacrosidase
Nateglinide	N/A
Pioglitazone	Bosentan Insulins Oral contraceptives Progestins
Repaglinide	Gemfibrozil Isophane insulin (NPH)
Rosiglitazone	Bosentan Insulins
Tolazamide	Methotrexate
Tolbutamide	Delavirdine Imatinib, STI-571 Methotrexate

1 Drugs screened for high- and very-high-severity interactions. Each medication has interactions not listed above. For more information, contact your physician and/or pharmacist.

Table A-4. Significant Drug Interactions of Diabetes

Common Inhibitors of CYP2C8, CYP2C9, and CYP3A4	Chlorpropamide (Diabinese)	Glipizide (Glucotrol)	Glimepiride (Amaryl)	Glyburide (DiaBeta)	Metformin (Glucophage) Renal elimination	Nateglinide (Starlix)	Pioglitazone (Actos)	Repaglinide (Prandin)	Rosiglitazone (Avandia)	Tolbutamide (Orinase)
Atazanavir (Reyataz)	X	X	X	X			X	X	X	X
Clarithromycin (Biaxin)						X	X	X		
Erythromycin						X	X	X		
Fluconazole (Diflucan)	X	X	X	X		X	X	X	X	X
Fluoxetine (Prozac)	X	X	X	X					X	X
Fluvastatin (Lescol)	X	X	X	X					X	X
Fluvoxamine (Luvox)	X	X	X	X		X	X	X	X	X
Gemfibrozil (Lopid)						X	X	X	X	
Grapefruit (large doses)						X	X	X		
Indinavir (Crixivan)						X	X			
Isoniazid (INH)	X	X	X	X		X	X		X	X
Itraconazole (Sporanox)						X	X	X		
Ketoconazole (Nizoral)						X	X	X		
Metronidazole (Flagyl)	X	X	X	X		X	X		X	X
Ritonavir (Norvir)						X	X	X		
Sulfamethoxazole	X	X	X	X		X	X	X	X	X
Voriconazole (Vfend)	X	X	X	X		X	X	X	X	X

Elimination Pathways for Oral Hypoglycemic Agents

Adapted from Hansten PD, Horn JR. 2004. *The Top 100 Drug Interactions: A Guide to Patient Management*, 157–169. H&H Publications: Edmonds, WA.

Table A-5.1. Drugs That May Cause Hyperglycemia Listed Alphabetically by Generic Name

Generic Name	Brand Name	Function
Abacavir	Ziagen	Anti-Infective
Abacavir; Lamivudine, 3TC	Epzicom	Anti-Infective
Abacavir; Lamivudine, 3TC; Zidovudine, ZDV	Trizivir	Anti-Infective
Acebutolol	Sectral	Cardiovascular Medication
Acetazolamide	Diamox	Cardiovascular Medication
Alosetron	Lotronex	Anti-Infective
Amiloride; Hydrochlorothiazide, HCTZ	Moduretic	Cardiovascular Medication
Amprenavir	Agenerase	Anti-Infective
Aripiprazole	Abilify	Psychiatric Medication
Arsenic Trioxide	Trisenox	Cancer Drug
Aspirin, ASA	Too Many to List	Pain Relief/Cardiovascular Medication
Aspirin, ASA; Butalbital; Caffeine	Fiorinal	Pain Relief
Aspirin, ASA; Butalbital; Caffeine; Codeine	Fiorinal with Codeine	Pain Relief
Aspirin, ASA; Caffeine; Dihydrocodeine	Synalgos-DC	Pain Relief
Atazanavir	Reyataz	Anti-Infective
Atenolol	Tenormin	Cardiovascular Medication
Atenolol; Chlorthalidone	Tenoretic	Cardiovascular Medication
Atovaquone	Mepron	Anti-Infective
Baclofen	Lioresal	Muscle Relaxant
Benazepril; Hydrochlorothiazide, HCTZ	Lotensin HCT	Cardiovascular Medication
Bendroflumethiazide; Nadolol	Corzide	Cardiovascular Medication
Betamethasone	Celestone	Anti-Inflammatory
Bexarotene	Targretin	Cancer Drug
Bicalutamide	Casodex	Cancer Drug
Bisoprolol	Zebeta	Cardiovascular Medication
Bisoprolol; Hydrochlorothiazide, HCTZ	Ziac	Cardiovascular Medication
Bumetanide	Bumex	Cardiovascular Medication
Busulfan	Myleran	Cancer Drug
Butalbital Compound	Fiorinal	Pain Relief
Caffeine	Keep Alert	Stimulant
Caffeine	Stay Awake	Stimulant

Generic Name	Brand Name	Function
Caffeine	NoDoz	Stimulant
Candesartan; Hydrochlorothiazide, HCTZ	Atacand HCT	Cardiovascular Medication
Captopril; Hydrochlorothiazide, HCTZ	Capozide	Cardiovascular Medication
Carvedilol	Coreg	Cardiovascular Medication
Cefditoren	Spectracef	Anti-Infective
Chlorothiazide	Diuril	Cardiovascular Medication
Chlorthalidone	Thalitone	Cardiovascular Medication
Choline Salicylate; Magnesium Salicylate		Pain Relief
Cilostazol	Pletal	Cardiovascular Medication
Clozapine	Clozaril	Psychiatric Medication
Codeine; Phenylephrine; Promethazine	Promethazine VC with Codeine	Cough Suppression
Conjugated Estrogens	Cenestin	Women's Health
Conjugated Estrogens	Premarin	Women's Health
Conjugated Estrogens; Medroxyprogesterone	Prempro	Women's Health
Cortisone		Anti-Inflammatory
Cyclosporine	Gengraf	Cancer Drug
Dexamethasone	Decadron	Anti-Inflammatory
Dexamethasone	DexPak	Anti-Inflammatory
Dextromethorphan; Promethazine	Prometh with Dextromethorphan	Anti-Inflammatory
Diazoxide	Proglycem	Cardiovascular Medication
Drospirenone; Estradiol	Angeliq	Women's Health
Emtricitabine; Tenofovir	Truvada	Anti-Infective
Enalapril; Hydrochlorothiazide, HCTZ	Vaseretic	Cardiovascular Medication
Enfuvirtide	Fuzeon	Anti-Infective
Eprosartan; Hydrochlorothiazide, HCTZ	Teveten HCT	Cardiovascular Medication
Esterified Estrogens	Menest	Women's Health
Esterified Estrogens; Methyltestosterone	Estratest HS	Women's Health
Estradiol	Climara	Women's Health
Estradiol	Estrace	Women's Health
Estradiol; Levonorgestrel	Climara Pro	Women's Health
Estradiol; Norethindrone	CombiPatch	Women's Health
Estradiol; Norethindrone	Activella	Women's Health
Estradiol; Norgestimate	Ortho-Cyclen	Women's Health

Generic Name	Brand Name	Function
Estradiol; Norgestimate	Ortho Tri-Cyclen Lo	Women's Health
Estradiol; Norgestimate	Ortho-Tri-Cyclen	Women's Health
Estrone	Primestrin	Women's Health
Estropipate	Ortho-Est	Women's Health
Ethacrynic Acid	Edecrin	Cardiovascular Medication
Ethinyl Estradiol	Estinyl	Women's Health
Fluoxetine; Olanzapine	Symbyax	Psychiatric Medication
Fosamprenavir	Lexiva	Anti-Infective
Fosinopril; Hydrochlorothiazide, HCTZ	Monopril-HCT	Cardiovascular Medication
Furosemide	Lasix	Cardiovascular Medication
Gatifloxacin	Tequin	Anti-Infective
Gemifloxacin	Factive	Anti-Infective
Green Tea		Herbal
Guarana	Oleomed Weight	Herbal
Hydralazine; Hydrochlorothiazide, HCTZ	Hydrazide	Cardiovascular Medication
Hydralazine; Isosorbide Dinitrate, ISDN	BiDil	Cardiovascular Medication
Hydrochlorothiazide, HCTZ	HydroDIURIL	Cardiovascular Medication
Hydrochlorothiazide, HCTZ; Irbesartan	Avalide	Cardiovascular Medication
Hydrochlorothiazide, HCTZ; Lisinopril	Zestoretic	Cardiovascular Medication
Hydrochlorothiazide, HCTZ; Losartan	Hyzaar	Cardiovascular Medication
Hydrochlorothiazide, HCTZ; Metoprolol	Lopressor HCT	Cardiovascular Medication
Hydrochlorothiazide, HCTZ; Moexipril	Uniretic	Cardiovascular Medication
Hydrochlorothiazide, HCTZ; Olmesartan	Benicar HCT	Cardiovascular Medication
Hydrochlorothiazide, HCTZ; Quinapril	Accuretic	Cardiovascular Medication
Hydrochlorothiazide, HCTZ; Spironolactone	Aldactazide	Cardiovascular Medication
Hydrochlorothiazide, HCTZ; Telmisartan	Micardis HCT	Cardiovascular Medication
Hydrochlorothiazide, HCTZ; Triamterene	Maxzide	Cardiovascular Medication
Hydrochlorothiazide, HCTZ; Valsartan	Diovan HCT	Cardiovascular Medication
Hydrocortisone	Cortef	Anti-Inflammatory

Generic Name	Brand Name	Function
Indapamide	Lozol	Cardiovascular Medication
Indinavir	Crixivan	Anti-Infective
Isoniazid, INH	Tubizid	Anti-Infective
Isotretinoin	Accutane	Dermatological Conditions
Labetalol	Trandate	Cardiovascular Medication
Lamivudine, 3TC	Epivir	Anti-Infective
Levalbuterol	Xopenex	Anti-Infective
Levonorgestrel	Norplant	Women's Health
Lopinavir; Ritonavir	Kaletra	Anti-Infective
Lovastatin; Niacin	Advicor	Hypercholesterolemia
Magnesium Salicylate	Doans	Pain Relief
Medroxyprogesterone	Depo-Provera	Women's Health
Medroxyprogesterone	Provera	Women's Health
Megestrol	Megace	Appetite Stimulant/Cancer
Methyclothiazide	Enduron	Cardiovascular Medication
Methylprednisolone	Methylpred	Anti-Inflammatory
Metolazone	Zaroxolyn	Cardiovascular Medication
Metoprolol	Lopressor	Cardiovascular Medication
Metoprolol	Toprol XL	Cardiovascular Medication
Metoprolol	Toprol	Cardiovascular Medication
Mirtazapine	Remeron	Psychiatric Medication
Modafinil	Provigil	Narcolepsy
Moxifloxacin	Avelox	Anti-Infective
Mycophenolate	CellCept	Immunosuppressant
Nadolol	Corgard	Cardiovascular Medication
Nelfinavir	Viracept	Anti-Infective
Niacin, Niacinamide	Niaspan	Hypercholesterolemia
Nilutamide	Nilandron	Cancer Drug
Nitric Oxide	INOmax	General Anesthesia
Norethindrone	Nora-BE	Women's Health
Norgestrel	Ovrette	Women's Health
Nystatin	Mycostatin	Anti-Infective
Nystatin; Triamcinolone	Mycogen	Anti-Infective
Ofloxacin	Ocuflox	Anti-Infective
Olanzapine	Zyprexa	Psychiatric Medication
Olanzapine	Zyprexa Zydis	Psychiatric Medication
Olanzapine; Fluoxetine	Symbyax	Psychiatric Medication
Oseltamivir	Tamiflu	Anti-Infective
Oxaliplatin	Eloxatin	Cancer Drug
Pantoprazole	Protonix	Indigestion
Penbutolol	Levatol	Cardiovascular Medication

Generic Name	Brand Name	Function
Pentamidine	NebuPent	Anti-Infective
Phenylephrine; Promethazine	Prometh VC Plain	Cough Suppression
Phenytoin	Dilantin	Anti-Seizure
Pindolol		Cardiovascular Medication
Pioglitazone	Actos	Diabetic Medication
Prednisolone	Orapred	Anti-Inflammatory
Prednisone	Deltasone	Anti-Inflammatory
Progesterone	Prometrium	Women's Health
Propranolol	Inderal	Cardiovascular Medication
Quetiapine	Seroquel	Psychiatric Medication
Risperidone	Risperdal M-Tab	Psychiatric Medication
Risperidone	Risperdal	Psychiatric Medication
Ritodrine		Cardiovascular Medication
Ritonavir	Norvir	Anti-Infective
Rituximab	Rituxan	Cancer Drug
Rosiglitazone	Avandia	Diabetic Medication
Salsalate	Salflex	Pain Relief
Saquinavir	Fortovase	Anti-Infective
Sevoflurane	Ultane	General Anesthesia
Somatropin, rh-GH	Saizen Click.Easy	Growth Hormone
Sotalol	Betapace	Cardiovascular Medication
Tacrolimus	Prograf	Immunosuppressant
Tenofovir, PMPA	Viread	Anti-Infective
Tigecycline	Tygacil	Anti-Infective
Timolol		Cardiovascular Medication
Tipranavir	Aptivus	Cardiovascular Medication
Torsemide	Demadex	Cardiovascular Medication
Ursodeoxycholic Acid, Ursodiol	Actigall	Treatment of Gallstones
Valproic Acid, Divalproex Sodium	Depakene	Anti-Seizure
Valproic Acid, Divalproex Sodium	Depakote	Anti-Seizure
Ziprasidone	Geodon	Psychiatric Medication

Table A-5.2. Drugs That May Cause Hyperglycemia Listed Alphabetically by the Most Common Brand Name

Brand Name	Generic Name	Function
Abilify	Aripiprazole	Psychiatric Medication
Accuretic	Hydrochlorothiazide, HCTZ; Quinapril	Cardiovascular Medication
Accutane	Isotretinoin	Dermatological Conditions
Actigall	Ursodeoxycholic Acid, Ursodiol	Treatment of Gallstones
Activella	Estradiol; Norethindrone	Women's Health
Actos	Pioglitazone	Diabetic Medication
Advicor	Lovastatin; Niacin	Hypercholesterolemia
Agenerase	Amprenavir	Anti-Infective
Aldactazide	Hydrochlorothiazide, HCTZ; Spironolactone	Cardiovascular Medication
Angeliq	Drospirenone; Estradiol	Women's Health
Aptivus	Tipranavir	Cardiovascular Medication
Atacand HCT	Candesartan; Hydrochlorothiazide, HCTZ	Cardiovascular Medication
Avalide	Hydrochlorothiazide, HCTZ; Irbesartan	Cardiovascular Medication
Avandia	Rosiglitazone	Diabetic Medication
Avelox	Moxifloxacin	Anti-Infective
Bayer	Aspirin, ASA	Pain Relief/Cardiovascular
Benicar HCT	Hydrochlorothiazide, HCTZ; Olmesartan	Cardiovascular Medication
Betapace	Sotalol	Cardiovascular Medication
BiDil	Hydralazine; Isosorbide Dinitrate, ISDN	Cardiovascular Medication
Bumex	Bumetanide	Cardiovascular Medication
Capozide	Captopril; Hydrochlorothiazide, HCTZ	Cardiovascular Medication
Casodex	Bicalutamide	Cancer Drug
Celestone	Betamethasone	Anti-Inflammatory
CellCept	Mycophenolate	Immunosuppressant
Cenestin	Conjugated Estrogens	Women's Health
Climara Pro	Estradiol; Levonorgestrel	Women's Health
Climara	Estradiol	Women's Health
Clozaril	Clozapine	Psychiatric Medication
CombiPatch	Estradiol; Norethindrone	Women's Health
Coreg	Carvedilol	Cardiovascular Medication

Brand Name	Generic Name	Function
Corgard	Nadolol	Cardiovascular Medication
Cortef	Hydrocortisone	Anti-Inflammatory
	Cortisone	Anti-Inflammatory
Corzide	Bendroflumethiazide; Nadolol	Cardiovascular Medication
Crixivan	Indinavir	Anti-Infective
Decadron	Dexamethasone	Anti-Inflammatory
Deltasone	Prednisone	Anti-Inflammatory
Demadex	Torsemide	Cardiovascular Medication
Depakene	Valproic Acid, Divalproex Sodium	Anti-Seizure
Depakote	Valproic Acid, Divalproex Sodium	Anti-Seizure
Depo-Provera	Medroxyprogesterone	Women's Health
DexPak	Dexamethasone	Anti-Inflammatory
Diamox	Acetazolamide	Cardiovascular Medication
Dilantin	Phenytoin	Anti-Seizure
Diovan HCT	Hydrochlorothiazide, HCTZ; Valsartan	Cardiovascular Medication
Diuril	Chlorothiazide	Cardiovascular Medication
Doans	Magnesium Salicylate	Pain Relief
Ecotrin	Aspirin, ASA	Pain Relief/Cardiovascular
Edecrin	Ethacrynic Acid	Cardiovascular Medication
Eloxatin	Oxaliplatin	Cancer Drug
Enduron	Methyclothiazide	Cardiovascular Medication
Epivir	Lamivudine, 3TC	Anti-Infective
Epzicom	Abacavir; Lamivudine, 3TC	Anti-Infective
Estinyl	Ethinyl Estradiol	Women's Health
Estrace	Estradiol	Women's Health
Estratest HS	Esterified Estrogens; Methyltestosterone	Women's Health
Factive	Gemifloxacin	Anti-Infective
Fiorinal	Aspirin, ASA; Butalbital; Caffeine	Pain Relief
Fiorinal with Codeine	Aspirin, ASA; Butalbital; Caffeine; Codeine	Pain Relief
Fortovase	Saquinavir	Anti-Infective
Fuzeon	Enfuvirtide	Anti-Infective
Gengraf	Cyclosporine	Cancer Drug
Geodon	Ziprasidone	Psychiatric Medication
	Green Tea	Herbal
Hydrazide	Hydralazine; Hydrochlorothiazide, HCTZ	Cardiovascular Medication

Brand Name	Generic Name	Function
HydroDIURIL	Hydrochlorothiazide, HCTZ	Cardiovascular Medication
Hyzaar	Hydrochlorothiazide, HCTZ; Losartan	Cardiovascular Medication
Inderal	Propranolol	Cardiovascular Medication
INOmax	Nitric Oxide	General Anesthesia
Kaletra	Lopinavir; Ritonavir	Anti-Infective
Keep Alert	Caffeine	Stimulant
Lasix	Furosemide	Cardiovascular Medication
Levatol	Penbutolol	Cardiovascular Medication
Lexiva	Fosamprenavir	Anti-Infective
Lioresal	Baclofen	Muscle Relaxant
Lopressor	Metoprolol	Cardiovascular Medication
Lopressor HCT	Hydrochlorothiazide, HCTZ; Metoprolol	Cardiovascular Medication
Lotensin HCT	Benazepril; Hydrochlorothiazide, HCTZ	Cardiovascular Medication
Lotronex	Alosetron	Anti-Infective
Lozol	Indapamide	Cardiovascular Medication
Maxzide	Hydrochlorothiazide, HCTZ; Triamterene	Cardiovascular Medication
Megace	Megestrol	Appetite Stimulant/Cancer
Menest	Esterified Estrogens	Women's Health
Mepron	Atovaquone	Anti-Infective
Methylpred	Methylprednisolone	Anti-Inflammatory
Micardis HCT	Hydrochlorothiazide, HCTZ; Telmisartan	Cardiovascular Medication
Moduretic	Amiloride; Hydrochlorothiazide, HCTZ	Cardiovascular Medication
Monopril-HCT	Fosinopril; Hydrochlorothiazide, HCTZ	Cardiovascular Medication
Mycogen	Nystatin; Triamcinolone	Anti-Infective
Mycostatin	Nystatin	Anti-Infective
Myleran	Busulfan	Cancer Drug
NebuPent	Pentamidine	Anti-Infective
Niaspan	Niacin, Niacinamide	Hypercholesterolemia
Nilandron	Nilutamide	Cancer Drug
NoDoz	Caffeine	Stimulant
Nora-BE	Norethindrone	Women's Health
Norplant	Levonorgestrel	Women's Health
Norvir	Ritonavir	Anti-Infective
Ocuflox	Ofloxacin	Anti-Infective
Oleomed Weight	Guarana	Herbal

Brand Name	Generic Name	Function
Orapred	Prednisolone	Anti-Inflammatory
Ortho Tri-Cyclen Lo	Estradiol; Norgestimate	Women's Health
Ortho-Cyclen	Estradiol; Norgestimate	Women's Health
Ortho-Est	Estropipate	Women's Health
Ortho-Tri-Cyclen	Estradiol; Norgestimate	Women's Health
Ovrette	Norgestrel	Women's Health
	Pindolol	Cardiovascular Medication
Pletal	Cilostazol	Cardiovascular Medication
Premarin	Conjugated Estrogens	Women's Health
Prempro	Conjugated Estrogens; Medroxyprogesterone	Women's Health
Primestrin	Estrone	Women's Health
Proglycem	Diazoxide	Cardiovascular Medication
Prograf	Tacrolimus	Immunosuppressant
Prometh VC Plain	Phenylephrine; Promethazine	Cough Suppression
Prometh with Dextromethorphan	Dextromethorphan; Promethazine	Anti-Inflammatory
Promethazine VC with Codeine	Codeine; Phenylephrine; Promethazine	Cough Suppression
Prometrium	Progesterone	Women's Health
Protonix	Pantoprazole	Indigestion
Provera	Medroxyprogesterone	Women's Health
Provigil	Modafinil	Narcolepsy
Remeron	Mirtazapine	Psychiatric Medication
Reyataz	Atazanavir	Anti-Infective
Risperdal M-Tab	Risperidone	Psychiatric Medication
Risperdal	Risperidone	Psychiatric Medication
	Ritodrine	Cardiovascular Medication
Rituxan	Rituximab	Cancer Drug
Saizen Click.Easy	Somatropin, rh-GH	Growth Hormone
Salflex	Salsalate	Pain Relief
Sectral	Acebutolol	Cardiovascular Medication
Seroquel	Quetiapine	Psychiatric Medication
Spectracef	Cefditoren	Anti-Infective
Stay Awake	Caffeine	Stimulant
Symbyax	Fluoxetine; Olanzapine	Psychiatric Medication
Synalgos-DC	Aspirin, ASA; Caffeine; Dihydrocodeine	Pain Relief
Tamiflu	Oseltamivir	Anti-Infective
Targretin	Bexarotene	Cancer Drug
Tenoretic	Atenolol; Chlorthalidone	Cardiovascular Medication

Brand Name	Generic Name	Function
Tenormin	Atenolol	Cardiovascular Medication
Tequin	Gatifloxacin	Anti-Infective
Teveten HCT	Eprosartan; Hydrochlorothiazide, HCTZ	Cardiovascular Medication
Thalitone	Chlorthalidone	Cardiovascular Medication
	Timolol	Cardiovascular Medication
Toprol	Metoprolol	Cardiovascular Medication
Toprol XL	Metoprolol	Cardiovascular Medication
Trandate	Labetalol	Cardiovascular Medication
Tricosal	Choline Salicylate; Magnesium Salicylate	Pain Relief
Trisenox	Arsenic Trioxide	Cancer Drug
Trizivir	Abacavir; Lamivudine, 3TC; Zidovudine, ZDV	Anti-Infective
Truvada	Emtricitabine; Tenofovir	Anti-Infective
Tubizid	Isoniazid, INH	Anti-Infective
Tygacil	Tigecycline	Anti-Infective
Ultane	Sevoflurane	General Anesthesia
Uniretic	Hydrochlorothiazide, HCTZ; Moexipril	Cardiovascular Medication
Vaseretic	Enalapril; Hydrochlorothiazide, HCTZ	Cardiovascular Medication
Viracept	Nelfinavir	Anti-Infective
Viread	Tenofovir, PMPA	Anti-Infective
Xopenex	Levalbuterol	Anti-Infective
Zaroxolyn	Metolazone	Cardiovascular Medication
Zebeta	Bisoprolol	Cardiovascular Medication
Zestoretic	Hydrochlorothiazide, HCTZ; Lisinopril	Cardiovascular Medication
Ziac	Bisoprolol; Hydrochlorothiazide, HCTZ	Cardiovascular Medication
Ziagen	Abacavir	Anti-Infective
Zyprexa	Olanzapine	Psychiatric Medication
Zyprexa Zydis	Olanzapine	Psychiatric Medication

Table A-6.1. Drugs That May Cause Hypoglycemia
Listed Alphabetically by Generic Name

Generic Name	Brand Name	Function
Acebutolol	Sectral	Cardiovascular Medication
Acetohexamide	Dymelor	Diabetic Medication
Alosetron	Lotronex	Antidiarrheal
Amphotericin B	Amphocin	Anti-Infective
Amphotericin B	Fungizone	Anti-Infective
Amphotericin B Lipid Formulations	Abelcet	Anti-Infective
Amphotericin B Lipid Formulations	AmBisome	Anti-Infective
Amphotericin B Lipid Formulations	Amphotec	Anti-Infective
Arsenic Trioxide	Trisenox	Cancer Medication
Aspirin, ASA	Too Many to List	Pain Relief/Cardiovascular Medication
Atenolol	Tenormin	Cardiovascular Medication
Atenolol; Chlorthalidone	Tenoretic	Cardiovascular Medication
Bendroflumethiazide; Nadolol	Corzide	Cardiovascular Medication
Betaxolol	Kerlone	Cardiovascular Medication
Bisoprolol	Zebeta	Cardiovascular Medication
Bortezomib	Velcade	Cancer Medication
Caffeine	NoDoz	Stimulant
Caffeine	Vivarin	Stimulant
Caffeine	Alert	Stimulant
Carteolol	Cartrol	Cardiovascular Medication
Carvedilol	Coreg	Cardiovascular Medication
Chlorpheniramine; Codeine		Allergies/Cough Suppressant
Chlorpropamide	Diabinese	Diabetic Medication
Choline Salicylate; Magnesium Salicylate	Tricosal	Pain Relief
Choline Salicylate; Magnesium Salicylate	Trilisate	Pain Relief
Clarithromycin	Biaxin	Anti-Infective
Dalfopristin; Quinupristin	Synercid	Anti-Infective
Daptomycin	Cubicin	Anti-Infective
Disopyramide	Norpace	Cardiovascular Medication
Duloxetine	Cymbalta	Psychiatric Medication/Diabetic Peripheral Neuropathy
Esmolol	Brevibloc	Cardiovascular Medication

Generic Name	Brand Name	Function
Ethionamide	Trecator	Anti-Infective
Exenatide	Byetta	Diabetic Medication
Flucytosine	Ancobon	Anti-Infective
Fluoxetine	Prozac	Psychiatric Medication
Fluoxetine	Sarafem	Psychiatric Medication
Gatifloxacin	Tequin	Anti-Infective
Ginseng, Panax ginseng	Ginsana	Herbal
Glimepiride	Amaryl	Diabetic Medication
Glimepiride; Rosiglitazone	Avandaryl	Diabetic Medication
Glipizide	Glucotrol	Diabetic Medication
Glipizide; Metformin	Metaglip	Diabetic Medication
Glyburide	Diabeta	Diabetic Medication
Glyburide	Glynase	Diabetic Medication
Glyburide	Micronase	Diabetic Medication
Glyburide; Metformin	Glucovance	Diabetic Medication
Green Tea		Herbal
Guarana	Oleomed Weight	Herbal
Horse Chestnut, Aesculus hippocastanum		Herbal
Indomethacin	Indocin	Pain Relief
Insulin Aspart	NovoLog	Diabetic Medication
Insulin Aspart; Insulin Aspart Protamine	NovoLog	Diabetic Medication
Insulin Detemir	Levemir	Diabetic Medication
Insulin Glargine	Lantus	Diabetic Medication
Insulin Glulisine	Apidra	Diabetic Medication
Insulin Lispro	Humalog	Diabetic Medication
Insulin Lispro; Insulin Lispro Protamine	Humalog	Diabetic Medication
Insulin, Inhaled	Exubera	Diabetic Medication
Isophane Insulin (NPH)	Humulin N	Diabetic Medication
Isophane Insulin (NPH)	Novolin N	Diabetic Medication
Labetalol	Trandate	Cardiovascular Medication
Lamivudine, 3TC	Epivir	Anti-Infective
Lente Insulin	Humulin L	Diabetic Medication
Lente Insulin	Novolin L	Diabetic Medication
Levofloxacin	Levaquin	Anti-Infective
Lomefloxacin	Maxaquin	Anti-Infective
Magnesium Salicylate	Doans	Pain Relief
Magnesium Salicylate	Momentum	Pain Relief
Magnesium Salicylate	Nuprin	Pain Relief
Mecasermin rinfabate	Iplex	Growth Hormone

Generic Name	Brand Name	Function
Mecasermin, Recombinant, rh-IGF-1	Increlex	Growth Hormone
Memantine	Namenda	Alzheimer's Medication
Metformin	Glucophage	Diabetic Medication
Metformin	Fortamet	Diabetic Medication
Metformin	Riomet	Diabetic Medication
Metformin; Pioglitazone	Actoplus Met	Diabetic Medication
Metformin; Rosiglitazone	Avandamet	Diabetic Medication
Metoprolol	Lopressor	Cardiovascular Medication
Metoprolol	Toprol XL	Cardiovascular Medication
Nadolol	Corgard	Cardiovascular Medication
Nateglinide	Starlix	Diabetic Medication
Nelarabine	Arranon	Cancer Medication
Norfloxacin	Noroxin	Anti-Infective
Ofloxacin	Floxin	Anti-Infective
Orlistat	Xenical	Weight Loss
Pegvisomant	Somavert	Growth Hormone
Penbutolol	Levatol	Cardiovascular Medication
Pentamidine	Pentam	Anti-Infective
Pentamidine	NebuPent	Anti-Infective
Pindolol		Cardiovascular Medication
Pioglitazone	Actos	Diabetic Medication
Polyethylene Glycol; Electrolytes	Colyte	Bowel Preparation
Polyethylene Glycol; Electrolytes	GoLYTELY	Bowel Preparation
Pramlintide	Symlin	Diabetic Medication
Propranolol	Inderal	Cardiovascular Medication
Propranolol	Pronol	Cardiovascular Medication
Propranolol	InnoPran XL	Cardiovascular Medication
Quinine		Anti-Infective
Ramipril	Altace	Cardiovascular Medication
Regular Insulin	Humulin R	Diabetic Medication
Regular Insulin	Novolin R	Diabetic Medication
Regular Insulin	Oralin	Diabetic Medication
Regular Insulin; Isophane Insulin (NPH)		Diabetic Medication
Repaglinide	Prandin	Diabetic Medication
Rituximab	Rituxan	Cancer Medication
Rosiglitazone	Avandia	Diabetic Medication
Salsalate	Amigesic	Pain Relief
Salsalate	Argesic SA	Pain Relief

Generic Name	Brand Name	Function
Sodium Ferric Gluconate Complex	Ferrlecit	Iron Replacement
Somatropin, rh-GH	Genotropin	Growth Hormone
Sotalol	Betapace	Cardiovascular Medication
Sotalol	Sorine	Cardiovascular Medication
Streptozocin	Zanosar	Cancer Medication
Sulfadiazine		Anti-Infective
Sulfamethoxazole; Trimethoprim, SMX-TMP	Bactrim	Anti-Infective
Sulfamethoxazole; Trimethoprim, SMX-TMP	Septra	Anti-Infective
Sulfasalazine	Sulfazine	Ulcerative Colitis
Sulfisoxazole	Gantrisin Pediatric	Anti-Infective
Tacrolimus	Prograf	Immunosuppressant
Tigecycline	Tygacil	Anti-Infective
Timolol		Cardiovascular Medications
Tolazamide	Tolinase	Diabetic Medication
Tolbutamide	Orinase	Diabetic Medication
Topiramate	Topamax	Anti-Seizure
Ultralente Insulin	Humulin U	Diabetic Medication
Varenicline	Chantix	Smoking Cessation Aid

Table A-6.2. – Drugs That May Cause Hypoglycemia, Listed Alphabetically by the Most Common Brand Names

Brand Name	Generic Name	Function
Sectral	Acebutolol	Cardiovascular Medication
Dymelor	Acetohexamide	Diabetic Medication
Lotronex	Alosetron	Antidiarrheal
Amphocin	Amphotericin B	Anti-Infective
Fungizone	Amphotericin B	Anti-Infective
Abelcet	Amphotericin B Lipid Formulations	Anti-Infective
AmBisome	Amphotericin B Lipid Formulations	Anti-Infective
Amphotec	Amphotericin B Lipid Formulations	Anti-Infective
Trisenox	Arsenic Trioxide	Cancer Medication
Bayer	Aspirin, ASA	Pain Relief/Cardiovascular Medication
Ecotrin	Aspirin, ASA	Pain Relief/Cardiovascular Medication
Tenormin	Atenolol	Cardiovascular Medication
Tenoretic	Atenolol; Chlorthalidone	Cardiovascular Medication
Corzide	Bendroflumethiazide; Nadolol	Cardiovascular Medication
Kerlone	Betaxolol	Cardiovascular Medication
Zebeta	Bisoprolol	Cardiovascular Medication
Velcade	Bortezomib	Cancer Medication
Alert	Caffeine	Stimulant
NoDoz	Caffeine	Stimulant
Vivarin	Caffeine	Stimulant
Cartrol	Carteolol	Cardiovascular Medication
Coreg	Carvedilol	Cardiovascular Medication
Codeprex	Chlorpheniramine; Codeine	Allergies/Cough Suppressant
Diabinese	Chlorpropamide	Diabetic Medication
Tricosal	Choline Salicylate; Magnesium Salicylate	Pain Relief
Trilisate	Choline Salicylate; Magnesium Salicylate	Pain Relief
Biaxin	Clarithromycin	Anti-Infective
Synercid	Dalfopristin; Quinupristin	Anti-Infective
Cubicin	Daptomycin	Anti-Infective
Norpace	Disopyramide	Cardiovascular Medication
Cymbalta	Duloxetine	Psychiatric Medication/Diabetic Peripheral Neuropathy
Brevibloc	Esmolol	Cardiovascular Medication

Brand Name	Generic Name	Function
Trecator	Ethionamide	Anti-Infective
Byetta	Exenatide	Diabetic Medication
Ancobon	Flucytosine	Anti-Infective
Prozac	Fluoxetine	Psychiatric Medication
Sarafem	Fluoxetine	Psychiatric Medication
Tequin	Gatifloxacin	Anti-Infective
Ginsana	Ginseng, Panax ginseng	Herbal
Amaryl	Glimepiride	Diabetic Medication
Avandaryl	Glimepiride; Rosiglitazone	Diabetic Medication
Glucotrol	Glipizide	Diabetic Medication
Metaglip	Glipizide; Metformin	Diabetic Medication
Diabeta	Glyburide	Diabetic Medication
Glynase	Glyburide	Diabetic Medication
Micronase	Glyburide	Diabetic Medication
Glucovance	Glyburide; Metformin	Diabetic Medication
	Green Tea	Herbal
Oleomed Weight	Guarana	Herbal
	Horse Chestnut, Aesculus Hippocastanum	Herbal
Indocin	Indomethacin	Pain Relief
NovoLog	Insulin Aspart	Diabetic Medication
NovoLog 70/30	Insulin Aspart; Insulin Aspart Protamine	Diabetic Medication
Levemir	Insulin Detemir	Diabetic Medication
Lantus	Insulin Glargine	Diabetic Medication
Apidra	Insulin Glulisine	Diabetic Medication
Humalog	Insulin Lispro	Diabetic Medication
Humalog 50/50	Insulin Lispro; Insulin Lispro Protamine	Diabetic Medication
Humalog 75/25	Insulin Lispro; Insulin Lispro Protamine	Diabetic Medication
Exubera	Insulin, Inhaled	Diabetic Medication
Humulin N	Isophane Insulin (NPH)	Diabetic Medication
Novolin N	Isophane Insulin (NPH)	Diabetic Medication
Trandate	Labetalol	Cardiovascular Medication
Epivir	Lamivudine, 3TC	Anti-Infective
Humulin L	Lente Insulin	Diabetic Medication
Novolin L	Lente Insulin	Diabetic Medication
Levaquin	Levofloxacin	Anti-Infective

Brand Name	Generic Name	Function
Maxaquin	Lomefloxacin	Anti-Infective
Doans	Magnesium Salicylate	Pain Relief
Momentum	Magnesium Salicylate	Pain Relief
Nuprin	Magnesium Salicylate	Pain Relief
Iplex	Mecasermin rinfabate	Growth Hormone
Increlex	Mecasermin, Recombinant, rh-IGF-1	Growth Hormone
Namenda	Memantine	Alzheimer's Medication
Fortamet	Metformin	Diabetic Medication
Glucophage	Metformin	Diabetic Medication
Riomet	Metformin	Diabetic Medication
Actoplus Met	Metformin; Pioglitazone	Diabetic Medication
Avandamet	Metformin; Rosiglitazone	Diabetic Medication
Lopressor	Metoprolol	Cardiovascular Medication
Toprol XL	Metoprolol	Cardiovascular Medication
Corgard	Nadolol	Cardiovascular Medication
Starlix	Nateglinide	Diabetic Medication
Arranon	Nelarabine	Cancer Medication
Noroxin	Norfloxacin	Anti-Infective
Floxin	Ofloxacin	Anti-Infective
Xenical	Orlistat	Weight Loss
Somavert	Pegvisomant	Growth Hormone
Levatol	Penbutolol	Cardiovascular Medication
NebuPent	Pentamidine	Anti-Infective
Pentam	Pentamidine	Anti-Infective
	Pindolol	Cardiovascular Medication
Actos	Pioglitazone	Diabetic Medication
Colyte	Polyethylene Glycol; Electrolytes	Bowel Preparation
GoLYTELY	Polyethylene Glycol; Electrolytes	Bowel Preparation
Symlin	Pramlintide	Diabetic Medication
Inderal	Propranolol	Cardiovascular Medication
InnoPran XL	Propranolol	Cardiovascular Medication
Pronol	Propranolol	Cardiovascular Medication
	Quinine	Anti-Infective
Altace	Ramipril	Cardiovascular Medication
Humulin R	Regular Insulin	Diabetic Medication
Novolin R	Regular Insulin	Diabetic Medication
Oralin	Regular Insulin	Diabetic Medication
Humulin 50/50	Regular Insulin; Isophane Insulin (NPH)	Diabetic Medication
Humulin 70/30	Regular Insulin; Isophane Insulin (NPH)	Diabetic Medication

Brand Name	Generic Name	Function
Novolin 70/30	Regular Insulin; Isophane Insulin (NPH)	Diabetic Medication
Prandin	Repaglinide	Diabetic Medication
Rituxan	Rituximab	Cancer Medication
Avandia	Rosiglitazone	Diabetic Medication
Amigesic	Salsalate	Pain Relief
Argesic SA	Salsalate	Pain Relief
Ferrlecit	Sodium Ferric Gluconate Complex	Iron Replacement
Betapace	Sotalol	Cardiovascular Medication
Sorine	Sotalol	Cardiovascular Medication
Zanosar	Streptozocin	Cancer Medication
Silvadene	Sulfadiazine	Anti-Infective
Bactrim	Sulfamethoxazole; Trimethoprim, SMX-TMP	Anti-Infective
Septra	Sulfamethoxazole; Trimethoprim, SMX-TMP	Anti-Infective
Sulfazine	Sulfasalazine	Ulcerative Colitis
Gantrisin Pediatric	Sulfisoxazole	Anti-Infective
Prograf	Tacrolimus	Immunosuppressant
Tygacil	Tigecycline	Anti-Infective
	Timolol	Cardiovascular Medications
Tolinase	Tolazamide	Diabetic Medication
Orinase	Tolbutamide	Diabetic Medication
Topamax	Topiramate	Anti-Seizure
Humulin U	Ultralente Insulin	Diabetic Medication
Chantix	Varenicline	Smoking Cessation Aid

Index

A

Abscesses, 277, S2

A1C
  described, 7
  levels, recommended, 71, 216
  measurements, 18, 306

Acanthosis nigricans, 283, 286, S4

Acarbose (Precose)
  described, 21, 413
  drugs to avoid, 414
  in hypoglycemia, 47–48
  in weight loss, 378

Accupril (quinapril), 60

Acetohexamide, 413–415

N-Acetylcysteine, 105

Actonel (risedronate), 293–294

Actos. *See* Pioglitazone (Actos)

Adipose tissue, 371–373

Adolescents, coping skills, 356, 365–366

Adult-onset diabetes mellitus (AODM), 5

Aftercataract, 140

Age, fractures and, 288, 289

Aggrenox, 118–119

Albuminuria, 93, 198

Alcohol
  cholesterol and, 80–81
  fractures and, 288
  heart disease and, 70
  neuropathy and, 163
  stroke and, 117

Alendronate (Fosamax), 293–294

Aliskiren (Tekturna), 94

Alpha glucosidase inhibitors
  described, 21, 413
  in hypoglycemia, 46
  in weight loss, 378

Altace (ramipril), 60

Alzheimer's disease, 347–351

Amaryl. *See* Glimepiride (Amaryl)

Amaurosis fugax, 143

Ambien (zolpidem), 333

American Cancer Society, 387

Amputation
  neuropathy and, 161
  post care, 188
  risk factors, 168
  statistics, 3, 103, 104

Amylinmimetic, 21

Analgesics, 165

Androgens, 254, 317–318

Anemia, 302–308

Angina, 55–56

Angiography, 114

Angioplasty, 61

Angiotensin-converting enzymes (ACE)
    inhibitors
  for CAD, 60, 70
  for CHF, 66
  for hypertension, 93, 99
  microalbuminuria, 213

Angiotensin-receptor blockers (ARB), 60, 66, 70, 93
Antibiotics, 338
Anticoagulants, 119–120
Antiepileptics, 165
Antiplatelet therapy, 118–119
Apidra (glulisine), 20, 48, 412
Apolipoprotein B, 19
A2 receptor blockers, 213
Arousal, 249, 254
Arsenic, 324
Arteries, measurements, 19
Arteriosclerosis, 169
Ascites, 213
Aspart (Novolog), 20, 36, 48, 412
Aspirin
    for CAD, 59, 75
    measurements, 19
    metabolic syndrome, 315
    for stroke, 118–119
Atacand (candesartan), 60
Atenolol (Tenormin), 59–60
Atherosclerosis, 54, 69, 112, 384
Atorvastatin (Lipitor), 81–83
Autonomic neuropathy, 45
Avandia. See Rosiglitazone (Avandia)
Avapro (irbesartan), 60

B

Baby aspirin, 315
Bacterial infections, 274–277, 286, 338–341, 345
Barbiturates, 333
Bariatric surgery, 14, 74, 238, 380–381
Beta-blockers (β-blockers), 59–60, 66, 94
Biguanides, 21, 46, 413
Bile acid resins, 21, 83–84
Biofeedback, 166
Bisacodyl (Dulcolax), 230
Bisphosphonates, 293–294
Bladder
    infection, 339, 341, 342
    neurogenic, 217
    neuropathy, 191–194

Blindness, temporary, 143
Blood glucose. See Glucose levels
Blood pressure
    control, benefits of, 117
    death, sudden, 198
    high (See Hypertension)
    instruments, 97–98
    levels, recommended, 98, 216
    measurements, 18
Body mass index (BMI), 371, 372
Bone overview, 288–289
Boniva (Ibandronate), 293–294
Breast cancer, 294
Bullosis diabeticorum (blisters), 281, 286
Bunions, 169, 171–172
Buproprion (Wellbutrin), 73, 387
Burnout, 363–364
Byetta. See Exenatide (Byetta)
Bypass surgery, PAD, 105–108

C

Calcitonin (Miacalcin), 294–295
Calcium, 291–292
Calcium channel blockers, 94
Calculus, 298
Cancer
    causes of, 322–325
    colorectal, 327
    described, 321–322
    diabetes effects on, 324–325
    endometrial, 326
    genetic factors, 322
    liver, 326
    lung, 324
    overview, 321
    pancreatic, 325–326
    prostate, 325–327
    treatment, 327–328
Candesartan (Atacand), 60
Candida infection (yeast), 271–273, 286, 338
Captopril (Capoten), 60
Carbuncles, 276

Cortisol-reducers, 379
Coumadin (warfarin), 118–120
Cozaar (losartan), 60
Creatinine, 389–390
Crestor (rosuvastatin), 81–83
Cryotherapy, 134, 136
Cystitis (bladder infection), 339, 341, 342

D

DASH diet, 94–95
Dementia
    Alzheimer's disease, 347–351
    case study, 347
    cognitive impairment, 352–354
    described, 347–348
    diabetes effects, 352–353
    prevention, 353–354
    risk, lowering, 353
    vascular (multi-infarct), 351–353
Depression, 19, 256
Desire, 249
Detemir, 20, 34, 48, 412
DiaBeta (Glyburide), 21, 413, 414, 416
Diabetes
    costs, 3, 8
    defined, 10
    statistics, 3–4, 7–8
    types of, 5
Diabetes Control and Complications
    Trial (DCCT), 148–149, 159
Diabetes Prevention Program (DPP),
    13, 95, 382
Diabetes team, 16–18
Diabetic dermopathy, 278–279, 286, S3
Diabetic diarrhea, 228–229
Diabetic ketoacidosis (DKA)
    case study, 29
    causes, 30–32
    described, 29–30
    prevention, 37–38
    progression, 38–39
    risk factors, 32–35
    symptoms, 36
    treatment, 36–37

Diagnosis, 4, 358–359
Dialysis, 218–220, 389
Diastolic dysfunction, 65
Diet. *See* Nutrition
Digitalis (Digoxin), 66
Diovan (valsartan), 60
Dipyridamole, 118–119
Diuretics, 66, 94
DNA, 150–154
Docusate (Colace), 230
Double vision, 142–143
DPP-IV inhibitors, 21, 46
Drug therapy. *See also specific medications*
    drugs to avoid, 414
    falls and, 293
    interactions, 409–410, 416
    pre-diabetes, 13
Drug use, stroke and, 117
Dual X-ray absorptiometry (DXA),
    290–291
Dulcolax (bisacodyl), 230
Dupuytren's contracture, 267, 286
Dyspareunia, 249

E

Education, 19
Elderly people, hypertension in, 98
Electrocardiogram (ECG), 57, 114
Emphysematous cholecystitis, 340, 345
Emphysematous pyelonephritis, 340
Enalapril (Vasotec), 60
Endarterectomy, 107, 120
Endometrial cancer, 326
Endorphins, 166
End-stage renal disease (ESRD), 212,
    215, 217–220, 389, 396
Enemas, 230–231
Entrapment neuropathy, 202–203
Epinephrine (adrenaline), 43–45, 200–
    201, 300–301
EPO analogues, 307–308
Erectile dysfunction (ED), 96, 240–245
Erysipelas, 275–276, 286
Erythrasma, 275, 286, S1
Erythromycin, 226

Glitazones. *See* Thiazolidinediones (TZDs)

Glomerular filtration rate (GFR), 214, 303

Glucagon, 43, 45, 50

Glucophage. *See* Metformin (Glucophage)

Glucose levels
 in bone health, 293
 in cognitive functioning, 353
 dental treatment and, 301
 drug therapy effects, 410–411
 fasting, recommended, 71
 infections and, 336–337
 lowering techniques, 19–22
 measurements, 18
 menstruation and, 251–252
 in neuropathy development, 160
 ranges of, 10, 31
 regulation of, 43–44
 uncontrolled, vision changes due to, 138–139

Glucotrol. *See* Glipizide (Glucotrol)

Glulisine (Apidra), 20, 48, 412

Glyburide (DiaBeta), 21, 413, 414, 416

Glycemic load, 374, 375

Granuloma annulare, 281, 286

Growth hormone, 44

Gynecologists, 256–257

H

Hammertoes, 162, 169–172

Heart attack
 causes, 54
 described, 62
 metabolic syndrome, 312, 313
 prevention, 93
 risk factors, 262
 silent, 197–198
 statistics, 3
 symptoms, 62–63
 treatment, 63–64

Heartburn, 227

Heart disease
 described, 53–54

risk factors, 69–76, 116, 330, 390–391

Heat stroke, 199

Hemodialysis, 218–220

Hemorrhages, vitreous, 121, 127, 133

Heparin, 220

Hepatitis, 326, 346

High-density lipoprotein (HDL)
 described, 78
 heart disease and, 55, 71–72
 levels, recommended, 81, 82
 measurements, 19
 menopause and, 262
 metabolic syndrome, 311, 312, 314
 smoking and, 384, 385

Hoodia, 379

Hormonal deficiency, 254

Hormonal replacement therapy (HRT), 261, 262, 294, 326

Humalog (lispro), 20, 36, 48, 412

Human Genome Project, 150

Humulin, 20, 408, 412

Hyperfiltration, 211, 212

Hyperglycemia
 drug reactions, 417–426
 heart disease and, 70–71
 menstruation and, 251–252

Hyperlipidemia, 213

Hyperosmolar hyperglycemic state (HHS), 29, 39–41, 111

Hypertension
 case study, 85
 causes of, 86–87, 196
 diagnosis, 87–90
 heart disease and, 55, 70
 monitoring, 86, 91, 97–98
 nephropathy in, 210, 216
 prevalence, 86
 as risk factor, 95, 113, 116
 symptoms, 86, 91
 treatment, 90–99
 white coat, 86

Hypoglycemia
 awareness training, 201
 drug reactions, 427–434
 drug therapy causes, 46–48, 251

Kidney stones, 292
Kumamoto study, 159

L

Lactaid, 229
Lactation, 259
Lactic acidosis, 32, 41–42, 217
Lactose intolerance, 229
Laser surgery, 122, 131–136
Laxatives, 230
Legs, circulation in, 102
Lente, 34
Lescol (fluvastatin), 81–83
Levemir, 20, 34, 48, 412
Lidocaine, 165
Lifestyle modifications
 benefits of, 319
 coping skills, 360–361
 glucose lowering techniques,
  20, 22
 heart disease and, 70
 in hypertension, 91–92, 94–95
 pre-diabetes, 12
Linkage analysis, 153–154
Lisinopril (Zestril, Prinivil), 60
Lispro (Humalog), 20, 36, 48, 412
Liver biopsy, 237
Liver cancer, 326
Lopid (gemfibrozil), 84
Lopressor (metoprolol, Toprol),
 59–60
Losartan (Cozaar), 60
Lovastatin (Mevacor), 81–83
Low-density lipoprotein (LDL)
 described, 78–79
 heart disease and, 71–72
 levels, recommended, 81, 82,
  314
 measurements, 19
 menopause and, 262
 smoking and, 384, 385
Lunesta (eszopiclone), 333
Lung cancer, 324
Lyrica (pregabalin), 165

M

Macrovascular complications, 10
Macular edema, 121–122, 125–126,
 133, 144
Magnetic resonance imaging arteriogram
 (MRA), 100
Management of diabetes. *See also specific*
 conditions/medications
 ABCDEs of, 266
 cancer in, 327–328
 coping skills (*See* Coping skills)
 drugs to avoid, 414
 heart health, 67–68
 individual responsibility in, 17–18,
  24, 96–97
 lifestyle modifications (*See* Lifestyle
  modifications)
 overview, 6–7
Meal-induced hypotension, 195, 196
Measurements, 18–19
Meglitinides, 21, 46, 47, 251
Menopause, 252, 254, 260–262
Menstruation, 251–252
Meridia (sibutramine), 378–379
Metabolic syndrome, 311–316
Metatarsals, 171
Metformin (Glucophage)
 described, 21, 413
 diabetic diarrhea and, 228
 drugs to avoid, 414
 in hypoglycemia, 47–48
 interactions, 416
 kidney damage by, 217
 pre-diabetes, 13
 in weight loss, 378
Methylcellulose (Citrucel), 230
Metoclopramide (Reglan), 225–226
Metoprolol (Lopressor, Toprol), 59–60
Mevacor (lovastatin), 81–83
Mexiletine, 165
Miacalcin (calcitonin), 294–295
Microalbuminuria, 211–213, 216
Microvascular complications, 10
Miglitol, 21, 413, 414

Polycystic ovary syndrome (PCOS), 11, 257, 317–320
Poly/monounsaturated fats, 78
Postural orthostatic bradycardia syndrome (POBS), 196
Postural orthostatic tachycardia syndrome (POTS), 196
Pramlintide (Symlin), 21, 414
Prandin. *See* Repaglinide (Prandin)
Pravastatin (Pravachol), 81–83
Pre-diabetes, 9–15, 55
Pregabalin (Lyrica), 165
Pregnancy
    diabetes effects on, 258–260
    gestational diabetes, 6, 11, 144–145, 260
    hypertension and, 98
    planning for, 24, 319
    retinopathy and, 144–145
Prinivil (lisinopril, Zestril), 60
Propranolol (Inderal), 59–60, 196
Prostate cancer, 325–327
Proteinuria, 216
Proto-oncogenes, 322
Psychosocial complications
    adolescents, 356, 365–366
    behavioral barriers, 357–358, 360–361
    coping skills, 358–366
    emotional barriers, 356, 359
    overview, 355
    social barriers, 356–357, 359, 361
Psyllium (Konsyl, Metamucil), 230
Pyelonephritis, 339, 340–342
Pyrazolopyrimidine (Sonata), 333

Q

Quinapril (Accupril), 60

R

Radiculopathy, 204
Radon, 324
Raloxifene (Evista), 294
Ramelteon (Rozerem), 333

Ramipril (Altace), 60
Reglan (metoclopramide), 225–226
Renal insufficiency. *See* Chronic kidney disease
Repaglinide (Prandin)
    described, 21, 413
    drugs to avoid, 414
    in hypoglycemia, 47
    interactions, 416
Restless leg syndrome, 331–333
Retina, 123–124
Retinopathy
    described, 124–125
    development of, 152–153
    diagnosis, 128–130
    examination, 127–128
    exercise and, 144
    genes, discovery of, 149–155
    genetic risk factors, 147–149
    hypertension and, 93, 95
    nonproliferative, 124, 130–131, 144
    post-treatment care, 135–136
    post-treatment vision changes, 137–138
    pregnancy and, 144–145
    prevention, 126, 145, 155–156
    proliferative, 122, 124–127, 131–135, 144
    risk factors, 126, 304, 385
    statistics, 3
    symptoms, 126–127
    treatment, 130–135
    type 1 *vs.* type 2 diabetes, 149
Rhinocerebral mucormycosis, 340, 344
Risedronate (Actonel), 293–294
Rosiglitazone (Avandia)
    as contraceptive, 257
    described, 21, 413
    drugs to avoid, 414
    fractures and, 289
    in hypoglycemia, 47–48
    interactions, 416
    pre-diabetes, 13–14
    side effects, 66–67, 377
Rosuvastatin (Crestor), 81–83
Rozerem (ramelteon), 333

S

Sandostatin (octreotide), 196, 229
Saturated fats, 77
Scleroderma, 267, 286
Selective estrogen receptor modulator (SERM), 294
Senna (Senna, senokot), 230
Sex, measurements, 19
Sexual health, men. *See* Erectile dysfunction (ED)
Sexual health, women
    case studies, 247–248
    contraception, 257–258
    diagnosis, 252–253
    difficulties, 248–249
    dysfunctions, 249–250
    menstruation, 251–252
    risk factors, 250–251
    symptoms, 250
    treatment, 253–257
Shingles, 346
Shoes
    importance of, 169–170
    inserts, 185–186
    therapeutic, 173, 176, 179–184, 186–188
Sibutramine (Meridia), 378–379
Sildenafil citrate (Viagra), 243
Simvastatin (Zocor), 81–83
Sitagliptin (Januvia)
    described, 21, 414
    for hypertension, 99
    hypoglycemia and, 47
    in weight loss, 378
Skin care, 268–269
Skin complications
    abscesses, 277, S2
    acanthosis nigricans, 283, 286, S4
    bullosis diabeticorum (blisters), 281, 286
    Candida infection (yeast), 271–273, 286, 338
    cellulitis, 276, 340, S2
    diabetic dermopathy, 278–279, 286, S3
    drug reactions, 283–284, 286
    dryness/itching, 268–270, 286, S1
    Dupuytren's contracture, 267, 286
    erysipelas, 275–276, 286
    erythrasma, 275, 286, S1
    folliculitis, 276, 286
    granuloma annulare, 281, 286
    impetigo, 275, 286
    infections, 270–277, 286, S1
    intertrigo, 278, 286
    joint mobility, 267, 286
    necrobiosis lipoidica diabeticorum (NLD), 279–280, 286, S3
    necrotizing fasciitis, 276–277, 286
    overview, 265–266, 286
    scleroderma, 267, 286
    scratching, 270
    skin tags, 278, 286, S2
    SSTIs, 340
    thick skin, 266
    treatment/self-care, 285–287
    ulcers (*See* Ulcers)
    xanthomas, 282, 286, S4
    yellow skin/nails, 267–268, 286
Skin/soft tissue infections (SSTIs), 340
Skin tags, 278, 286, S2
Sleep apnea, 331–333
Sleep disturbances, 329–334
Smoking
    cancer and, 323
    diabetes effects, 384–385
    fractures and, 288, 293
    heart disease and, 72–73
    hypertension and, 87
    measurements, 19
    metabolism effects, 384, 385
    osteoporosis risk, 264
    overview, 383–384, 388
    quitting, 386, 387
    as risk factor, 386
    stroke and, 117
Social support, benefits of, 357, 361, 363
Socks, 184–185
Sonata (pyrazolopyrimidine), 333

classification of, 5
described, 6
DKA in, 34, 35
glucose lowering techniques, 19–22
hyperfiltration, 211, 212
nephropathy in, 207
PCOS and, 319
retinopathy in, 149
smoking as risk factor, 386

U

Ulcers
case study, 167
causes of, 173–174
healing, problems with, 176–177
infections and, 169 174–175, 177
neuropathy and, 161, 168–169
overview, 167–168, 277–278
prevention, 177–180
risk factors, 103, 168–170
symptoms, 172–174, S2
treatment, 174–176
Ultralente, 34, 412
Ultrasonography, 129–130
United Kingdom Prospective Diabetes
Study (UKPDS), 159
Urethral suppositories, 243–244
Urinary tract infection (UTI), 193, 262,
338, 339, 341–342

V

Vaccinations, 345–346
Vacuum erection devices (VEDs), 244
Vaginitis, 251
Valium, 333
Valsalva maneuver, 197
Valsartan (Diovan), 60
Vardenafil (Levitra), 243
Varenicline (Chantix), 73, 387

Vascular (multi-infarct) dementia,
351–353
Vasotec (enalapril), 60
Viagra (sildenafil citrate), 243
Viral infections, 338–340
Vitamin D, 291–292
Vitrectomy, 134–137
Vitreous hemorrhages, 121, 127, 133

W

Waist circumference, 371
Walker boots, 175–176
Warfarin (Coumadin), 118–120
Water pills, 66, 94
Weight loss, 373–374, 378–379
Weight measurements, 19
Wellbutrin (buproprion), 73, 387
Whooping cough (pertussis), 346
Withdrawal, 359

X

Xanthelasma palpebrarum, 282
Xanthomas, 282, 286, S4
Xerostomia (dry mouth), 300

Y

Yeast infection, 271–273, 286, 338
Yellow skin/nails, 267–268, 286
Yoga, 166, 262

Z

Zelnorm (tegaserod), 226, 231
Zestril (lisinopril, Prinivil), 60
Zetia (ezetimibe), 83, 316
Zocor (simvastatin), 81–83
Zolpidem (Ambien), 333

OTHER TITLES FROM THE
AMERICAN DIABETES ASSOCIATION

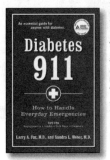

Diabetes 911: How to Handle Everyday Emergencies
by Larry A. Fox, MD, and Sandra L. Weber, MD
When it comes to a condition as serious as diabetes, the best way to solve problems is to prevent them from ever happening. Do you know what to do in case of an emergency? With *Diabetes 911*, you will learn the necessary skills to handle hypoglycemia, insulin pump malfunctions, natural disasters, travel, depression, and sick days.
Order no. 4887-01; Price $12.95

Diabetes & Heart Healthy Meals for Two
by the American Diabetes Association and the American Heart Association
If you or a loved one has diabetes, you need to eat heart-healthy meals. The simple, flavorful recipes were designed for those looking to improve or maintain their cardiovascular health. Each recipe is for two people, making this book perfect for adults without children in the house or for those who want to keep leftovers to a minimum. With over 170 recipes, there are countless options to keep you heart at its healthiest and your blood glucose under control.
Order no. 4673-01; Price $18.95

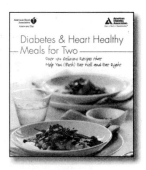

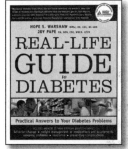

Real-Life Guide to Diabetes
by Hope S. Warshaw, MMSc, RD, CDE, BC-ADM, and Joy Pape, RN, BSC, CDE, WOCN, CFCN
Real-Life Guide puts everything you need to know about diabetes into a one-of-a-kind book packed with the information you won't find anywhere else. Learn to prevent long-term complications, understand the ins and outs of health insurance, work physical activity into your daily life, and control your blood glucose, cholesterol, and blood pressure. Bring a realistic approach to your diabetes care plan.
Order no. 4893-01; Price $19.95

Your First Year with Diabetes
by Theresa Garnero, CDE, APRN, BC-ADM, MSN
Diabetes happens. It can happen to anyone—even you. If diabetes has left you feeling confused or angry, then it's time to turn to Theresa Garnero. Straightforward and easy to read, *Your First Year with Diabetes* will help you manage and deal with your diabetes—day to day, week to week, and month to month. You'll learn about medication, exercise, meal planning, and lifestyle and emotional issues at a pace that suits you.
Order no. 5024-01; Price $16.95

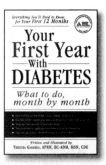

To order these and other great American Diabetes Association titles, call **1-800-232-6733** or visit ***http://store.diabetes.org***. American Diabetes Association titles are also available in bookstores nationwide.